To Act As A Unit

THE STORY OF
THE CLEVELAND CLINIC

To Act As A Unit

THE STORY OF
THE CLEVELAND CLINIC

Fourth Edition

John D. Clough, M.D., Editor

CLEVELAND CLINIC PRESS

To Act As A Unit: The Story of the Cleveland Clinic   ISBN 1-59624-000-8

Copyright © 2004 The Cleveland Clinic Foundation

9500 Euclid Avenue, NA32
Cleveland, Ohio 44195

Printed in the United States of America

10 9 8 7 6 5 4

CONTENTS

PREFACE TO THE FOURTH EDITION   11

FOREWORD   15

SECTION ONE: THE EARLY YEARS

1. **THE FOUNDERS**   19
   The Earliest Beginnings   19
   Early Practice   23
   The World War I Years   25
   Return to Practice   29

2. **THE FIRST YEARS, 1921-1929**   33
   Building the New Clinic   33
   Charter and Organization   36
   The Grand Opening   39
   The Clinic's Work Begins   43

3. **THE DISASTER, 1929**   49
   The Explosions   49
   Emergency and Rescue   51
   Sorting It All Out   56

4. **THE PHOENIX RISES FROM THE ASHES, 1929-1941**   59
   The Great Depression   59
   Growth and Maturation   62

5. **TURBULENT SUCCESS, 1941-1955**   69
   The Torch Passes   69
   Success and Maturation   73
   Grumbling and Unrest   76

SECTION TWO: THE BOARD OF GOVERNORS ERA

6. THE LeFevre Years, 1955-1968   83
   Into a New Era   83
   Trustees and Governors   85
   Commitment and Growth   86

7. THE Wasmuth Years, 1969-1976   89
   The Winds of Change   89
   Confined Expansion and Community Reaction   92

8. THE Kiser Years, 1977-1989   95
   A Gentler Style   95
   New Managerial Approaches   97
   Changing Times   99
   Building for the Future   101
   A Move to the South   105

9. THE Loop Years (Part I), 1989-1995   111
   Turnaround Time   111
   The New Team   113
   Full Steam Ahead   118

SECTION THREE: SYSTEM AND CONSOLIDATION

10. THE Loop Years (Part II), 1995-2004   127
    Assembly of the Cleveland Clinic Health System   128
    The Cleveland Clinic Health System's   134
       Physicians' Organization
    Deployment of Family Health Centers   136
       and Ambulatory Surgery Centers
    New Buildings: Acquisitions   139
       and New Construction
    The Academic Enterprise and   144
       the Medical School
    Information Technology and the   145
       Electronic Medical Record
    Strengthening of Management   148
    Taking Stock: A Progress Report   152

SECTION FOUR: DIVISIONS, DEPARTMENTS, INSTITUTES, AND CENTERS

11. DIVISION OF MEDICINE 157
    Beginnings 157
    Nephrology and Hypertension 161
    Cardiovascular Medicine 163
    Pulmonary and Critical Care Medicine 164
    Endocrinology 166
    Dermatology 167
    Gastroenterology 169
    Neurology 170
    Psychiatry and Psychology 172
    Rheumatic and Immunologic Disease 173
    Hematology and Medical Oncology 175
    General Internal Medicine 176
    Infectious Disease 179
    Emergency Medicine 180
    Conclusion 181

12. DIVISION OF PEDIATRICS 183
    Pediatrics Begins 183
    Relationship with Obstetrics 184
    Pediatric Specialization 185
    The Children's Hospital at The Cleveland Clinic 191
    The Division of Pediatrics 192

13. DIVISION OF SURGERY 195
    General Surgery 196
    Colorectal Surgery 202
    Otolaryngology 204
    Neurological Surgery 206
    Orthopedic Surgery 209
    Urology and the Glickman Institute 212
    Obstetrics and Gynecology 214
    Plastic Surgery 216
    Dentistry 217
    Vascular Surgery 218
    Thoracic and Cardiovascular Surgery 220
    Conclusion 226

14. **DIVISION OF ANESTHESIOLOGY AND CRITICAL CARE MEDICINE**   229
    The Hale Years, 1946-1967   230
    The Wasmuth Years, 1967-1969   230
    The Potter-Viljoen Years, 1970-1977   230
    The Boutros Years, 1977-1986   231
    The Estafanous Years, 1986-   231
    Cardiothoracic Anesthesiology   232
    General Anesthesiology   233
    Pain Management   235
    Clinical Engineering and Information Technology Center   235
    Education Center   236
    Research Center   237

15. **CENTERS, INSTITUTES, AND EMERGING DIVISIONS**   239
    The Cleveland Clinic Spine Institute   240
    Mellen Center for Multiple Sclerosis   242
    Transplant Center   244
    Taussig Cancer Center   253
    Cole Eye Institute and Division of Ophthalmology   258
    Division of Post-Acute Care   261
    Division of Clinical Research   262
    Division of Regional Medical Practice   263
    Conclusion   263

16. **DIVISION OF PATHOLOGY AND LABORATORY MEDICINE**   265
    Anatomic Pathology   267
    Clinical Pathology   270
    The Cleveland Clinic Reference Laboratory   275
    Laboratory Information Systems   276
    Conclusion   277

17. **DIVISION OF RADIOLOGY**   279
    Diagnostic Radiology   283
    Radiation Oncology   287
    Nuclear Medicine (Molecular and Functional Imaging)   288
    Conclusion   289

18. **DIVISION OF NURSING**   291
    In the Beginning   291

The Danielsen Era, 1981-1986   292
The Coulter Era, 1987-1997   293
The Ulreich Era, 1998-2003   296
Looking Ahead   304

19. DIVISION OF EDUCATION   307
The Early Years, 1921-1944   307
The Leedham Years, 1955-1962   310
The Zeiter Years, 1962-1973   311
The Michener Years, 1973-1991   311
The Fishleder Years, 1991-   313

20. LERNER RESEARCH INSTITUTE   317
Early Activities   317
The Page Era, 1945-1966   318
The Bumpus Era, 1966-1985   324
The Healy Era, 1985-1991   325
The Stark Era, 1992-2002   328
The DiCorleto Era, 2002-   330

21. CLEVELAND CLINIC FLORIDA   333
Florida Beckons   333
Preliminary Red Tape   335
Grand Opening and Pushback   337
Progress   339
Expansion to Weston   340
A Bi-Coastal Presence   342
Maturation and New Leadership   346

SECTION FIVE: TRUSTEES, GOVERNORS, AND ADMINISTRATION

22. ADMINISTRATION: THE "GRAY COATS"   351
In the Beginning   352
The Post-War Era   353
The Turbulent 1960s and 1970s   355
The Clinic Side   359
Alphabet Soup, the 1970s and 1980s   360
The Bean Counters   362

A National Health Resource   363
Further Education of Those Who Serve   364
Marketing the Brand   365
Human Resources   366
Automated Information   367
Visitors from Other Lands   367
A Commitment to Cleveland   368
Legal Contributions   369
A City within a City   370
East 93rd Street and Beyond   371

23. TRUSTEES, GOVERNORS, AND STAFF   375
Trustees and Governors   375
The Professional Staff   378

INDEX   385

PREFACE
TO THE FOURTH EDITION

An army of sheep led by a lion would defeat
an army of lions led by a sheep.
—Arab Proverb

LESS THAN A DECADE HAS PASSED SINCE THE CLEVELAND CLINIC PUBLISHED the third edition of *To Act as a Unit*, but the pace of change has accelerated to the point where the third edition is already hopelessly outdated. Since 1996, the Clinic's 75th anniversary year, the organization has dedicated three major buildings on the main campus, established the Cleveland Clinic Health System, opened or acquired 14 regional satellite facilities, expanded the Florida operation to new campuses in Weston and Naples, begun a major service improvement initiative based on leadership development, and announced plans for a new medical school. Through it all, the staff has continued to grow at an exponential rate.

Although the focus of the organization is solidly on the future, some reflections on the past are in order. The phrase "to act as a unit," which serves as the title of this book, has become a second motto for The Cleveland Clinic Foundation. It was extracted from the journal of George W. Crile, later known as George Crile, Sr., who wrote it as he was reminiscing about his professional relationship with his partners, surgeons Frank Bunts and William Lower, in France during World War I.

Over the years, the phrase has taken on an egalitarian connotation that has become engrained in the culture of the organization, expressing the cooperative spirit of group practice. Crile viewed this salubrious concept with a touch of cynicism, however. In fact, he

11

was once quoted as having said, "mediocrity well organized is more efficient than brilliancy combined with strife and discord."[1] Crile's apparent assumption that these two attributes—organization and brilliancy—are mutually exclusive is interesting, and the institution he helped found may have proved him erroneous in this assumption.

It is most likely that what Crile had in mind on that battlefield in France was a military "unit" whose predictable function was assured by the fact that its members were used to following orders. It also implies that strong leadership is a *sine qua non* for success.

Crile, himself, was used to providing strong leadership. As Chief of Surgery at Lakeside Hospital, he led a team of Cleveland's best surgeons of the time. When war broke out, he organized and led the Lakeside unit, which set up an army hospital in France, where he found himself when he coined the famous phrase. He became enthralled with the team approach to patient care that characterized military medicine in that setting and resolved to apply it in his peacetime practice after the war.

The Cleveland Clinic, a group practice that has always had strong leadership since its inception in 1921, was the result. Democracy came to the Clinic more than 30 years later, in the form of the Board of Governors, which did not exist until 1955. The Board of Governors has varied in its importance in the daily life of the Clinic, depending on the style of leadership in place at the time. In reality, the power of the mostly elected Board of Governors, which receives its authority from the Board of Trustees, derives from the Governors' annual duty to (re)appoint the top leadership (i.e., the officers of the Foundation: Chief Executive Officer, Chief Operating Officer, Chief Financial Officer, and Chief of Staff), subject to ratification by the Trustees. Historically, the Clinic's leadership stays in place at the pleasure of the Board of Governors, the composition of which is determined by the staff. This approach has worked very well over the years.

Thus, the relevant meaning of the phrase "to act as a unit" has evolved over the years to something possibly more powerful than its original intent. There is no question that the group practice model, as it exists at The Cleveland Clinic, has been successful beyond the wildest dreams of the founders. Those familiar with the organization's professional staff recognize a level of collegiality and teamwork, both in patient care and in academic pursuits, that transcends disciplinary borders and belies the concept of simply following orders efficiently. The ideal of "organized brilliancy," which Crile's statement implied was impossible, may have come as close to full realization at The Cleveland Clinic as it does anywhere.

To return to the matter at hand, this fourth edition is structured similarly to the third. Some chapters have changed but little, while others are entirely new. We have specifically attributed chapter authorship in this edition, the better to recognize the efforts of the many contributors to this work. Many of the quotations at the heads of chapters (a new feature in the third edition) are retained, but some have been changed by special request. Each chapter is now divided into sections, as in the Internet edition. I have edited all the chapters, heavily in some cases, more lightly in others, and I assume sole responsibility for any errors that have crept in during this process. I thank the Clinic's archivists, Carol Tomer and Fred Lautzenheiser, for once again critically reviewing this work for accuracy and style, and for being a limitless source of good ideas and information, particularly about the Clinic's early years. I also thank Peter Studer, head of the Department of Scientific Publications and publisher of the *Cleveland Clinic Journal of Medicine*, Kathy Dunasky of the Department of Scientific Publications, Robert Kay, M.D., the Clinic's Chief of Staff, and Floyd D. Loop, M.D., the Clinic's Chief Executive Officer, for their careful review of the manuscript prior to publication. This book could not have been completed in its present form without their help.

—JOHN D. CLOUGH, M.D.
February 7, 2004

---

[1] Clapesattle HB. *The Doctors Mayo.* Garden City, NY, Garden City Publishing Co., Inc., 1943, p 561.

FOREWORD

CREDO: *The singular purpose of The Cleveland Clinic Foundation is to benefit humanity through the efficient, effective, and ethical practice of medicine, by advancing scientific investigation and medical education, by maintaining the highest standard of quality, and by honoring creativity and innovation. Each member of the organization is a guardian of this enterprise and is responsible for assuring that the Cleveland Clinic is synonymous with the finest health care in the world.*

FOR THE PAST 83 YEARS, THE CLEVELAND CLINIC HAS LIVED UP TO THE tenets of this credo and upheld the highest standards of medical practice, research, and education. A number of factors contribute to our ability to do so. These include physician leadership, our not-for-profit, group practice model, the skill and experience of our physician staff, academic achievement, and an institutional culture that places a premium on hard work and professional accomplishment. The four founders of The Cleveland Clinic left us a model of medicine that not only served them well in their own time, but has emerged as an optimal institutional framework for medicine in the 21st century.

Since the last edition of *To Act as A Unit*, The Cleveland Clinic has continued to evolve. Among many new developments, we have opened the Cleveland Clinic Lerner College of Medicine of Case Western Reserve University, which is devoted to the education of physician investigators. We have improved our clinical quality measurement through our Quality Institute and begun a genetics institute and stem-cell center. We are moving in a favorable direction toward the construction of a new Cleveland Clinic Heart Center and growing in a thousand ways to meet the health, science, and educational needs of the coming century.

This fourth edition of *To Act as A Unit* is compiled by John Clough, M.D., a writer and editor whose consummate skills have added inestimably to the value of its contents. Through his contributions and those of his valued predecessors, we can have the pleasure of tracking The Cleveland Clinic's growth from a small group practice to the second largest private medical center in the world. We can see how The Cleveland Clinic has remained true to its core values while pursuing the most advanced clinical practices and scientific knowledge.

To Act as A Unit reminds us that we are only the temporary stewards of an enduring public trust and that we are accountable for maintaining its tradition of excellence. The Cleveland Clinic has been a beacon of health to people everywhere in times of illness and wellness, crisis and confidence. We hope that *To Act as A Unit* will inspire us as we write the future of medicine and create The Cleveland Clinic of tomorrow.

—FLOYD D. LOOP, M.D.
January 5, 2004

section one

THE EARLY YEARS

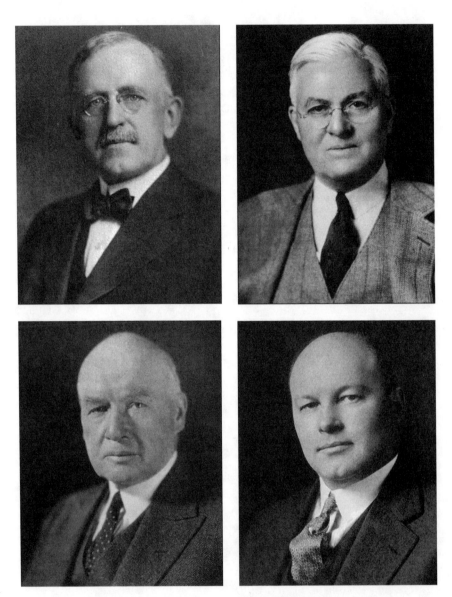

The Founders (clockwise from upper left): Frank E. Bunts, M.D.,
George W. Crile, M.D., John Phillips, M.D., and William E. Lower, M.D.

1. THE FOUNDERS

By Alexander T. Bunts and George Crile, Jr.

Remove not the ancient landmark, which thy fathers have set.
—Proverbs 22:28

THE EARLIEST BEGINNINGS

ON AUGUST 27, 1918, DR. GEORGE W. CRILE (KNOWN AS GEORGE CRILE, Sr.), who at the time was with the Lakeside Hospital Unit in France, wrote in his journal:

> "What a remarkable record Bunts, Crile and Lower have had all these years. We have been rivals in everything, yet through all the vicissitudes of personal, financial and professional relations we have been able to think and act as a unit."[1]

This sense of cooperation and unity, shared by three of the four future founders of The Cleveland Clinic, made it possible to create the group practice model that still forms the basis for the institution.

Dr. Frank E. Bunts was the senior member of the three surgeons who had been so closely associated for many years before the founding of The Cleveland Clinic. After a brief career in the Navy, he attended medical school for three years at Western Reserve University and graduated in 1886 as valedictorian of his class. After a year of internship at St. Vincent Charity Hospital in Cleveland, he entered the office of Dr. Frank J. Weed, then Dean and Professor of Surgery at the Wooster University Department of Medicine, Cleveland, Ohio. Wooster University's medical school was located

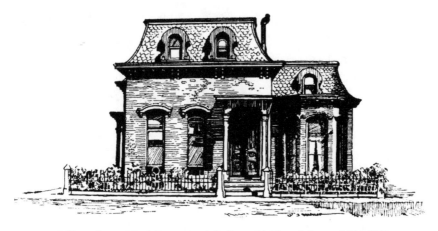

Offices of Drs. Weed, Bunts, and Crile at 16 Church Street, 1886-1889
(artist's drawing)

at what would now be East 14th Street (formerly Brownell) and Central Avenue in Cleveland, if that intersection still existed. An interstate highway now occupies that location. The school was closed and absorbed into Western Reserve University in 1896.

Crile was born in 1864 on a farm in Chili, Ohio. He worked his way through Northwestern Ohio Normal School (later known as Ohio Northern University) in Ada by teaching in elementary schools. After receiving a teaching certificate in 1884, he was appointed Principal of the Plainfield (Ohio) Schools. Soon his interest turned to medicine, mainly as a result of his contacts with a local physician, Dr. A. E. Walker, who loaned him books and with whom he visited patients.[2] Some of the events of this period are related in his autobiography, among them the fascinating details of "quilling" an obstetric patient by blowing snuff through a goose quill into her nose. The sneezing that this induced led to prompt delivery of the baby. In March 1886, Crile enrolled at Wooster, and in July 1887, after only 15 months, he received his M.D. degree. It is doubtful that Crile spent the entire 15 months there since the Wooster Medical School operated summer sessions only, and Crile continued his work as principal of the Plainfield Schools during the winter. He received a master's degree from the Northwestern Ohio Normal School in 1888, the year after he got his M.D.

Crile served his internship at University Hospital under Dr. Frank J. Weed, and after that he joined Bunts as an assistant to Weed in his large office practice. Crile described the origin of University Hospital (not to be confused with University Hospitals of Cleveland, established in 1931) in his autobiography. "In 1882, three years before I first came to Cleveland, Dr. Weed and the group of associates who had revived Wooster Medical School, having no hospital privileges for their students except for the county poorhouse, established University Hospital in two old residences on Brownell Street 'in juxtaposition,' as the catalogue stated in a high-sounding phrase, to Wooster Medical School. This simple hospital had a capacity of perhaps thirty beds."

Then, tragically, at age 45 and at the peak of his professional career, Weed contracted pneumonia and died. At that time, Bunts was not yet 30 years old and Crile was three years younger. Crile expressed their feelings as follows:

"Wearied by loss of sleep, worry and constant vigil, we left Doctor Weed's house on that cheerless March morning and walked to Doctor Bunts's for breakfast. In our dejection, it seemed to us that everything had suddenly come to an end. Our light had gone out. We had no money, no books, no surgical instruments. The only instrument either of us owned, other than my microscope, was a stethoscope. But we agreed to carry on together, to share and share alike both the expenses and the income from the accident practice, each to reserve for himself the income from his private patients."

After talking with Mrs. Weed, Bunts and Crile decided to buy, from the estate, Dr. Weed's goods, chattels, and instruments. Excerpts from the bill of sale are listed below. This property represented the embryo from which The Cleveland Clinic was born.[3]

Bill of Sale
From Estate of Dr. Frank J. Weed
to
Dr. Frank E. Bunts and Dr. George Crile

Small brown mares (Brown Jug and Roseline)	$125.00
Small sorrel horse (Duke)	100.00
Bay horse (Roy)	75.00
Top buggy	50.00

Bill of Sale (*continued*)

Top buggy, very old	$10.00
Open buggy	20.00
2 Cutters, one very old	20.00
4 sets single harness	20.00
Lap robes	15.00
Miscellaneous articles in barn	3.00
Shed, old stoves, battery, etc.	50.00
Articles on stand	20.00
Milliamperes	10.00
Contents of case (silk, bandages, and dressings)	15.00
Contents of desk (hand mirror, 6 sprinklers, medicine case)	8.00
Medicine on desk	25.00
3 McCune chisels	3.75
4 Small chisels	2.00
14 Pairs scissors	2.50
3 Large pairs shears	1.50
2 Pairs retractors	2.00
2 Forceps	2.50
3 Nasal saws	1.50
2 Intestinal clasps	1.00
1 Chain saw	2.00
2 Hayes saws	1.50
1 Small met. saw	.50
7 Needles	1.00
4 Wire twisters	1.00
6 Sponge holders	1.50
1 Clamp	2.00
3 Bullet forceps	2.00
2 Large retractors	2.00
4 Small nasal dilators	1.25
1 Throat forcep	1.50
1 Head reflector	2.50
4 Self retaining female catheters	1.75
2 Tools	.50
5 Bone elevators	2.00
5 Bone forceps	6.00
1 Chain saw guide	.75
1 Bone drill with three tips	.75
1 Hamilton bone drill with four tips	3.00
1 Emergency bag No. 2	5.00
1 Emergency bag No. 3	11.00
1 Box—3 knives and 3 pairs scissors	1.50
1 Stomach pump in box	6.00
1 Stone set in case	8.00
1 Horse shoe turnica	1.00
1 Cloven clutch	4.00
1 Small aspirating set	2.00
1 Kelley pad	.75
1 Syringe	.50
1 Microscope	40.00
2 Syringes	1.50
Total	$1778.10

Bill of Sale (*continued*)

Cleveland, O., Apr. 10th, 1891

In consideration of seventeen hundred and seventy eight 10/100 dollars I have this day sold to Drs. F. E. Bunts and G.W. Crile all the goods, chattels, instruments and other articles contained in brick house and barn in rear at No. 380 Pearl Street as per inventory marked Exhibit A attached to bill of sale.

C. H. Weed, Administrator of Frank J. Weed

EARLY PRACTICE

The practice of the new partners grew rapidly, and by 1892 they needed an associate. Crile engaged his cousin, Dr. William E. Lower. Both had attended district schools. Lower, too, had been reared on a farm and from an early age had developed a sense of independence as well as the importance of hard work and the necessity of thrift and frugality. Lower had attended the Medical Department of Wooster University, from which he was graduated in 1891; he served as house physician in City Hospital, and then set up practice in Conneaut, Ohio. Bunts and Crile had little difficulty in persuading him to leave there to share their office practice. By 1895, Bunts, Crile, and Lower were full partners, equally sharing the expenses and the income from emergency work but remaining competitors in private practice. Mutual trust and confidence became a keystone for their future accomplishments.

With the continued growth of their practices, Bunts, Crile, and Lower moved their office in 1897 from the west side of Cleveland downtown to the Osborn Building, at the junction of Huron Road and Prospect Avenue. A year later, this collaboration was interrupted by the Spanish-American War; Bunts was surgeon to the First Ohio Volunteer Cavalry Unit of the Ohio National Guard, and Crile was surgeon to the Gatling Gun Battery in Cleveland, also a unit of the Guard. When they volunteered for active duty, Lower was left alone with the office practice. Not long after the war was over and his partners had returned, he retaliated by volunteering to help quell the Boxer Rebellion in China, entering the Army as a first lieutenant. By the time he reached China, the rebellion was over, so he served as surgeon to the 9th U.S. Cavalry in the Philippines, 1900-1901.

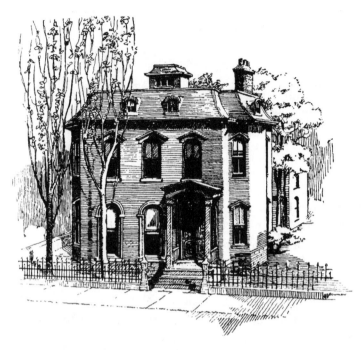

*Offices of Drs. Bunts, Crile, and Lower at 380 Pearl Street
(now West 25th Street), 1890-1897 (artist's drawing)*

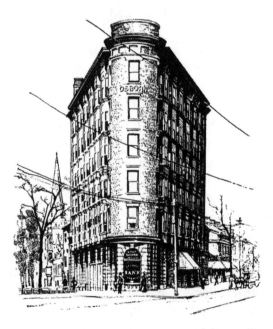

*Offices of Drs. Bunts, Crile, and Lower, Osborn Building at East 9th Street
and Huron Road, 1897-1920 (artist's drawing)*

By 1901, the various wars were over, and Bunts, Crile, and Lower were reunited in the Osborn Building office, where they remained until World War I separated them again. The period immediately before World War I was productive. In addition to their large trauma and private practices, Bunts became professor of principles of surgery and clinical surgery at the Western Reserve University School of Medicine. He was also the first president of the newly formed Academy of Medicine of Cleveland. Crile was professor of surgery at Western Reserve. Lower, whose major interest soon became urology, was associate professor of genito-urinary surgery at Western Reserve. Both Crile and Lower also served as presidents of the Academy of Medicine during its first decade.

During these years, Crile maintained his interest in physiology and applied to clinical practice the principles that he discovered in the laboratory in the fields of shock, transfusion, and anesthesia. Lower collaborated in some of Crile's early works, but neither he nor Bunts shared Crile's consuming and lifelong interest in basic laboratory research.

As the practice expanded, Dr. Harry G. Sloan, a surgeon, was added to the staff, and Dr. John D. Osmond was sent to the Mayo Clinic to observe the newly developed techniques of radiology. Osmond returned to establish, in 1913, the group's first X-ray Department. Dr. Thomas P. Shupe also joined the staff as an associate of Lower in urology.

At that time, Crile was helping to form the American College of Surgeons. The purposes of this organization were to improve the standards of surgical practice in the United States and Canada, as well as to provide postgraduate education, improve ethics, raise the standards of care in hospitals, and educate the public about medical and surgical problems.

THE WORLD WAR I YEARS

In 1914, Europe was ablaze with war. In December of that year, Crile, who was then Chief Surgeon at Lakeside Hospital, was asked by Clevelander Myron T. Herrick, then Ambassador to France, to organize a team to work in France. Crile accepted, for even at that time he realized that the United States would be drawn into the war and that experience in military surgery would be valuable. As Crile prepared to leave for France, Lower drafted a report to be presented to the office staff. The final report is less interesting than this draft, here reproduced with some minor editing to correct errors. Both versions are in the Archives of The Cleveland Clinic Foundation.

Partial Report for the Year 1914

In behalf of Drs. Bunts, Crile, and Lower, I want to make a necessarily incomplete report for the year 1914, incomplete because the year is not entirely ended and because the rush of extra work at this time has made it impossible to get all the necessary data ready. It is only by summing up of the year's work that we can get a keen appreciation of what we have accomplished. I wish you to particularly hear this because of the important part you all have taken in the work.

Your loyalty, zeal, enthusiasm, and devotion we have all recognized throughout the year, and we wish to take this occasion to tell you how keenly we appreciate it and also to get your suggestions, if any, for the coming year.

The great European conflict has had its effect upon practically every line of public endeavor in every country of the globe and will continue to do so, more or less, until the war is ended. This means personal sacrifice, more economy, and greater efficiency if we wish to hold our place. Our work is particularly trying because it deals solely with others' afflictions. It means great tact, every consideration for the comfort of our patients, the application of the latest and best scientific and practical means for the alleviation of their ailments; special research and laboratory work, reviewing of the literature, the development of new methods of treatment, and the careful computing of our clinical results, which is a guide as to the value of any method of treatment.

The following statistics show approximately what we have done.

Number of cases seen in 1913	8,467
Number of cases seen in 1914	9,245

Number of examinations for the Railroad Companies in 1913	3,185
Number of examinations for the Railroad Companies in 1914	2,378
Number of laboratory tests	
Wasserman Reactions	113
Complement Fixation Tests	192
Cystoscopies	105
Ureteral Catheterizations	31
Number of papers read at different meetings	30
Number of articles published in the Medical Journals	30+
Number of reprints sent out	10,000
Number of books published	2

This office has always felt equal to any emergency or occasion that might arise. During the breaking out of the Spanish-American war, when we were just beginning to feel our way, and trying to take our place in the professional world, Drs. Bunts and Crile gave up their work to serve during the war. It was a big office sacrifice. Upon their return I went into our foreign service for a period of nearly one year. Now the opportunity has again arisen to do our part in the great European war and again we are ready. Dr. Crile with his traditional enthusiasm and resources goes to take charge of a division in the American Ambulance Hospital in Paris. With him goes our great aide-de-camp, Miss Rowland, whose ability and capacity for work we all know. With this important division away, the lesser of us must try all the harder to keep the good work going. It means for the rest of us no let down if the coming year is to make anywhere near as good a showing as this one has.

After three months of treating casualties at Neuilly, the group returned, and Crile organized a base-hospital unit.

When the United States entered the war, the Lakeside Unit (U.S. Army Base Hospital No. 4) was the first detachment of the American Expeditionary Forces to arrive in France, taking over a British general hospital near Rouen on May 25, 1917. Crile was the hospital's Clinical Director, but later was given a broader assignment as Director of the Division of Research for the American Expeditionary

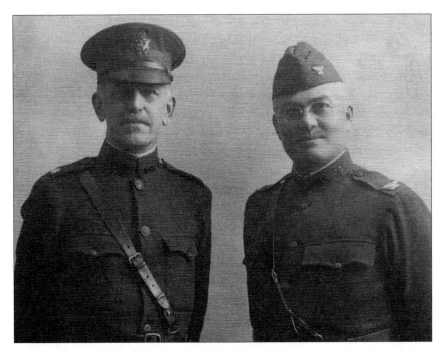

Lt. Col. Frank E. Bunts and Col. George W. Crile at Rouen, France, 1918

Forces, a post that permitted him to move about and visit the stations wherever the action was.

Lower was with Crile in the Lakeside Unit, and soon Bunts, a reservist, was ordered to Camp Travis, Texas, leaving only Sloan and Osmond to keep the practice going. Both were able to pay the office expenses, but Bunts, concerned about the future, wrote to Lower in France as follows:

> "I feel very strongly that we ought to hold the office together at all hazards, not only for ourselves, but for the younger men who have been with us and whose future will depend largely on having a place to come back to. If Sloan and Osmond go, I think we could at least keep Miss Slattery and Miss Van Spyker. It would be quite an outlay for each of us to ante up our share for keeping the office from being occupied by others, but I for one would be glad to do it. We haven't so very many years left for active work after this war is over, and it would seem to be almost too much to undertake to start afresh in new offices, and the stimulus and friendship of our old associations mean much more than money to me."

Bunts succeeded Lower as commanding officer of the hospital near Rouen in August 1918. After the armistice, November 11, 1918, activities at the Base Hospital gradually subsided, tensions eased, and soldiers found time to engage in nonmilitary pursuits and conversations. The long and friendly association of the three Cleveland surgeons is apparent in the following letter written in December 1918 and addressed to Lower in Cleveland from Bunts in France.

"It's getting around Christmas time, and while I know this won't reach you for a month, yet I just want to let you know that we are thinking of you and wishing we could see you. Crile has been here for a couple of weeks, but left again for Paris a few days ago, and evenings he and I have foregathered about the little stove in your old room, leaving G. W.'s door open wide enough to warm his room up too, and there we have sat like two old G.A.R. relics, smoking and laughing, telling stories, dipping back into even our boyhood days and laughing often til the tears rolled down our cheeks. It has been a varied life we three have had and filled with trials and pleasures without number. I have dubbed our little fireside chats the 'Arabian Nights,' and often we have been startled when the coal gave out and the fire died down that it was long past midnight and time for antiques to go to bed."

During those nocturnal chats at Rouen, an idea that eventually led to the founding of The Cleveland Clinic took shape. The military hospital experience impressed these men with the efficiency of an organization that included every branch or specialty of medicine and surgery. They recognized the benefits that could be obtained from cooperation by a group of specialists. Before their return to the United States they began to formulate plans for the future.

RETURN TO PRACTICE

Bunts and Crile returned to Cleveland early in 1919 and were once more united with Lower in their Osborn Building offices. They began to rebuild their interrupted surgical practices and soon found themselves as busy as they had been before the war.

Although the military hospital was used as a model for their future plan, elements of the pattern were furnished also by the Mayo Clinic, founded by close professional friends. Bunts, Crile, and Lower were surgeons, and in order to develop a broader field of medical service they resolved to add an internist to organize and head a department of medicine. They were fortunate to obtain the enthusiastic cooperation of Dr. John Phillips, who was at that time a member of the faculty of the School of Medicine of Western Reserve. He, too, had served in military hospitals during the war and held the same broad concept of what might be accomplished by a clinic organization.

John Phillips was born in 1879 on a farm near Welland, Ontario. He was a quiet, serious-minded youth who nevertheless had a keen sense of humor. After obtaining his teacher's certificate, he taught for three years in a district school. He then entered the Faculty of Medicine in the University of Toronto, where in 1903 he received the M.B. degree with honors. After graduation he served for three years as intern and resident in medicine at Lakeside Hospital in Cleveland. He then entered practice as an associate in the office of Dr. E. F. Cushing, professor of pediatrics at Western Reserve. During the years before the founding of The Cleveland Clinic, Phillips held assistant professorships in both medicine and therapeutics at the Western Reserve University School of Medicine. Simultaneously, he had hospital appointments at Babies' Dispensary and Hospital and Lakeside Hospital. He was also consulting physician to St. John's Hospital. Phillips had a large private and consulting practice and was highly regarded for his ability as clinician and teacher in internal medicine and the diseases of children. During World War I, he served as a captain in the Medical Corps of the United States Army.

In 1920, most private physicians did not like the idea of group practice. Some felt that the large resources available to a group might give them an unfair competitive advantage. Many were openly critical of the concept and might have attempted to block the establishment of The Cleveland Clinic if the founders had not been so highly regarded in the medical community. All were professors in one or more of the Cleveland medical schools. Crile was a major national and international figure in surgery and in national medical organizations; Lower was already well known nationally as a urologic surgeon; Phillips had a solid reputation locally and nationally in internal medicine; and Bunts's professional and personal reputation was of the highest order. As previously noted, Bunts, Crile, and Lower had all been presidents of the Academy of Medicine, and Phillips was the president-elect.

The founders' reputation was not based solely on the medical schools; it also was well established in the community hospitals. They held appointments at Cleveland General, University, City, St. Alexis, St. Vincent Charity, Lutheran, St. John's, Lakeside, and Mt. Sinai hospitals. Moreover, many of the community's business leaders were their patients and friends. It would have been difficult to stand in the way of any legitimate enterprise that these physicians decided to organize. This point is underscored by a thumbnail sketch of their personalities as Dr. George Crile, Jr., remembered them.

"Crile was the dynamo of the group, imaginative, creative, innovative, and driving. It is possible that some considered him inconsiderate of others in his overriding desire to get things done. For this reason, and because he occasionally was premature in applying to the treatment of patients the principles learned in research, he had enemies as well as supporters. Yet most of his contemporaries would have readily admitted that Crile was one of the first surgeons in the world to apply physiologic research to surgical problems, that he was one of the country's leaders in organizing and promoting medical organizations such as The American College of Surgeons of which he became the president, and that it was largely as a result of Crile's energy, prestige, and practice that The Cleveland Clinic was founded.

"If Crile was the driver, Lower was the brake. He was a born conservative, even to the point of the keyhole size of his surgical incisions. No one but he could operate through them. His assistants could not even see into them. He was a technician of consummate skill and an imaginative pioneer in the then new field of urology. Lower was also a perfect treasurer. He checked on every expenditure, thus compensating for Crile's tendency to disregard the Clinic's cash position. Later in life, Doctor Lower even went around the buildings, in the evenings, turning out lights that were burning needlessly. He was no miser, but his conservatism afforded a perfect balance to Crile's over-enthusiasm. Despite the differences in their personalities, no one ever saw them quarrel.

"I never knew Bunts as well as the others, for he died early, but I do recall that he never, in my presence at least, displayed the exuberant type of humor that Crile and Lower did. I have seen the latter two almost rolling on the floor in laughter as they reminisced on how they dealt with some ancient enemy, but I could not imagine Bunts doing that. He had the presence and dignity that one associates with the image of an old-time senator. 'Bunts was invaluable in our association,' my father once told me. 'He was the one that gave it respectability.'

"Phillips, like Bunts, died early, so that I knew him only as my childhood physician rather than as a personal friend. My impression was of a man who was silent, confident, and imperturbable. I am sure that his patients and colleagues shared this confidence in him and that was why he was able to organize a successful department of internal medicine.

"Although the personalities of the Clinic's founders were so different from one another, there were common bonds that united them. All had served in the military, all had taught in medical schools, all were devoted to the practice of medicine. As a result of these common backgrounds and motivations, there emerged a common ideal—an institution in which medicine and surgery could be practiced, studied, and taught by a group of associated specialists. To create it, the four founders began to plan an institution that would be greater than the sum of its individual parts."

---

[1] An important source for *To Act as a Unit* was *George Crile, An Autobiography*, edited with sidelights by Grace Crile, Philadelphia, J.B. Lippincott, 1947. George Crile was the author of 650 publications, including several books.

[2] The State of Ohio recently commemorated this phase of Crile's career by placing a historical marker in Plainfield on June 3, 2001. Near the marker is the grave of Dr. Walker, Crile's earliest medical mentor.

[3] This document is now located in the Archives of The Cleveland Clinic.

2. THE FIRST YEARS
1921-1929

BY ALEXANDER T. BUNTS AND GEORGE CRILE, JR.

Life is a petty thing unless it is moved by the indomitable
urge to extend its boundaries. Only in proportion as we
are desirous of living more do we really live.
—José Ortega y Gasset, 1925

BUILDING THE NEW CLINIC

IN OCTOBER 1919, THE FOUNDERS, WITH THE AID OF BUNTS'S SON-IN-LAW Mr. Edward C. Daoust, an able attorney, formed the Association Building Company to finance, erect, and equip an outpatient medical building. Organized as a for-profit corporation, the company issued common and preferred stock, most of which was bought by the founders and their families, and leased a parcel of land on the southwest corner of East 93rd Street and Euclid Avenue. At the time of construction, the corporation acquired the land under the original building from Ralph Fuller through a 99-year lease (also referred to as a "perpetual lease") beginning October 29, 1919. This lease eventually passed, through inheritance, into the hands of the Worthington family, from whom The Cleveland Clinic bought it, as authorized by the Board of Trustees, on October 5, 1970. Ironically, this bit of land was the last in the block to be acquired by The Cleveland Clinic!

The architectural firm of Ellerbe and Company estimated that a suitable building could be constructed for $400,000. Excavation

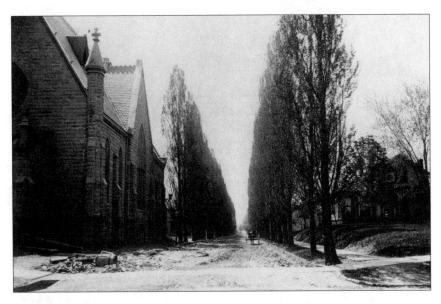

Oakdale Street (later East 93rd), looking south from Euclid Avenue, circa 1887
(Courtesy: Cleveland Public Library)

began in February 1920, and a year later the building was completed. Although the Crowell-Little Company was the contractor, Crile said in his autobiography that "the real builder of the Clinic was Ed Lower, he knew each brick and screw by name and was on hand early enough every morning to check the laborers as they arrived."

The Clinic Building (now known as the "T Building") had four stories, of which the upper three were built around a large central well extending from the second floor up to a skylight of tinted glass. The main waiting room, handsome with tiled floors and walls and with arched, tiled doorways and windows, was at the bottom of the well on the second floor. The offices, examining rooms, and treatment rooms opened onto the main second-floor waiting area and onto corridors consisting of the balconies that surrounded the central well on the third and fourth floors. On the first floor were the x-ray department, the clinical laboratories, and a pharmacy. On the fourth floor were the art and photography department, editorial offices, a library, a boardroom in which the founders met, offices for administrators and bookkeepers, and Dr. Crile's biophysics laboratory. Thus, from the beginning there were departments representing not only the cooperative practice of medicine, but also education and research.

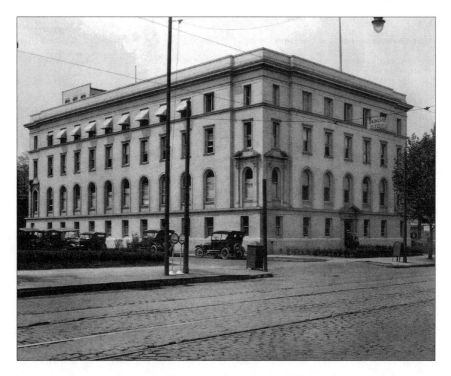

Original Clinic Building, 1921

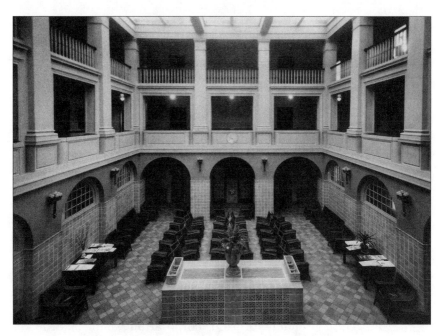

Waiting room, original Clinic Building, 1921

From the time of The Cleveland Clinic's formation as a not-for-profit corporation, there were no shareholders, and no profits accrued to the founders. All of them received fixed salaries set by the trustees. Likewise, all other members of the Clinic staff received salaries that were not directly dependent on the amount of income they brought into the Clinic.

The founders had donated substantially to the Clinic's capital funds, and in the formative years they had taken the risk of personally underwriting the Clinic's debts in order to establish a nonprofit foundation dedicated to service to the community, medical education, and research. To ensure there would be no future deviation from these aims, the founders empowered the Board of Trustees, at its discretion, to donate all assets of the organization to any local institution incorporated "for promoting education, science, or art." These assets could, thus, never contribute to anyone's personal enrichment.

At the first meeting of the incorporators on February 21, 1921, the signers were elected Trustees of the new institution, and provision was made for increasing the number of trustees to as many as fifteen if this became desirable. Bunts, Crile, Lower, and Phillips were designated Founders.

CHARTER AND ORGANIZATION

The Cleveland Clinic's charter is an extraordinary document for its time because the scope of medical practice it defined was so liberal. The document, reproduced below, also raised the issue of the corporate practice of medicine, much criticized at the time. The charter granted by the State on February 5, 1921, reads as follows:

These Articles of Incorporation of the
Cleveland Clinic Foundation

WITNESSETH: That we, the undersigned, all of whom are citizens of the State of Ohio, desiring to form a corporation, not for profit, under the general corporation laws of said State, do hereby certify:

FIRST: The name of said corporation shall be The Cleveland Clinic Foundation.

SECOND: Said corporation and its principal office is to be located at Cleveland, Cuyahoga County, Ohio, and its principal business there transacted.

THIRD: The purpose for which said corporation is formed is to own and conduct hospitals for sick and disabled persons; and in connection therewith, owning, maintaining, developing and conducting institutions, dispensaries, laboratories, buildings and equipment for medical, surgical, and hygienic care and treatment of sick and disabled persons, engaging in making scientific diagnoses and clinical studies in, carrying on scientific research in, and conducting public lectures on, the sciences and subjects of medicine, surgery, hygiene, anatomy, and kindred sciences and subjects, accepting, receiving and acquiring funds, stocks, securities and property by donations, bequests, devises or otherwise, and using, holding, investing, reinvesting, conveying, exchanging, selling, transferring, leasing, mortgaging, pledging and disposing of, any and all funds, stocks, securities and property so received or acquired, charging and receiving compensation for services, care, treatment, and accommodations for the purpose of maintaining said hospitals not for profit and the doing of all acts, exercising all powers and assuming all obligations necessary or incident thereto.

IN WITNESS WHEREOF, We have hereunto set our hands, this 5th day of Feb. A.D. 1921

> Frank E. Bunts
> George W. Crile
> William E. Lower
> John Phillips
> Edward C. Daoust

The practice of medicine in the United States has traditionally been founded on the sanctity of the doctor-patient relationship. A somewhat questionable and clearly self-serving economic corollary is that, to preserve this relationship, an individual patient must pay a fee for medical service directly to the doctor of his or her choice. Organized medicine has always resisted attempts to change the basis of this relationship, and the legal system has generally been supportive of this view. Similarly, lawyers have sought to preserve the lawyer-client relationship, threatened by large corporations, such as banks, that set out to sell legal services to customers through the offices of their salaried lawyers. If a corporation were allowed to do the same with the services of physicians, i.e., engage in corporate medical practice, by analogy a precedent dangerous to the status of lawyers might be established. For this reason, most state legislatures, being dominated by lawyers, passed laws prohibiting the corporate practice of medicine, and most group practices, whether operating for profit or not, were obliged to include within their structure some sort of professional partnership in order to bill patients and to collect fees legally. The properties of the Mayo Clinic, for example, have always been held by a nonprofit foundation. The physicians, however, were organized first as a partnership and then as an association from 1919 to 1969. The doctors received salaries from the fees paid by patients and turned over to the Mayo Foundation the excess of receipts over disbursements. This "landlord-tenant" relationship between the Mayo Foundation and its medical staff was changed in 1970 when, as a result of corporate restructuring, all interests came under the Mayo Foundation. Thus, in most nonprofit clinics, devious means have been used to achieve what The Cleveland Clinic accomplishes directly; the organization itself collects fees and pays the salaries of its staff. Today, with the strong trend toward group practice, the right of a nonprofit organization like the Clinic to "practice medicine" is unlikely to be challenged. The charter of 1921 remains a source of wonder to lawyers.

Thirteen members made up the professional staff of The Cleveland Clinic in its first year. Joining Bunts and Crile were Dr. Thomas E. Jones and Dr. Harry G. Sloan in surgery. Lower was joined by Dr. Thomas P. Shupe in urology. With Phillips in medicine were Dr. Henry J. John, Dr. Oliver P. Kimball, and Dr. John P. Tucker. Henry John was also head of the clinical laboratories. Dr. Justin M. Waugh was the otolaryngologist, Dr. Bernard H. Nichols was the radiologist, and Hugo Fricke, Ph.D., was the biophysicist.

Crile was elected the first president of The Cleveland Clinic Foundation; Bunts, vice president; Lower, treasurer; and Phillips, secretary. Daoust, who had so skillfully handled the Clinic's legal needs, was designated a life member of the Board of Trustees.

THE GRAND OPENING

At 8:00 P.M. on February 26, 1921, 500 local members of the medical profession and many physicians from outside the city attended the opening of The Cleveland Clinic. This event was modestly noted in the *Bulletin of the Academy of Medicine of Cleveland* as follows:

"CLINIC BUILDING OPENS
"Drs. Frank E. Bunts, George W. Crile and W.E. Lower and their associates, Dr. H.G. Sloan, T.P. Shupe, Bernard H. Nichols, Thomas E. Jones and Justin M. Waugh, announce the removal of their offices from the Osborn Building to the Clinic Building, Euclid Avenue at East 93rd Street, effective March 1st, 1921."

Among those from other cities were Dr. William J. Mayo of Rochester, Minnesota, who delivered the main address of the evening; Dr. Joseph C. Bloodgood of Baltimore, Maryland; and Dr. J. F. Baldwin of Columbus, Ohio. The program included talks by each of the founders and by Charles Howe, president of the Case School of Applied Science. Mayo gave the main address.

Crile described the incorporation of The Cleveland Clinic and outlined its purposes and aims as follows:

"With the rapid advance of medicine to its present-day status in which it evokes the aid of all the natural sciences, an individual is no more able to undertake the more intricate problems alone, without the aid and cooperation of colleagues having special training in each of the various clinical and laboratory branches, than he would be today to make an automobile alone. We have, therefore, created an organization and a building to the end that in making a diagnosis or planning a treatment, the clinician may have at his disposal the advantages of the laboratories of the applied sciences and of colleagues with special training in the various branches of medicine and surgery.

"Another reason for establishing this organization is that of making permanent our long-time practice of expending for research a goodly portion of our income. On this occasion we are pleased to state that we and our successors are pledged to give not less than one-fourth of our net income toward building up the property and the endowment of The Cleveland Clinic Foundation. It is through The Cleveland Clinic Foundation under a state charter that a continual policy of active investigation of disease will be assured. That is to say, we are considering not only our duty to the patient of today, but no less our duty to the patient of tomorrow.

"It is, moreover, our purpose, also pursuant to our practice in the past, that by reason of the convenience of the plant, the diminished overhead expense, and the accumulation of funds in the Foundation, the patient with no means and the patient with moderate means may have at a cost he can afford, as complete an investigation as the patient with ample means.

"The fourth reason for the establishment of this Clinic is educational. We shall offer a limited number of fellowships to approved young physicians who have had at least one year of hospital training, thus supplementing the hospital and the medical school. In addition there will be established a schedule of daily conferences and lectures for our group and for others who may be interested.

"This organization makes it possible to pass on to our successors experience and methods and special technical achievements without a break of continuity.

"Since this organization functions as an institution, it has no intention either to compete with, nor to supplant the individual practitioner who is the backbone of the profession and carries on his shoulder the burden of the professional work of the community. We wish only to supplement, to aid, and to cooperate with him.

"Since this institution is not a school of medicine, it cannot, if it would, compete in any way with the University, but what it proposes to do is to offer a hearty cooperation in every way we can with the University.

"Our institution is designed to meet what we believe to be a public need in a more flexible organization than is possible for the University to attain, because the University as a teaching organization must of necessity be departmentalized. As compared with the University, this organization has the advantage of plasticity; as compared with the individual practitioner it has the advantage of equipment.

"The result of such an organization will be that the entire staff—the bacteriologist, the pathologist, the biochemist, the physicist, the physiologist, and radiologist, no less than the internist and the general surgeon, each, we hope and believe, will maintain the spirit of collective work, and each of us will accept as our reward for work done, his respective part in the contribution of the group, however small, to the comfort, and usefulness, and the prolongation of human life.

"Should the successors seek to convert it into an institution solely for profit or personal exploitations, or otherwise materially alter the purpose for which it was organized, the whole property shall be turned over to one of the institutions of learning or science of this city."

Bunts reviewed the concepts underlying the Clinic's unique organizational structure and outlined the founders' aims and hopes for the future. He stated that the founders hoped that, when their associates took the places of their predecessors, they would "carry on the work to higher and better ends, aiding their fellow practitioners, caring for the sick, educating and training younger men in all the advances in medicine and surgery, and seeking always to attain the highest and noblest aspirations of their profession."

Phillips reemphasized the fact that the founders had no desire for the Clinic to compete with the family physician. Instead, they sought to make it a place to which general practitioners might send patients for diagnostic consultations.

Lower explained the design of the building and its plan of construction, which was intended to ensure the greatest efficiency for each department, resulting in the most salutary operation of the Clinic as a whole, for the ultimate welfare of the patients.

Mayo's speech was entitled "The Medical Profession and the Public." Its content was significant, and it contained many truths and ideas that are still worthy of consideration. He spoke in part as follows:

"On every side we see the acceptance of an idea which is generally expressed by the loose term 'group medicine,' a term which fails in many respects to express conditions clearly. In my father's time, success in the professions was more or less dependent on convention, tradition, and impressive surroundings. The top hat and the double-breasted frock coat of the doctor, the wig and gown of the jurist, and the clerical garb of the ecclesiastic supplied the necessary stage scenery. The practitioner of medicine today may wear a business suit. The known facts in medicine are so comprehensive that the standing of the physician in his profession and in his community no longer depends on accessories.

"So tremendous has been the recent advance of medicine that no one man can understand more than a small fraction of it; thus, physicians have become more or less dependent on the skill, ability, and specialized training of other physicians for sufficient knowledge to care for the patient intelligently. An unconscious movement for cooperative medicine is seen in the intimate relation of the private physician to the public health service made possible by the establishment of laboratories by the state board of health and similar organizations. On every hand, even among laymen, we see this growing conception of the futility of the individual effort to encompass the necessary knowledge needed in treating the simplest and most common maladies because of the many complications which experience has shown are inherent possibilities of any disease."

Mayo went on to discuss some of the fundamental political and professional aspects of medical care and ended by stating:

"[O]f each hundred dollars spent by our government during 1920, only one dollar went to public health, agriculture and education, just one percent for life, living conditions, and national progress. . . . The striking feature of the medicine of the immediate future will be the development of medical cooperation, in which the state, the community, and the physician must play a part.

"[P]roperly considered, group medicine is not a financial arrangement, except for minor details, but a scientific cooperation for the welfare of the sick.

"Medicine's place is fixed by its services to mankind; if we fail to measure up to our opportunity, it means state medicine, political control, mediocrity, and loss of professional ideals. The members of the medical fraternity must cooperate in this work, and they can do so without interfering with private professional practice. Such a community of interest will raise the general level of professional attainments. The internist, the surgeon, and the specialist may join with the physiologist, the pathologist, and the laboratory workers to form the clinical group, which must also include men learned in the abstract sciences, such as biochemistry and physics. Union of all these forces will lengthen by many years the span of human life and as a byproduct will do much to improve professional ethics by overcoming some of the evils of competitive medicine."

With these instructive and challenging remarks, Mayo highlighted the fundamental aims of the founders of The Cleveland Clinic: better care of the sick, investigation of their problems, and further education of those who serve. Although Mayo emphasized that The Cleveland Clinic was organized for "better care of the sick, investigation of their problems, and further education of those who serve," he did not phrase it in such a succinct manner. The earliest documented use of this phrase was in 1941 on a plaque dedicated to the founders that was hung at the entrance to Crile's museum and can now be seen in the lobby of the original Clinic Building.

On Sunday, February 27, 1921, the Clinic held an open house for some 1,500 visitors. On the following day it opened to the public, and 42 patients registered.

THE CLINIC'S WORK BEGINS

The public accepted the Clinic so enthusiastically that it soon became apparent to the founders that they needed an adjacent hospital, even though the staff continued to have hospital privileges at Lakeside, Charity, and Mt. Sinai hospitals. Crile had agreed with the trustees of Lakeside that he would retire as professor of surgery at Western Reserve in 1924, and Lower had consented to a similar agreement with the trustees of Mt. Sinai. Considering the prevailing attitude toward group practice and the corporate practice of medicine, there was ample cause for concern about whether the hospitals would continue to make available a sufficient number of beds to the staff of the new clinic.

With the prospect of being frozen out of hospital beds a real possibility, the Clinic purchased two old houses on East 93rd Street just

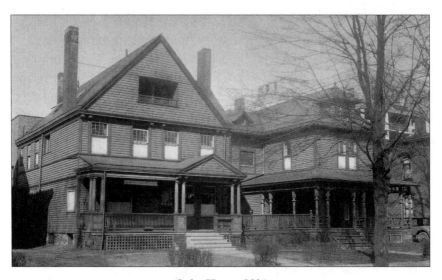

Oxley Homes, 1924

north of Carnegie Avenue and converted them into a 53-bed hospital, the Oxley Homes, named for the competent English nurse who was put in charge. In 1928, Lower wrote, "Dr. Crile suggested one day if we could get two houses near together on 93rd Street, not too far from the Clinic, we could fix them up and use [sic] for a temporary hospital. The suggestion was made at noon. At 2 P.M. a patient of Lower's— a real estate agent—came in to see him professionally. After dispensing with the professional visit, Lower incidentally asked if she knew of any property on 93rd Street which might be bought or leased— preferably the latter as we had no money. She said she would find out. She returned in an hour reporting that two maiden ladies down the street had two houses they would be glad to lease as they wanted to go to California to live. Lower gave the agent $100 to go and close the deal. About 5 P.M. of the same day, Dr. Lower asked Dr. Crile about the property he thought he should have. He replied 'Two houses near together on E. 93rd Street.' Lower said, 'I have them!' Crile said, 'The hell you have!' Thus closed the second land deal on 93rd Street and the first step in the formation of a hospital."

Another house was used by Dr. Henry John to treat diabetes, not easy in those days, since insulin had just been discovered and reactions to it were not yet well understood. A fourth house, "Therapy House," was used for radiation therapy, and a fifth for serving luncheons to the medical staff.

At first, Oxley Homes was considered to be essentially a nursing home. Soon, however, an operating room for major operations was installed. This presented some difficulties because there were no elevators in the buildings. Orderlies, nurses, and doctors had to carry patients up and down the stairs of the old houses. In the meantime, plans were made to build a modern 184-bed hospital on East 90th Street. It opened June 14, 1924, and Miss Charlotte E. Dunning was put in charge. The seventh floor contained operating rooms, living quarters for several residents, and anatomic and clinical pathology laboratories. Although 237 beds were now available, between the Oxley Homes and the new hospital, the demand for beds continued to exceed the supply. Two years later two floors of the Bolton Square Hotel, located one block west on Carnegie Avenue, were equipped for the care of 40 medical patients.

With the successful completion of the Hospital building in 1924, the Association Building Company had fulfilled its useful life. It had provided the founders with the legal and financial means to construct both the clinic and hospital buildings. Since 1921, the Clinic had gradually bought up the stock of the Association Building Company. By December 31, 1925, the Clinic owned all common and preferred shares that had at one time represented equity in the old Association Building Company. The founders instructed Daoust to merge all interests into The Cleveland Clinic Foundation. The Association Building Company passed out of existence. Its assets formed the nucleus of an endowment fund that was used to help support research and to finance the charitable services of the organization.

The Cleveland Clinic's experience with hospital beds can be summarized in the phrase, "too few and too late." By 1928, the shortage was again acute, and construction began on an eastward extension of the Hospital to 93rd Street to provide a total of 275 beds, excluding Oxley Homes and the hotel rooms. Increasing need for supplementary services necessitated installation of a machine shop in a penthouse atop the Clinic building and construction of a power plant, laundry, and ice plant. Parking of cars became increasingly problematic, and the Clinic bought and razed a number of nearby houses to provide space. Lower wrote: "The purchase of these . . . houses created a land boom on 93rd Street between Euclid and Carnegie Avenue and no other property was for sale at the prices paid for the parcels already purchased . . . . When we decided to build a hospital unit, we had an agent buy land on East 90th Street, ostensibly for garage purposes. We succeeded in getting enough land on East 90th Street for the first unit of the Cleveland Clinic Hospital. From then on trading in land became an interesting game of chess for the Clinic and the property owners on East 93rd Street between Euclid and Carnegie."

By 1928, the biophysics laboratory in the Clinic building had become inadequate because of the expansion of research, and a narrow, eight-story research building was constructed between the Hospital and the Clinic.

In that same year, Bunts, who had appeared to be in good health and had been carrying on his practice as usual, died suddenly of a heart attack. The event saddened all who knew him.

At a special meeting of the Board of Trustees on Wednesday December 5, 1928, the following resolution was passed:

"Resolved: That we, members of the Board of Trustees of The Cleveland Clinic Foundation, wish to place on record our appreciation of our association with Dr. Frank E. Bunts, who died November 28, 1928.

"Dr. Bunts was one of the four members who laid this Foundation, and who helped to carry it forward to its present condition of power and of influence. The relations of its members to each other have been long and intimate. To one, that relation covered more that two score years of precious meanings. With the others, either through professional or professional co-working, he held closest relations. To another, Dr. Bunts was a father by marriage.

"In Dr. Bunts were united qualities and elements unto a character of the noblest type. Richly endowed in intellect, he was no less rich in the treasures of the heart. Dr. Bunts had an outspoken religion which was evident in his daily life. His intellectual and emotional nature gave support to a will which was firm without being unyielding, forceful yet having full respect for others' rights. He graciously gave happiness to others, as well as gratefully received happiness from them. His smile, like his speech, was a benediction. A sympathetic comrade, he shared others' tears and others' anxieties, and still he

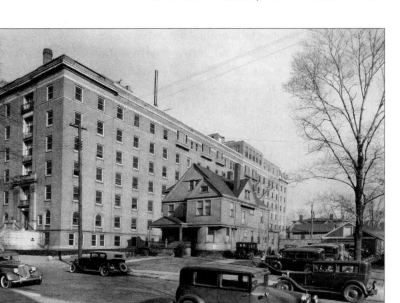

Cleveland Clinic Hospital, East 90th Street (photographed 1930s)

was glad and hopeful. Faithful to the immediate duty, his interest was world-wide, covering seas and many lands. Recognized by his professional colleagues as of the highest type of excellence and of service, he was yet humble before his own achievements. Richly blessed in his own home, he helped to construct and reconstruct other homes ravaged by disease. Gratitude for his rare skill and for the gentleness of his devoted ministries is felt in thousands of lives restored unto health and usefulness. He loved people and was loved as very few men are by the multitudes.

"His thoughtful judgment and rare kindliness was always evident at Board meetings, and his gracious manner will ever be remembered.

"If, however, we would see his monument, we ask ourselves to look about. Seeking for evidence of the beauty of his character, of the happiness which he gave like sunshine, or of the usefulness of his service, we turn instinctively to our own grateful, loving and never-forgetting hearts." [Punctuation in the foregoing quotation has been edited.]

During the memorial meeting held in the Clinic auditorium to honor Bunts's memory, Dr. C. F. Thwing, president of Western Reserve University and a member of The Cleveland Clinic's Board of Trustees, remarked that Bunts had always been "responsive, heart to heart, mind to mind, and added to this responsiveness was a constant sense of restraint; he never overflowed; he never went too far. There was an old set of philosophers called the Peripatetics who were of this type. He held himself together. He was a being in whom integrity had unbounded rule and control."

Fortunately, the expanding workload of the Clinic had enabled Bunts to appoint a young associate whom he had taught in medical school and residency and who now stood ready to take over his practice. This was Dr. Thomas E. Jones, who was destined to become one of the most brilliant technical surgeons of his time.

In response to continually rising demand for both outpatient and inpatient services, the Clinic increased the professional staff and strengthened the existing departments. Using the remains of the building fund, the Clinic purchased a gram of radium and installed a radium emanation plant. This plant made radon seeds for use in the treatment of cancer in the Therapy House. This was the first such plant in the region. In 1922, the Clinic also added an X-ray therapy unit of the highest available quality and put Dr U. V. Portmann, a highly trained specialist in radiation therapy, in charge. Portmann, in conjunction with Mr. Valentine Seitz, the brilliant engineer who headed the machine shop, and Otto Glasser, Ph.D., of the Biophysics Department, made the first dosimeter capable of accurately measuring the amount of radiation administered to a patient. Jones, who was by then on the surgical staff, had received special training in the use of radium and radon seeds and was well prepared to take advantage of the new radiation facilities.

The Clinic also added new departments, including endocrinology, which was still in its infancy but growing fast. At the same time, surgery was becoming more and more specialized, requiring the formation of such departments as orthopedic surgery and neurological surgery. The Clinic took full advantage of the development of the specialties and of the prosperity that characterized the '20s. The future appeared bright, and life was good.

3. THE DISASTER
1929

By ALEXANDER T. BUNTS

That which does not kill me makes me stronger.
—Nietzsche, 1888

THE EXPLOSIONS

ON WEDNESDAY, MAY 15, 1929, IN THE COURSE OF WHAT BEGAN AS A normal, busy working day at the Clinic, disaster struck, resulting in great loss of life and threatening the very existence of the institution. Incomplete combustion of nitrocellulose X-ray films, which at that time were stored in an inadequately ventilated basement room of the Clinic building, generated vast quantities of toxic fumes, including oxides of nitrogen and carbon monoxide. At least two explosions occurred. Toxic gases permeated the building, causing the deaths of 123 persons and temporary illness of about 50.

The first explosion took place about 11:30 A.M. when about 250 patients, visitors, and employees were in the building. Fire did not present a major threat because the building was fireproof. The danger lay in inhalation of toxic gases. The occupants of the nearby research building and hospital experienced no problems. A fire door closed the underground tunnel connecting these buildings, confining the gas to the Clinic building.

The room in which old films were stored was located on the west side of the basement next to the rear elevator shaft. There was direct communication between this room and a horizontal pipe tun-

49

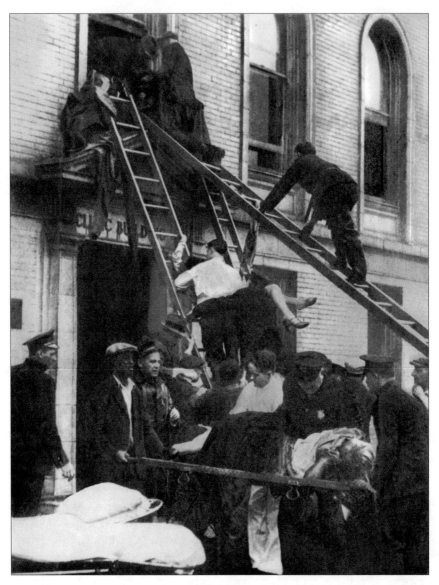

The Disaster, May 15, 1929

nel or chase, which made a complete circuit of the basement and from which nineteen vertical pipe ducts extended through partitions to the roof. These provided the principal routes for the passage of gases throughout the building.

Old nitrocellulose X-ray films, still in use despite their known safety hazards, were stored in manila envelopes (averaging three films to the envelope), on wooden shelves and in standard steel file cabinets. No one knew the exact number of films in the room, but it was estimated that there were about 70,000 films of all sizes, equivalent to about 4,200 pounds of nitrocellulose. Some estimates were as high as 10,000 pounds. Water pipes and three insulated steam lines were located below the ceiling of the room. One steam line, pressurized at about 65 pounds per square inch, passed within seven and one-half inches of the nearest film shelf. The room had no outside ventilation. Electrical wiring was in conduit, and there were several pendant lamps. There were no automatic sprinklers.

Several hours before the disaster, a leak had been discovered in the high-pressure steam line in the film storage room. A steam fitter, who was called to make repairs, arrived about 9:00 A.M. and removed about 14 inches of insulation, allowing a jet of steam about three feet long to issue from the pipe in the direction of the film rack against the north wall. He went to the power house to close the steam line and then returned to his shop to allow the line to drain and cool. Upon returning to the film room about 11:00 A.M., the workman discovered a cloud of yellow smoke in one upper corner of the room. He emptied a fire extinguisher in the direction of the smoke, but was soon overcome by the fumes and fell to the floor. Revived by a draft of fresh air, he crawled toward the door on hands and knees. A small explosion flung him through the doorway into a maintenance room, where another workman joined him. Together they made their way through a window and out of the building. Another explosion occurred while the men were still at the window. The custodian spread the alarm.

EMERGENCY AND RESCUE

Alarms were telephoned in from several locations. The first was officially recorded at 11:30 A.M., and two others were recorded by 11:44 A.M. A fire company based on East 105th Street just north of Euclid Avenue was the first to respond. When it arrived, most of the building was obscured by a dense, yellowish-brown cloud. Two more alarms brought more fire-fighting equipment and rescue squads. Ladders were raised on each side of the building in an effort to reach and evacuate the people who appeared at the windows. About eight minutes after the arrival of the first fire company, an explosion blew out the skylights and parts of the ceiling of the fourth story, liberating an immense cloud of brown vapor and partially clearing the building of gas. Rescue work then began in earnest. Firemen and volunteers manned stretchers, removed people from inside the building, and helped them down the ladders. A rescue squad wearing gas masks tried to enter the front door on the north side but was forced out of the building by the concentration of gases. Battalion Chief Michael Graham and members of Hook and Ladder Company No. 8 entered the building from the roof. Fire hoses were trained on the flaming gas visible through windows in the rear stair shaft and some of the basement windows.

Many people died trapped in the north elevator and in the north stairway. Descending the stairway in an effort to escape through the Euclid Avenue entrance, they encountered an ascending mass of frantic people who had found the ground-floor entrance blocked by flames. Many died in the ensuing melee. Some reached safety by going down ladders from window ledges. Others, by climbing up through the broken skylight, made it to the roof of the building and then descended by ladder to the ground.

Dr. A. D. Ruedemann, head of the Department of Ophthalmology, perched on the ledge of his office window on the western side of the fourth floor and supported himself by holding a hot pipe inside the room. He managed to grab a ladder when it reached his level and made his way to the ground.

Dr. E. Perry McCullagh has left the following account:

"It was customary in those days for one of the Staff or a Fellow to accompany the patient to another department. I had gone to the front of the fourth floor with a lady and had introduced her to Dr. Ruedemann. As I approached the balustrade, I heard a rumbling explosion and saw a high mushroom of dense rust-colored, smoke-like gas arise from the center ventilator. I thought at first of bromine. It was clear to me that the masonry building could not burn and that the staff should help the people out and avoid panic.

"The ventilating system connected the basement with all the rooms individually, so that within a minute or so they were filled with the poisonous smoke. The elevator near the front stair was stopped when someone in the power house turned off the electricity, and those in the crowded elevator died. The front stairway was crowded with frightened, choking people beginning to panic. Those near the bottom were shouting, 'Go back, you can't get out here—there's fire down here.' There were flames across the front doorway where the partially oxidized fumes met the oxygen of the open air. Most and perhaps all of the people who remained in the stairway died there. A few escaped through the skylight to die later, as did the neurosurgeon, Dr. C. E. Locke, Jr.

"I left the stairway and went into the thick gas on the fourth floor. Those who reached an open window on the west were pretty well off because the breeze was from that direction. I stumbled against a door on the east corridor, and Dr. Edward Sherrer, who was then a young staff member, pulled me in and helped me to hang my head out of the window, which did little good as the fumes were mushrooming out the window. With the help of firemen we were able to get down one of the first ladders to be put up.

"After helping with what emergency care could be given in our own hospital, we searched for our friends, some of whom were alive and many dead at Mt. Sinai Hospital. Many were located at the County Morgue; others were visited at their homes. Dr. Sherrer and I were admitted to the Cleveland Clinic Hospital late that evening with shortness of breath, very rapid respirations and cyanosis. After a few days in oxygen tents, we were discharged, only to be readmitted about ten days after the disaster, and were in oxygen tents again for most of six weeks. This relapse was the result of interstitial edema of the lungs which occurred late in all of those who were badly gassed but survived the first few days.

"Among many of us who were most severely ill, courage and calmness seemed to play an important role in recovery. The lack of oxygen caused loss of judgment and encouraged restless activity, so that those who fought against instructions and the use of oxygen died. The courage and complete disregard of fear in the case of my roommate, Dr. Conrad C. Gilkison, was amazing. We both believed we were dying because everyone up to that time who had developed cyanotic nail beds had died, and we could see our blue nails plainly enough. At 1:00 or 2:00 A.M., both of us unable to sleep, Gilk said 'Perry, if you're here in the morning and I'm not, get old Bennett to take me to the ball game.' Mr. Bennett was the undertaker at the corner of East 90th and Euclid Avenue, a block from where we lay.

"Dr. Sherrer, Dr. Gilkison and I were finally able to return to work about November 15. Recovery of pulmonary function was complete."

During the confusion of that tragic morning, those trapped within the building were unaware of the nature of the gas that filled the halls, corridors, and examining rooms. They only knew that it severely irritated the throat and lungs, causing coughing and difficulty breathing. Those who reached the examining rooms at the sides of the building and closed the doors behind them had a chance of survival. They opened the windows widely and leaned into the fresh air. When the ladders reached them, many made their way safely to the ground. A few jumped. Dr. Robert S. Dinsmore of the Department of Surgery broke his ankle leaping from a second floor window on the east side of the building.

A number of non-Clinic physicians came to the hospital and spent many hours assisting members of the Clinic staff with their overwhelming task. Many survivors were cyanotic and short of breath, and it rapidly became evident that the problem was toxic gas inhalation. Respiration became more difficult, cyanosis increased, and severe pulmonary edema developed. Fluid caused by gas-induced irritation of the airways filled the pulmonary alveoli. Many of these persons, including Locke and Hunter, died in two or three hours. Edgar S. Hunter, M.D., was a neurosurgery resident working with Dr. Locke. Some died later that afternoon or that night, among them Mr. William Brownlow, artist, and John Phillips, one of the Clinic's founders and head of the medical department. Phillips had reached the ground by a ladder on the east side of the building. He sat for a while on the steps of the church across 93rd Street and finally was taken by car to his apartment at the Wade Park Manor on

East 107th Street. There his condition worsened as the afternoon wore on. About 7:00 P.M. a transfusion team, headed by Crile, went to his room and performed a transfusion, but to no avail. Phillips died at about 8:30 P.M. He was only 50 years old, and the loss of such a talented physician and leader was a particularly sad event for the Clinic and for Cleveland's medical community.

In his book with the grisly title *They Died Crawling and Other Tales of Cleveland Woe* (Gray & Company, Cleveland, 1995), John Stark Bellamy, II, noted "Dr. Crile himself was at his best throughout the disaster, a veritable battlefield general who tirelessly marshalled [sic] resources to heal the wounded and console the grieving."[1]

On the day after the disaster, Dr. Harvey Cushing, a distinguished neurosurgeon in Boston and an old friend of Crile's, arrived in Cleveland to offer his services. Locke, his former assistant, who was the first neurologic surgeon on the Clinic staff (1924-1929), had died of gas inhalation the previous day. Crile asked his first assistant, Dr. Alexander T. Bunts, to take Cushing around the hospital to see those with any possible neurologic injuries.

A few days later, Crile wrote to all surviving family members who could be identified. For example, in a letter to Mr. A. Lippert of Barberton, Ohio, dated May 23, 1929, he wrote, "Because of our sad lack of definite information regarding the family connections of Mr. and Mrs. Carl Long, who lost their lives in the Cleveland Clinic disaster, we are asking you to extend to his family our deepest sympathy in their great sorrow. Only our duty to the surviving has kept us from giving them more promptly this assurance that we sorrow with them."

Crile and others who had had first-hand experience in treating gassed patients during the war in France commented upon the similarities of the clinical effects of the gas to those observed in soldiers who had inhaled phosgene gas ($COCl_2$) at the front. After the disaster, Major General Gilchrist, Chief of the Chemical Warfare Service, came to Cleveland and initiated a thorough investigation of its possible causes. Decomposition of the nitrocellulose film may have been caused (a) by the rise in temperature produced by the leaking and uncovered steam line, (b) by ignition of the film from an incandescent lamp attached to a portable cord close to the shelves, or (c) by a lighted cigarette on or near the films. None of these theories was ever proved. The investigations conducted by the Chemical Warfare Service did determine the nature of the gases produced by the burning or decomposition of nitrocellulose films: carbon monoxide and "nitrous fumes" (NO, NO_2, and N_2O_4). Carbon monoxide breathed in high concentrations causes almost instant death. "Nitrous fumes," which comprised most of the brownish gases, became nitric acid on contact with moisture in the lungs. This led to acute rupture of the alveolar walls, pulmonary congestion, and edema. The Clinic disaster resulted in worldwide adoption of revised safety codes for storing films and led to the mandatory use of safety film that would not explode.

A commemorative booklet, *In Memoriam*, was issued by the Board of Trustees in June 1929, eulogizing the victims of the disaster. It reads in part, "The integrity of the Cleveland Clinic Foundation could receive no more severe test than that of the recent disaster. Each member of the medical staff, as well as every employee in every department, has faithfully carried on his or her own task, knowing that the Clinic was not destroyed, but rather that from the ruins will arise an even better institution which will be dedicated as a sacred memorial to the dead."

SORTING IT ALL OUT

After the disaster many problems confronted the two remaining founders. Miss Litta Perkins, executive secretary to the founders and the Board of Trustees and in whose photographic memory existed most of the records of the Foundation, had died. The Clinic building, although still structurally sound, could not be used. The interior was badly damaged, brownish stains were present everywhere, and there was a rumor that lethal fumes were still escaping. Some advised razing the building, fearing that patients would never again be willing to enter it. Lower and Crile, however, adopted a wise position. "They'll talk for a while," Crile said, "and then, when they forget it, we'll start again to use the building." That is exactly what happened.

A frame house that stood directly across Euclid Avenue from the Clinic had been used as a dormitory for the girls of Laurel School. This house was made available to the Clinic by Mrs. Lyman, headmistress of the school and a lifelong friend of Crile's. The house was transformed into a temporary clinic. For four days after the disaster, the staff and personnel of the Clinic worked unceasingly, aided by carpenters and movers and by a committee of civic leaders headed by Mr. Samuel Mather and Mr. Roger C. Hyatt. Desks, chairs, tables, lamps, x-ray equipment, files, records, and all other necessities were carried across Euclid Avenue and placed on all three floors of the loaned house. Telephone and power lines were installed. On Monday morning, May 20, 1929, just five days after the disaster, the building was opened for the examination of patients.

Liability insurance coverage for such carnage was inadequate, but it did provide eight thousand dollars per person plus funeral or hospital expenses. State industrial insurance gave what Crile termed "cold comfort" to the personnel. The medical staff, however, took on the task of paying the families of the members of the staff who died full salary for the first six months and half salary for the next six. The founders suffered no personal liability because the Foundation, which owned everything, was a nonprofit corporation of which the founders were salaried employees. Expressions of sympathy and offers of financial assistance were received from many Clevelanders as well as from colleagues or patients as far away as India, China, and Australia. More than $30,000 poured in as gifts. Then Crile said, "When Lower and I found we still possessed the

---

[1] The sentiment of a Cleveland physician, Dr. Frank A. Rice, who was one of the many local doctors who helped in the efforts to save victims on the day of the disaster, is well expressed in the following letter addressed to Dr. Lower:

"May 18, 1929

"My dear Doctor Lower:

"Our hearts are wrung and we are bowed in sorrow over the loss of your associates, whom we have all learned to love and respect. We feel, too keenly, the pain it has caused you and those of your group who were spared, but we are justly proud of your undaunted spirit to carry on, and out of the ashes of yesterday to erect an institution bound by traditions, to be a worthy monument to lives and ambitions of its sturdy founders.

"I cannot let the opportunity pass without a word of praise and admiration for your nursing staff. I arrived at your hospital as the first of the injured were brought in. Throughout the day, and into the night, I have never seen, not even in 17 consecutive days in the Argonne, such perfect organization. With death increasing horror at every turn, your nursing staff functioned with alacrity, coolness and decision which marked them as masters of their art—truly a remarkable tribute to their institution and your years of instruction.

"Yours most sincerely,

"Frank A. Rice"

Another letter, this one to Dr. Crile, was from Boston's Dr. Ernest A. Codman, the father of quality assessment in medicine, excerpts of which follow:

"I am writing to ask a question.

confidence of the public, of our own staff, and of the members of our institution, we knew we could finance our own way. So, after holding these gifts for a few months of security, we returned them all with their accumulated interest."

After operating in the Laurel School quarters throughout the summer of 1929, the equipment and functions of the Clinic were transferred in September to the newly completed addition to the hospital, which had just been extended to East 93rd Street. The rooms on several floors were arranged and equipped as examining rooms for outpatients. For the next two years the Clinic's work was carried out here. Although the quarters were cramped, the patients continued to come in increasing numbers.

"I always think of you as an eagle able to look directly into the sun, looking down, perhaps, on the rest of us common birds, who are controlled by our sympathies, petty desires, and emotions.

"You have climbed the ladder of surgical ambition high into the skies of Fame. You have done more good by your introduction of blood pressure measurements, of transfusion, anoci-association, and gas-oxygen anesthesia than could be counteracted by the death of every patient who entered your clinic in a whole year. In the haste of your upward progress you have known that some wings would break and lives be lost.

"Now comes this accident which is not the least your fault, and which will do untold good, as every x-ray laboratory in the world will be safer for it.

"And now, my question: Since you have known both 'Triumph and Disaster'—did you 'treat those two Impostors just the same'?"

To this query Dr. Crile replied:

"Referring to our own terrible blow, the only thing that hurts me, and that will always be, is the loss of life. I saw nothing in France so terrible. It was a crucible. Almost four hundred people were in the building at the time.

"You have always been a close friend. I appreciate you, especially now."

In the June 1929 issue of the *Bulletin of the Academy of Medicine of Cleveland* the disaster was acknowledged, and the following paragraphs summed up the Academy's sentiments:

"The Academy of Medicine bows in sorrow with the rest of the city. The suddenness and tremendous import of it all was brought home to us all the more forcibly by the fact that five of our own members lost their lives. They were all men either prominent in their specialties or starting in on careers which promised well for themselves and for the profession.

"The Academy members who died in this disaster are as follows:

John Phillips, M.D.

C.E. Locke, Jr., M.D.

Harry M. Andison, M.D.

Roy A. Brintnall, M.D.

George W. Belcher, M.D."

A later issue noted two additional deaths, those of Miriam K. Stage, M.D. (one of the leaders of Women's Hospital), and J.H. Swafford, M.D. (radiology).

4. THE PHOENIX RISES FROM THE ASHES

1929-1941

By Alexander Bunts and George Crile, Jr.

Fate loves the fearless;
Fools, when their roof-tree
Falls, think it doomsday;
Firm stands the sky.
—James Russell Lowell, 1868

THE GREAT DEPRESSION

In October 1929, five months after the disaster, the stock market crashed, heralding the Great Depression of the 1930s. It was at this time—with three million dollars of lawsuits filed not only against The Cleveland Clinic but also against Lower, Crile, and the estates of Bunts and Phillips—that the surviving founders decided to build a new three-story Clinic building with foundations to support fourteen stories (eventually known as the "S Building"). They planned to connect this new structure with the original Clinic Building, and to remodel the latter so that it would not remind people of the disaster. At the time of this decision, Crile was 66 years old and Lower was 63. They reasoned that if the court decision went against them and the Foundation, they would all go bankrupt, and there would be nothing to lose.

Crile and Lower did not think that there would be any liability. Storage of the films had been in accordance with the fire laws, and

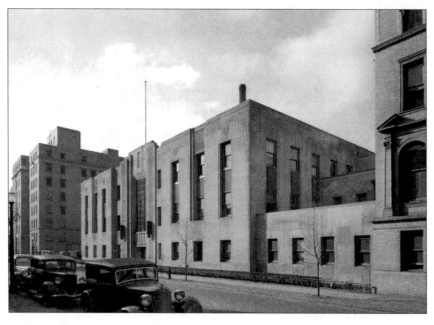

Cleveland Clinic, 2020 East 93rd Street (Left to right): Hospital addition, 1929;
Research Building, 1928; Main Clinic (three stories); Original Clinic Building
(southeast corner showing), 1921 (Photographed in 1935)

the fumes from films had not been recognized as potentially fatal. In 1928, however, eight persons had died in a similar fire in Albany, New York. Suffocation was believed to have been the cause of several of those fatalities.

The two founders started to raise money for the new building with trepidation, facing the difficulties posed by this task. "Every day Ed and I spent the lunch hour in the board room discussing them," Crile wrote. "I was able to convince Ed that we would weather our difficulties; but the next day he would appear so exhausted and excited over a new angle, which had occurred to him while he was fighting out the lawsuits overnight, that I told him if someone struck a match near him he would explode. But he was always a joy, appearing one morning with the suggestion that perhaps there would be Christian Scientists on the jury."

From a professional standpoint, 1929 was a good time to start building. The earnings of both Crile and Lower were at their peak. Phillips, lost in the disaster, was replaced as head of the medical department by Dr. Russell L. Haden, a nationally known physician from the University of Kansas. He began to develop subspecialty departments in internal medicine and soon accumulated a large practice in his own specialty, diseases of the blood. There were able young physicians in all departments, and the reputation and practice of the Clinic were growing rapidly. Indebtedness and the voluntarily assumed burden of paying the salaries of the staff members who had died in the disaster made it difficult to meet the payroll, and Lower once sent a telegram to Crile, who was attending a meeting in New York, "Just across without reserve."

The financial success of the Clinic at this time depended mainly on the fact that some of the physicians' earnings were more than four times as great as their salaries, the excess going to the Foundation. But in order to borrow the $850,000 required for the new building, Crile and Lower had to put up their personal life insurance policies to guarantee $150,000 of the loan. Three million dollars in lawsuits resulting from the disaster were settled out of court for about $45,000, for the pragmatic reason that The Cleveland Clinic had no liquid or negotiable assets that would make it worthwhile for the plaintiffs to bring the cases to court.

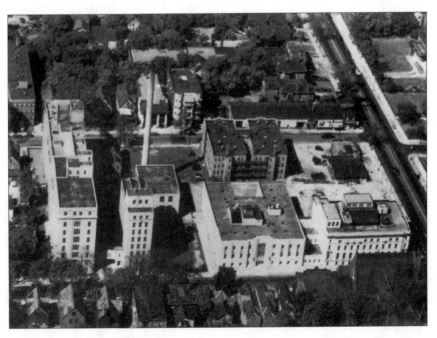

Aerial view of The Cleveland Clinic (Euclid Avenue at right) in 1931

In September 1932, in order to help repay the debt incurred by the disaster and the cost of the new building, all employees, including the medical staff, took a 10 percent pay cut. This financial curtailment was accepted graciously, if not enthusiastically, because everyone was aware of the Clinic's crisis. At that time, no one predicted the severity of the Great Depression that would cloud the years to come. Instead, there was a confident expectation about the future.

"Late in February 1933, while Grace and I were attending a dinner in Cleveland," Crile wrote in his autobiography, "one of the guests, a prominent industrialist and director of one of Cleveland's largest banks, was called to the telephone just as we were seated. He did not return until dinner was nearly over and, when he returned, he seemed deeply perturbed, was without conversation, and soon left." The next day the Maryland banks closed; the following day most Cleveland banks announced that only 5 percent withdrawals were allowed. The economic depression deepened. The banks failed while the Clinic was still heavily in debt. A second 10 percent reduction in salaries had been necessary one month before the banks closed. Four months later there was an additional 25 percent cut. Circulating money had almost ceased to exist, but its absence did not impede the incidence of disease. The sick still required treatment, and somehow many of them managed to pay something for it. The staff and employees remained loyal; their choice, in those days of unemployment, lay between a low-paying job and no job at all. Crile wrote in 1933, "[T]he one abiding comfort, as I looked at our beautiful cathedral for service, was that during the years that I had needed least and could give most I had been able to earn in such excess of my salary that we had been able to accomplish that of which we had dreamed."

The Clinic survived.

GROWTH AND MATURATION

In 1934, the depression was still in its depths. Although Crile was then 70 years old, his surgical practice continued to provide a major part of the Clinic's income. His interest had gradually shifted from thyroid surgery, which had attracted patients from all over the world, to surgery of the adrenal glands, a field that he was exploring to treat such diverse conditions as hypertension, peptic ulcer, epilepsy, hyperthyroidism, and neurocirculatory asthenia. The results of these operations were sometimes promising, but rarely spectacular. The field was so controversial that Crile's personal practice began to shrink. During that time he underwent surgery on his eyes for glaucoma, and soon thereafter he began to develop cataracts.

Fortunately, Crile had able young associates in the Department of Surgery, including Dr. Robert S. Dinsmore, who continued his interest in surgery of the thyroid and breast, and Dr. Thomas E. Jones, who had already become nationally famous for abdominal surgery, particularly for cancer of the rectum and colon. The surgical specialties were headed by capable surgeons, and under Haden's leadership, the Department of Medicine was expanding rapidly. Therefore, Crile began to disengage himself from conventional surgery and to spend more of his time researching the energy systems of man and animals, traveling twice to Africa to collect and study the brains, thyroids, and adrenals of various species of African wildlife.

Crile's research into the energy systems of animals was supported in part by an endowment received from Sarah Tod McBride. In 1941, the Museum of Intelligence, Power, and Personality was built adjacent to the old Clinic Building, to exhibit the specimens that Crile had collected. Dr. Alexander T. Bunts wrote in 1965, "Many parties of school children visited the museum and were fascinated by the mounted specimens of lion, alligator, elephant, gazelles, giraffe, shark, porpoise, manatee, zebra, and many other interesting creatures. Models of the hearts of race horses and whales, fashioned of paraffin or plaster, and wax models of the sympathetic nervous systems, brains, thyroids, and adrenal glands attracted the interest of the curious and challenged the logical thinking of visiting scientists and physicians . . . . Those of us who were working at the clinic in those days were never surprised to encounter a dead lion or alligator in the freight elevator of the Research building or occasionally even a live one, as well as a battery of vats filled with viscera of various animals. In the study of this material, emphasis was placed on the relative weight of thyroid, adrenals, liver, and brain, and the complexity of the autonomic nervous systems."

Mr. Walter Halle, later to become one of the Clinic's trustees, recalled the following episode:

"I got a call from Doctor Crile one day asking if I would come down to the Clinic and serve in some sort of protective capacity, armed with my Mauser 3006, while they were attempting to uncrate a lion sent to him from the Toledo Zoo. The lion was brought up on an elevator in a cage, in a very irritable condition, and moved into the room where he was supposed to be dispatched in some fashion that had not been too thoroughly worked out. After much thrashing around the lion was quieted and someone gave him a shot to put him away peacefully. I hesitate to think what would have happened had the lion broken out of the cage, which he was attempting to do. Fortunately for everyone we did not have to use our firearms because firing a high-powered rifle in a room 14 x 18, with Doctor Crile and three other doctors, would have made it problematical just who would get drilled.

"I can't tell you what an interesting session I had afterwards watching him dissect the lion and listening to his marvelous running-fire commentary about the glands and various parts of the anatomy."

On the way home from Florida in 1941, Dr. and Mrs. Crile and the Clinic's anatomist, Dr. Daniel Quiring, were injured when their airplane hit a tornado and crashed in a swamp near Vero Beach.

"It had been a great day, a manatee was dissected and cast," Dr. Crile wrote, "and we had also stored away in jars the energy organs of a marlin, a sailfish and a barracuda, so we decided to take the early morning plane to Daytona Beach, visit Marineland and catch our train at midnight. This was Quiring's first flight.

"When the steward told us that there were a few thunderheads beyond, Grace remarked that Quiring was going to see a little of every kind of weather. We had left the usual beach route and were flying over marshland that looked like the waterhole country in Africa. The mist became thicker. Suddenly I was conscious of an abrupt vertical upsurge; we had entered the thunderheads and were shrouded in darkness and a violent hail storm, pierced by zigzag lightning that flashed from every bit of metal in the plane. We must have resembled a Christmas tree hurling through space.

"A deafening roar as of a high pressure wind under a powerful drive beat on our ear drums. Blankets, hats, pillows, trays were sucked to the ceiling, then flew in all directions about the cabin. I did not suspect it at the time but we were in an active tornado and were actually observing its mechanism at work. The plane seemed to be whirling. Blackness spun before my eyes. Everything was tipping—I recall how difficult it was to pull my tilting body to the left.

"A lurch! A feeling of gratitude that Grace got off our manuscript to the publisher. Then oblivion!"

Quiring's shoulder was dislocated; Grace Crile suffered two broken ribs, a broken sternum, and a cracked vertebra; and Crile, the most seriously injured of any of the passengers (his seat was at the point where the plane buckled), had three fractures of the pelvis, three broken ribs, and fractures of the transverse processes of two vertebrae as well as severe contusions. Despite these injuries, he was the first to break the silence after the crash. As the chill marsh mire began to rise in the cabin he imagined himself at home in a bathtub. "Grace," he called to his wife, "Grace, would you mind turning on the hot water please?"

Miraculously, no one in that accident died. Crile then made the following observation: "After the experience of everyone in the plane it seems clear to me that the cause of the blackout in aviation must be the failure of the blood to return to the brain and the heart because of the rapid ascent of the plane. Had I been standing on my head or lying flat with feet elevated and head down—the position used in surgical shock when the blood pressure fails, probably I would not have lost consciousness . . . . Were an aviator encased in a rubber suit and the pneumatic pressure established, the suit in itself would prevent the pooling of the blood in the large vessels in the abdomen and extremities and would maintain the conscious state. I believe that an aviator thus equipped would be protected against the failure of the blood to return to the heart and hence would have protection against blackout."

Crile thought of the pneumatic suit that he had developed years before to treat shock. Why not use such a suit to prevent blackouts that occurred when pilots "pulled out" after dive-bombing? The suggestion was passed on to appropriate officers in the Army, Navy, and Air Force. Crile at the age of 77 was made an honorary Consultant to

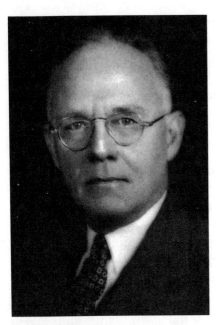

Henry S. Sherman, President, The Cleveland Clinic Foundation, 1941-42

the Navy, and in cooperation with engineers of the Goodyear Tire and Rubber Company produced the first G-suit for military use.

Although Crile had remained president of The Cleveland Clinic until 1940, more and more of the executive duties had been turned over to an Administrative Board composed of four staff physicians. They were responsible for the professional aspects of administration. The Board of Trustees, then composed exclusively of laymen, was responsible for properties and finance. Prosperity had returned to the country, and it seemed that the Clinic was out of its financial straits. But there were still other troubles ahead, many of them arising from conflicts of personalities.

For the Clinic, governed as it had been by the founders for many years with no thought of succession planning, the transfer of authority was bound to be difficult. As the old leaders faltered or stepped down, there ensued a struggle for power among the next generation of leaders. As Dr. Joseph Hahn put it many years later under similar circumstances, "Let the games begin!" It was at this point that the Board of Trustees, which had previously acted mainly in support of the founders' decisions, showed their value. Without them it is doubtful that the institution could have survived. Much of that part of the history of the Clinic is recounted later. It is sufficient to say here that able physicians and surgeons are not necessarily the best administrators.

By 1940, Crile's eyesight was failing badly, and he retired from the position of president of the Clinic. His brother-in-law, Mr. Henry S. Sherman, a former industrialist who at the time was president of the Society for Savings (a Cleveland financial institution) and one of the Clinic's trustees, succeeded him as president. Sherman married Crile's sister-in-law, Edith McBride. He was a trustee of The Cleveland Clinic Foundation from 1936 to 1956. He is remembered not only for his wise counsel in the affairs of the Clinic but also for his friendly concern for the professional staff, many of whom he knew personally. Sherman's son-in-law is James A. Hughes, who was chairman of the Board of Trustees from 1969 to 1984 (with the exception of a two-year interruption from 1973 through 1974). Although Lower was still active in an advisory capacity in 1940, he, too, was by then in his seventies and was equally anxious to turn over the administrative responsibilities to the next generation.

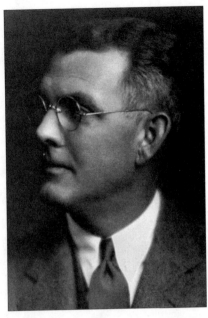

Edward C. Daoust, LL.B., President, The Cleveland Clinic Foundation, 1943-1947

Three years later, Mr. Edward C. Daoust, who had participated so effectively in the founding of the Clinic, was elected to the full-time presidency of the Foundation. Sherman became Chairman of the Board of Trustees.

The Cleveland Clinic had been growing steadily ever since the financial depression began to lift, and the number of employees had increased from 216 in 1930 to 739 in 1941. In September 1941 the Foundation was able to repay the last $180,000 of its indebtedness. The founders then relinquished the last of their administrative duties with the comment, "The child has learned to walk." But the road still led uphill.

5. TURBULENT SUCCESS
1941-1955

By Alexander Bunts and George Crile, Jr.

> *The dogs bark, but the caravan moves on.*
> *—Arabic Proverb*

THE TORCH PASSES

Although the "child" was walking, the problems of adolescence still had to be met. No firm leadership, autocratic or democratic, capable of replacing that of the founders had as yet developed. The dominant personalities on the staff were men like Dr. William V. Mullin, head of the Department of Otolaryngology; Dr. A. D. Ruedemann, head of the Department of Ophthalmology; Dr. Russell L. Haden, head of the Department of Medicine; and Dr. Thomas E. Jones, who replaced Crile as head of the Department of Surgery in 1940. Problems arose as a result of the conflicts among these brilliant and competitive personalities. Sadly, some of their arguments were settled by Mullin's untimely death in 1935 and by Ruedemann's resignation from the Clinic in 1947.

One factor that helped to distract attention from the difficulties of the early 1940s was the sheer weight of work. The military draft had reduced the staff by more than 20 percent and the number of residents by one third. Since most of the young physicians in the area had been drafted, many of their patients came to the Clinic. Surgical schedules and new patient registrations rose to an all-time high. In 1942 there were 21,500 new patients, and by 1944 the number had increased to 27,900. Everyone was too busy to spend much time discussing administrative affairs. Daoust was an effective and respected chief executive, and Sherman, chairman of the Board of Trustees, had a unique insight into the problems of the Clinic in which he had been interested since its inception.

The Clinic's Naval Reserve Unit was called to active duty in the spring of 1942. Two months of training were spent on Pier No. 14 of the Brooklyn Naval Yard in New York, a bleak, barn-like structure in which, as Crile, Jr., recalled, there was very little to do but read *The New York Times*. The Unit then sailed for New Zealand to establish Mobile Hospital No. 4, the first of its kind in the South Pacific. In the Unit were Drs. George Crile, Jr., William J. Engel, A. Carlton Ernstene, W. James Gardner, Roscoe J. Kennedy, Joseph C. Root, William A. Nosik, and Edward J. Ryan, as well as Guy H. Williams, Jr. (a neuropsychiatrist from City Hospital, Cleveland), and Don H. Nichols (a Cleveland dentist).

Construction of the portable hospital, all of which was shipped from the United States, was a race against time, for the landing on Guadalcanal was being planned, and there would have to be a hospital ready to receive the casualties. For three weeks, the physicians and corpsmen labored in the mud of a cricket field on the outskirts of Auckland to put the hospital together. Marie Kennedy, widow of Dr. Roscoe "Ken" Kennedy, recalls that, "Someone accidentally walked across what was to be the ceiling of a large ward, from one corner to another. The footprints dried, and they wouldn't come off. That turned out to be the ceiling of a psychiatric ward! Allegedly the admiral said, 'If you weren't nuts when you were brought in, you would be nuts when you came out!'"

Miraculously they succeeded and were ready when the hospital ship Solace brought its first load of wounded. Most of them had had excellent attention, and there was little left to do except give them convalescent care. But there was a lot to be learned about tropical diseases. A young Marine, strong and apparently well, fell sick one day and the next day was dead with convulsions and the meningeal manifestations of malaria. In his journal Kennedy noted, "What Sherman said about war ('War is hell') still holds."

Mobile Hospital No. 4 was based in New Zealand for 18 months and dealt more with tropical diseases and rehabilitation of the sick n with wounds. Thereafter its officers were dispersed to other stations. As soon as the war was over, the Clinic physicians returned home. After their tours of active duty, the Clinic paid the returning men their full salaries less the amount paid them by the Navy.

Crile was 77 years old when the United States entered World War II. In 1940, after a cataract operation made difficult by a previous operation for glaucoma, he lost an eye. Remaining vision had failed to the point where he could no longer easily recognize people by sight, and he had become subject to occasional spells of unconsciousness. Crile then contracted bacterial endocarditis, and, after an illness of several months, he died in January 1943.

Lower expressed the feelings of many when he wrote on the occasion of Crile's death, "George Crile had a quest and a vision that he pursued throughout his entire adult life with a devotion amounting almost to mystic fervor. This is the striking thing that distinguished him from other surgeons and that gave special meaning to his life. He was not content to make use of known truths, but was forever searching for the answer to 'What is Life?' This was the stream into which his tremendous energies flowed, and all his activities and observations were purposeful and tributary to this."

Crile died with his major quest unfulfilled: he had failed to divine the unfathomable mystery of life. Nonetheless, he left The Cleveland Clinic, complete with its own hospital, research, and educational facilities, to stand as a memorial to its founders. The institution's prosperity in the early 1940s made possible many improvements in its facilities. There were troubles ahead, however, and tumultuous times were to characterize the late 1940s.

On January 1, 1943, Daoust retired from his law practice and became the full-time president of The Cleveland Clinic and its chief administrative officer, responsible to the trustees. He had been associated with the founders and the Clinic for more than 20 years. On that date, Sherman became chairman of the Board, and Mr. John Sherwin, whose activities as a trustee were to be so important to the Foundation through the years, joined Daoust and Sherman as the third member of a new executive committee of the Board of Trustees. In Sherwin's words, "While formal meetings were infrequent, luncheon meetings and telephone conversations took place often, and a closer rapport was established with the Administrative Board then composed of Daoust and Drs. Thomas Jones, Russell Haden, A. D. Ruedemann, W. James Gardner, and E. P. McCullagh."

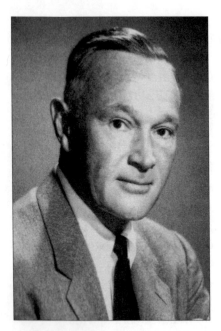

John Sherwin, President, The Cleveland Clinic Foundation, 1948-1957

The Administrative Board referred to by Sherwin was established to represent the professional staff at the same time the new Executive Committee was established. The new Administrative Board had its first meeting in January 1943. The meetings of that body in earlier years have been described as always interesting and frequently almost frightening. Lower would sometimes leave the meeting trembling visibly. Impressions of the meetings of the Administrative Board were recalled by McCullagh, the youngest member of the Board. "The original Medical Administrative Board was formed in February 1937, and was composed of Dr. Crile, Dr. Lower, Dr. Russell Haden, Dr. Thomas E. Jones, Dr. A. D. Ruedemann, and Dr. Bernard H. Nichols with Mr. Edward Daoust attending. These were exciting meetings, for Dr. Ruedemann, Dr. Jones, and Dr. Haden often reacted suddenly. Sometimes this, added to a hot temper, would threaten physical violence. Drs. Haden and Jones, it seemed to me, always disagreed, apparently on general principles. Dr. Ruedemann had no favorites, disagreeing with everyone in turn. This concerned Dr. Crile and Dr. Lower very much, and I'm sure caused them anxiety for fear that no plans for satisfactory Clinic administration were evolving."

The two most powerful figures on the Administrative Board in the 1940s were Jones, Chief of Surgery, and Haden, Chief of Medicine. According to Mrs. Janet Winters Getz, who attended some of the meetings of the Administrative Board in a secretarial capacity, it seemed that these two brilliant and attractive men had agreed to disagree. Sometimes their shouting could be heard over the entire floor. Often the fiery Ruedemann would add his bit. He was a particularly colorful and outspoken man, as exemplified by a story that old about him when he was in medical school. When asked about the blood count of a patient with leukemia, he reported that the white cell count was 500,000. "Did you count them?" his professor asked. "Hell no, I weighed them," said Ruedemann.

SUCCESS AND MATURATION

During the war and immediately thereafter, the Clinic enjoyed prosperity and reached professional maturity. Specialization was increasing in both medical and surgical divisions. New patient registrations continued to increase, rising to 31,504 by 1947, nearly three times the number served a decade earlier. This growth necessitated further building, and seven stories were added to the new Clinic building in 1945. One year later, a wing was added to the hospital, connecting it to the research building. Few beds were added by the new wing, however, as much of the space was taken up by elevator shafts designed to serve future additions. The turbulence of the post-war years required the steady hand of Daoust in administering the growing organization, and his accidental death in June 1947 was a serious blow to the Foundation. The airliner on which Daoust was a passenger crashed into a mountaintop. All on board were killed.

The trustees promptly confronted the administrative crisis precipitated by Daoust's death. Sherwin's own account states that on the morning following the airplane crash, Lower, Sherman, and Sherwin met to determine how to best assume Daoust's responsibilities. There had already been many discussions about how to administer the organization after its founders retired. Conversations had taken place with the management consulting firm of Booz, Allen and Hamilton with an idea of engaging that firm to study the Clinic and its operations and to make recommendations.

Sherman, Sherwin, and Lower agreed to recommend to the Board of Trustees that:
- the position of president would be left vacant for the time being;
- the responsibilities of the president would be assumed by the Executive Committee;
- Sherwin would become chairman of the Executive Committee;
- recently elected trustees John R. Chandler, Benjamin F. Fiery, Walter M. Halle, and John C. Virden would join Sherman and Sherwin on the Executive Committee;

- the Executive Committee in conjunction with the Administrative Board would employ Booz, Allen and Hamilton to make a study and recommend (a) how the Foundation should be administered and (b) how the compensation of the professional staff should be determined.

These recommendations were adopted by the Board of Trustees on June 26, 1947, and a new Administrative Board composed of Drs. Dickson, Ernstene, Gardner, Jones, and Netherton was appointed. That same day the staff assembled to learn of these actions.

During the ensuing four months, the Executive Committee and Administrative Board met almost weekly, usually from five o'clock in the afternoon through dinner and on to ten o'clock or later. Representatives of Booz, Allen and Hamilton attended most of these meetings. They reviewed the entire operation of the institution and developed a plan for the organization and operation of the Foundation. The plan of August 14, 1947, had the unanimous support of the trustees and the Administrative Board. It was during the last year of Lower's life that Booz, Allen and Hamilton gathered data for their report to the trustees.

The idea of spending money for this sort of thing annoyed Lower, and ever the frugal and conservative founder, he finally refused to talk with the management consultants. Mrs. Janet Winters Getz, who at that time served as Dr. Lower's secretary, stated that he refused to allow their representatives on his floor or to permit any of the personnel on his corridor to talk with them. Yet the firm's report, when it finally came, was constructive. Although it was not accepted in full (the staff was opposed to the suggestion that there be a medical director), it paved the way for the development of a committee system. The death of Lower in June 1948 at the age of 80 years severed the last of the personal ties to the origins of the Clinic. The era of the founders had passed, and the Clinic was on its own.

During these sessions, everyone realized the need for an administrative head. A search started for such a person, and, in October, Mr. Clarence M. Taylor, recently retired as executive vice president of Lincoln Electric Company, was invited to become executive director. He assumed the office on January 1, 1948, but spent the balance of 1947 acquainting himself with the Booz, Allen and Hamilton report and the Clinic's operations. Sherwin continued to handle the ies and responsibilities of executive director until Taylor's arrival.

The new plan of organization and operation and the appointment of Taylor were announced at a special meeting of the staff on September 19, 1947. Jones described the plan as the staff's "Magna Charta" and the new executive director as a "welder—formerly of metals, now of people." Both statements proved to be accurate. On September 19, 1947, the Executive Committee, in cooperation with the Administrative Board, made appointments of professional administrative officers: (1) Thomas E. Jones, chief of staff, surgery; (2) Russell L. Haden, chief of staff, medicine; (3) Irvine H. Page, director of research; and (4) Edwin P. Jordan, director of education. A professional policy committee was organized to "consult with, advise and make recommendations to the Board of Trustees or the Executive Committee on major professional policies regarding the operation and activities of the hospital and the clinical, research, and allied departments of the Foundation." The first membership of that committee consisted of Jones, Haden, Ernstene, Gardner, Page, and Jordan. Although some staff members had misgivings, the plan was, on the whole, enthusiastically accepted. The plan provided that administration and policy were the responsibility of lay trustees and that the entire professional operation was the responsibility of a professional staff organization. It was then that Sherwin was elected president of the Clinic.

A member of the professional staff observed many years later that one of the most extraordinary events in the Clinic's history took place at that time. Without salary or remuneration of any kind, the Executive Committee of the Board of Trustees, and Sherwin in particular, devoted many hours a week to meeting with representatives of the professional staff and with the management consultants. The issue was how to manage the Clinic. All of the board members were busy executives with full-time careers of their own. At that critical time, they were not figurehead trustees. They shouldered the full responsibility of their office, bringing to it the organizational skills, the patience, and the understanding that characterize top-flight executives. To these men, the Clinic owes an enormous debt of gratitude. The trustees became more active in Clinic affairs than previously, in an effort to establish better rapport with the staff. The Executive Committee of the trustees and the Professional Policy Committee held frequent joint meetings. Subcommittees of trustees and staff members considered many of the problems involving property, facilities, research budgets, and the hospital. A fundamental feature of the new plan of organization was that committees established policies. For nine years this form of administration continued.

GRUMBLING AND UNREST

At the time of Daoust's death in 1947, there was little harmony among the members of the staff and no organization in which the democratic process could function. The president had been empowered to conduct the Clinic's business affairs; each department head was an autocrat in charge of the professional policies of his own department, and the sometimes tumultuous sessions of the Administrative Board have already been described. The composition of the board was altered in 1947, when Ruedemann resigned from the staff, and in 1949, when Haden retired and Jones died. Jones fell dead in the surgeons' locker room of a ruptured aneurysm of the heart. These events, though traumatic at the time, helped set the stage for the development of a more democratic organization of the professional staff.

Sometimes aging renders leaders too rigid in outlook. Several persons remaining in key positions were in their sixties. In the early 1950s there was hardening of the lines of authority. One department chairman noted that it was impossible to run a department and, at the same time, win a popularity contest. Some of the younger members of the staff began to feel that there was no democratic process allowing them to register either protests or preferences. In those days, one of the ethical principles of the American Medical Association stated that "a physician should not dispose of his professional attainment or services to a hospital, body, or organization, group or individual by whatever name called or however organized under terms or conditions which permit exploitation of the physician for financial profit of the agency concerned." This historic principle made it unethical for any physician to permit a third party to intervene in the relationship between the doctor and his patient. Members of the staff were also members of the American Medical Association, and some began to feel insecure under a plan of organization that seemed sometimes to infringe upon this ethical principle. The complex relationships ong the consumer, provider, and payer that now characterize erican health care were only foreshadowed in the 1950s.

With the purpose of investigating this and related problems, the trustees of the Clinic and the Professional Policy Committee met on October 13, 1954, at which time they appointed a Medical Survey Committee.[1] After several months of careful deliberation and consultation with every member of the staff, the Medical Survey Committee issued a report recommending changes in both administrative and professional affairs of the Foundation.

The preamble of the report states that "The Cleveland Clinic Foundation is celebrating its 34th Anniversary this year (1954). Under the leadership of its four dynamic founders it pioneered in the practice of group medicine and laid the groundwork that has brought it world renown. Many changes have taken place since the Clinic's founding days. Its physical plant has expanded immeasurably and is in the process of further expansion. From the original four men has grown a medical staff approaching 100. Instead of four successful rugged individualists, the staff now consists of 25 times that number, perhaps less successful, perhaps less rugged, but nonetheless individualist. In many organizations faced with the loss of the leaders who were their creators, a time for appraisal comes somewhere around the 30th year of their history. It is desirable to pause then for some serious thought as to whether the institution continues to carry on the ideals which made it great, and if so, whether it is doing only that or is actually continuing to aggressively meet the challenge of the future."

The Medical Survey Committee suggested that many of the Clinic's problems could be solved if the trustees delegated certain responsibilities to an elected Board of Governors composed of members of the professional staff. They recommended that a Planning Committee of trustees and staff be charged to study the administrative structure of the Clinic.

The Medical Survey Committee identified administrative and medical practice issues they felt were critical to the continued success of the Clinic's development. The report recommended that:
- the government of The Cleveland Clinic Foundation must become more democratic, so that every member of the staff will feel a greater responsibility for the welfare of the institution and have a more definite stake in its future;
- the legal status of the Clinic must be clarified;
- the Clinic research and educational programs must be reevaluated and strengthened where possible, since the professional emi-

nence of the institution depends in large measure upon their accomplishments;

- the financial well-being of the professional staff must be evaluated to determine whether or not it is adequate;
- the Clinic should evaluate the medical needs of the area served, and modify its services to fit these needs;
- the Clinic must make a vigorous effort to improve its relations with patients and with physicians both in local and outlying areas;
- the Clinic must increase its efforts to keep the public informed about its services, facilities, and achievements;
- patient care in the Cleveland Clinic Hospital must be improved.

The Planning Committee met frequently during the summer of 1955, and as a result of its deliberations the Board of Trustees adopted a new plan of organization. The new organization provided that all professional matters pertaining to the practice of medicine be under the jurisdiction of the Board of Governors. Provision was made also to form elected committees within the divisions of medicine, surgery, and pathology. The plan also proposed formation of committees for research, the hospital, properties, education, and planning. The committees would be composed of trustees and members of the professional staff.

The divisional committees were to manage the professional affairs within their respective domains under the authority of a Board of Governors. During the early deliberations of the Planning Committee, it became quite clear that there were certain ancillary professional services that could not be separated from professional responsibility. These areas included the central appointment desk, routing desk (including information and patient registration), professional service personnel (including clinic nurses, medical secretaries, and desk receptionists), records and statistics, telephone operators, and patient relations.

The work of the Planning Committee was greatly facilitated by a study of the structure and operation of the Mayo Clinic, in which a board of governors had been the responsible body of government since 1919. From this study, with due regard for the differences that existed between the two institutions, a plan of organization was developed and adapted to the corporate structure of the Cleveland Clinic. The posed plan delegated responsibility for medical practice to a Board overnors to be composed of seven members of the professional staff. These were to be elected by the staff for staggered terms of five years. To prevent self-perpetuation, no member would be eligible for re-election for one year after expiration of the term. To prevent election of members of the board by cliques, an indirect method was devised. Each year, the staff would elect a Nominating Committee. After deliberation, this committee would nominate a member of the staff to fill each vacancy. The entire staff would then vote on the nominees, and if 60 percent approved each candidate, he or she would be elected. Only twice in the years since this system was introduced has the staff failed to support the nominating committee's candidates.

The Board of Governors was given authority to select and appoint new members of the staff, but the setting of the salaries for these and all other members of the staff remained a function of the Compensation Committee of the Board of Trustees. To aid this committee in evaluating the performance of each member of the staff, the Board of Governors was authorized to discuss each member and rate his or her performance. The focus of the evaluation was not to be only the number of patients seen or money earned, but also his or her scientific and other achievements, so that, in effect, the performance of each staff member would be judged by peers.

On the professional side, an effort was made to diminish the authority of the chiefs and to encourage individual initiative. Thus, the Chiefs of Medicine and Surgery, who previously had absolute authority in their divisions, became chairmen, respectively, of the Medical and the Surgical Committees that were elected annually by the members of their respective divisions. The Board of Governors appointed these chairmen for a period of one year, but almost without exception the appointments were renewed annually. Short of illness or mismanagement, the divisional chairmen had what amounted to tenure in their offices. Yet they did not have total control, for they had no authority to act completely independently of their committees. They could be out-voted. Moreover, the actions of the committees were subject to review by the Board of Governors. This afforded protection to the individual staff member from capricious or unfair treatment by the chiefs.

Since the Division of Research was supported by endowment funds, earnings of the Clinic, and outside grants, its administrative problems were to be the responsibility of the Board of Trustees. For this purpose, the Committee on Research Policy and Administration was established. A Research Projects Committee, appointed by the Board of Governors from the members of the Division of Research and from members of the clinical divisions who had special knowledge of or interest in research problems, was put in control of all research projects undertaken by members of the clinical divisions. The long-range program of research, devoted largely to the study of hypertension and arteriosclerosis, remained under the control of the Director of Research, Dr. Irvine H. Page, who reported only to the Board of Trustees. It was not until 1969 that the Division of Research was brought under the control of the Board of Governors.

As a memorial to Bunts, an educational foundation was established and named for him some years after his death. The Bunts Fund, established shortly after Bunts's death in 1928, was changed to an education fund in 1935 at the time the educational foundation was created. The same Board of Trustees that directed The Cleveland Clinic Foundation also directed the Cleveland Clinic Educational Foundation. The original endowments and also the profits of the Cleveland Clinic Pharmacy (incorporated as a taxable, profit-making company) supported the Educational Foundation.

The report of the Planning Committee was a significant document that addressed many issues and had far-reaching consequences. The months of effort in 1955 were rewarded by a truly new system of governance for the Foundation. At a meeting of the professional staff it was unanimously recommended that the professional members of the Planning Committee nominate the first Board of Governors. The names of the nominees were sent to the staff for approval, and thus was created the first Board of Governors, composed of Drs. Fay A. LeFevre (chairman), William J. Engel (vice chairman), George Crile, Jr., A. Carlton Ernstene, W. James Gardner, E. Perry McCullagh, and Irvine H. Page. Dr. Walter J. Zeiter was elected executive secretary, and Mrs. Janet Winters Getz was elected recording secretary. The first meeting was held on Thursday, December 8, 1955, at 12:15 p.m. in the Board Room of the Main Clinic Building. In attendance by invitation were Richard A. Gottron, business manager of the Foundation, and James G. Harding, director of the Hospital. Thus began a new era.

---

[1] The members of the Medical Survey Committee were Mr. Richard A. Gottron (chairman), Drs. Robin Anderson, Victor G. deWolfe, C. Robert Hughes, Alfred W. Humphries, Fay A. LeFevre, Ausey H. Robnett, John F. Whitman, Walter J. Zeiter, and Clarence M. Taylor (ex officio).

section two

THE BOARD OF GOVERNORS ERA

6. THE LEFEVRE YEARS
1955-1968

By Shattuck Hartwell

The physician must have at his command a certain ready wit,
as dourness is repulsive both to the healthy and the sick.
—Hippocrates, about 400 B.C.

INTO A NEW ERA

LITTLE DID THE GROUP OF PHYSICIANS WHO FIRST MET AS GOVERNORS IN December 1955 realize the magnitude of the responsibilities they would come to assume and the importance of the decisions they and future Boards of Governors would make. Nor, obviously, did LeFevre know that he would serve as chairman for the next 13 exciting and formative years. Following months of discussion and deliberation, the Planning Committee recommended, and the Board of Trustees approved, the policy that delegates responsibility for all professional matters to the Board of Governors.

Fay A. LeFevre, M.D., became the first chairman of the Board of Governors on December 7, 1955, just four months before his 51st birthday. A lifelong Clevelander and son of a physician, LeFevre was a graduate of Cleveland Heights High School, the University of Michigan, and the Western Reserve University School of Medicine. His postgraduate training included an internship at St. Luke's Hospital and further training in cardiovascular disease at The Cleveland Clinic. After a few years of private practice, he joined the Clinic's staff in 1942, and in 1947 he founded the Department of Peripheral Vascular

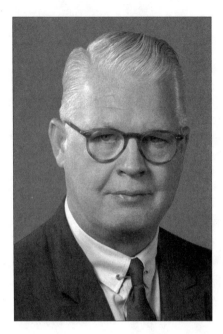

Fay A. LeFevre, M.D., Chairman, Board of Governors, 1955-1968

Disease, now the Section of Vascular Medicine. In addition to chairing that department for eight years, he served a four-year stint as the Clinic's Director of Education beginning in 1952. LeFevre's gentlemanly demeanor, impeccable integrity, and reputation as an outstanding physician made him the ideal choice for the chairmanship of the new board.

Besides LeFevre, the first Board of Governors consisted of W. James Gardner, M.D. (neurosurgeon), William J. Engel, M.D. (urologist), George Crile, Jr., M.D. (general surgeon), E. Perry McCullagh, M.D. (endocrinologist), A. Carlton Ernstene, M.D. (cardiologist), and Irvine H. Page, M.D. (research). It was their responsibility to plan and coordinate all professional activities. Among their most important duties were the appointment, promotion, and termination of members of the professional staff. With the growth of the institution, this became increasingly crucial and difficult. Members of the Board also reviewed criticisms and complaints concerning relationships with patients and initiated corrective measures. In addition, it was their responsibility to review and establish fees for professional services and to review at regular intervals the financial results of professional activities. As the Clinic expanded, planning and policy-making were tasks that took increasing amounts of time. The success of these efforts required the cooperation and collaboration of trustees and governors.

LeFevre had for many years served as a director of the Chesapeake and Ohio Railroad and was knowledgeable in business and finance. Although he was chairman of the Board of Governors, he wished to continue the part-time practice of medicine. He believed that by keeping in touch with his medical practice roots he would be in a better position to understand issues and problems associated with them. For some time LeFevre was able to do this, and he found it both satisfying and stimulating. "It was also a great protective mechanism for me," he said. "When things got 'too hot' in the first floor administrative offices, Janet Getz would call me and say that my patients were ready on the third floor. This gave me an ideal opportunity to excuse myself. Likewise, when some patients became too long-winded, I could politely say that an urgent problem had occurred in the administrative office that would require my immediate attention. This best of two worlds did not last long, however, for it was necessary to spend more and more time in the administrative office."

TRUSTEES AND GOVERNORS

In the early years, some of the trustees thought that the administration of medical affairs by the Board of Governors would not succeed. The responsibility for professional affairs had been delegated to a professional group, and business affairs were under the direction of a business manager. The weakness in this arrangement was that no one person or group had the final authority to make a major decision when professional and business issues were both involved.

Throughout this era, the trustees kept a tight rein on the management of the Clinic by placing their representatives in key authoritative roles—those of business manager and hospital administrator.

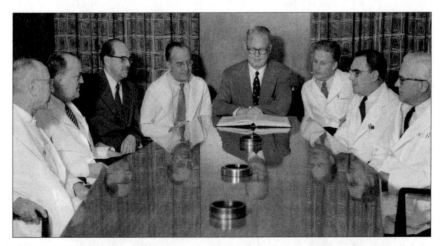

Board of Governors, 1956 (Left to right): Drs. W. James Gardner, E. Perry McCullagh, Walter J. Zeiter (Executive Secretary), Irvine H. Page, Fay A. LeFevre (Chairman), George Crile, Jr., A. Carlton Ernstene, William J. Engel

Nonetheless, the Board of Governors had plenty to do. There were pressures to provide new facilities, to expand existing services, and to subspecialize clinical practice to meet both the demands of patients and the opportunities of practice. These pressures led to the growth of the professional staff and ultimately to the need to acquire property and build new facilities. The impetus for these changes (growth and increasing numbers of patients) lay with the professional staff, but it was for the Board of Governors to interpret and present the needs of patients and staff so that the trustees could understand and respond.

Between 1956 and 1968, the trustees were ably led first by John Sherwin and then by George Karch. James A. Hughes became chairman in 1969 and, except for the period when Arthur S. Holden, Jr., served in that post (1973-1974), continued his leadership through 1984. The first members of the professional staff to serve on the Board of Trustees were Drs. W. James Gardner, Fay A. LeFevre, and Irvine H. Page, and since 1956, members of the staff have always been included in that body. This representation quickened the tempo of decision-making and the rudimentary planning process of that time, but decision making was still not easy. Investment in new property, buildings, and equipment led to increased amounts of work and therefore to increases in revenues, staff, and the total number of employees. The Board of Governors looked to the trustees for authorization of its plans and allocation of the money necessary to fund them. The money for all these expansion projects was in hand. There was no debt financing, and funds set aside from operational revenues were adequate for payment in full. Long-term financial obligations would not be incurred until a later era.

COMMITMENT AND GROWTH

Several construction projects undertaken during LeFevre's administration laid to rest a nagging issue for the Clinic, i.e., whether or not to abandon the inner-city location of the Clinic and move the entire operation into or even beyond the eastern suburbs of Cleveland. A bequest from Martha Holden Jennings financed the Education Building, and that was followed by additions to the Clinic and Hospital buildings and by the construction of a hotel (now called the P Building) to lodge out-of-town patients and their families.

Parking garages were built, and the trustees authorized the acquisition of real estate adjoining the Clinic to allow for future expansion. The die was cast: the Clinic would remain in the city.

The Board of Governors made a decision in December 1965 that was to have an impact far beyond what they imagined. This was the decision to close the obstetrical service, which then occupied the south wing of the hospital's sixth floor. Behind this move was a steadily mounting pressure for space and facilities for cardiac surgery. Something had to give, and a declining national birth rate and low obstetrics-unit occupancy eased the decision. The winner of the institutional support sweepstakes was the heart disease program.

Obstetrical services in American hospitals, as decreed by the Joint Commission on Accreditation of Hospitals, must be isolated from the rest of the hospital. Therefore, delivery rooms, newborn nurseries, and the rooms for mothers were separated from rooms for medical and surgical patients and the general operating rooms of The Cleveland Clinic. The Department of Thoracic and Cardiovascular Surgery moved their inpatient functions into this area, thereby consolidating the operating rooms, recovery room, intensive care unit, and convalescent wards into what would become the most productive and renowned department in the Division of Surgery.

During the LeFevre era, two sets of issues generated conflict in matters of governance and authority. Conflict was inevitable because Mr. Richard A. Gottron, the business manager of the Clinic, and Mr. James G. Harding, the administrator of the Hospital, reported to the Board of Trustees and not to the Board of Governors or its chairman. Sitting *ex officio* with the Board of Governors was helpful to Gottron and Harding in the exercise of their duties and provided them the opportunity to be sympathetic with the wishes and the ideas of the governors, but their sympathy could not have been expected to endure, and it didn't.

The main issue was institutional growth and its capital cost. The trustees were anxious that the ambitions of the staff might launch the institution on a breakneck pace of development in which the prudence of businesslike standards could easily be cast aside. Gottron nourished that fear, and his pessimism respecting the growth of the Foundation irreconcilably alienated him from the governors by the summer of 1968. Gottron was ill at this time, suffering from an unrecognized serious depression.

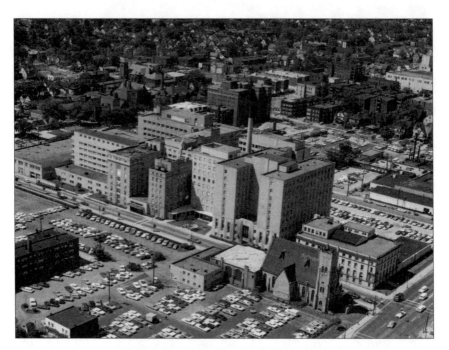

Aerial view of The Cleveland Clinic, 1968

The second and subtler issue had to do with management, authority, and control in what by then had become a large enterprise. By 1968, it had been nearly 13 years since the first meeting of the Board of Governors, and that body had successfully faced matters of policy, planning, and professional practice. Under LeFevre's leadership, the governors had worked together and had discovered that they represented the strength of the professional staff. Governance of the organization was beginning to take on a new meaning. The governors could not take the next step, however, without the willingness of the trustees to recognize them as a responsible body and to delegate the operations of the Clinic and the Hospital to them. Dialogue between trustees and governors in the summer of 1968 led to that next step. Mr. James H. Nichols replaced Gottron as business manager, and both he and Harding were directed to report to the chairman of the Board of Governors. When Nichols replaced him, Gottron received the job of president of the Bolton Square Hotel Company, a subsidiary operation of the Clinic. Not long thereafter he took his own life. LeFevre, who was ready to retire, would be succeeded by a chairman who was destined to function like a chief executive officer of a large corporation.

7. THE WASMUTH YEARS
1969-1976

BY SHATTUCK HARTWELL

> More history's made by secret handshakes
> than by battles, bills, and proclamations.
> —John Barth, 1960

THE WINDS OF CHANGE

CARL E. WASMUTH, JR., M.D., LL.B., BECAME THE SECOND CHAIRMAN OF THE Board of Governors on January 2, 1969, about six weeks before his 50th birthday. A native of Pennsylvania, he had received his undergraduate and medical degrees from the University of Pittsburgh and interned at Western Pennsylvania Hospital (Pittsburgh) followed by nine years of private practice. He then completed a fellowship in anesthesiology at The Cleveland Clinic and joined the staff in 1951. Wasmuth obtained his LL.B. degree, on his own initiative and at his own expense, from the Cleveland-Marshall Law School in 1959 and taught there until 1974. He became chairman of the Department of Anesthesiology in 1967, a post he held until he was appointed chairman of the Board of Governors. He was elected president of the American Society of Anesthesiologists in 1968.

Wasmuth's chairmanship was the outgrowth of a struggle between the non-physician administration (led by Gottron), who wanted to constrain the organization's growth, and the medical staff, who wanted the Clinic to grow. Although he was never elected to the Board of Governors, Wasmuth was chosen to lead the staff because he

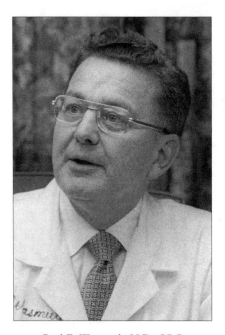

Carl E. Wasmuth, M.D., LL.B.,
Chairman, Board of Governors,
1969-1976

was viewed as the toughest proponent of the staff's viewpoint. His law degree lent credibility to this perception. In a secret meeting at Cleveland's Union Club, from which LeFevre was excluded, a small group of Clinic leaders made the decision to put the administrative functions of the organization, which had previously reported to the trustees, under the Board of Governors.

According to the recollections of Dr. Ralph Straffon and Dr. Thomas Meaney, those present at the meeting were Mr. James Hughes, Mr. John Sherwin, Mr. George E. Enos, Meaney, and Straffon. Gottron was removed as business manager and placed in charge of subsidiaries, as noted in the previous chapter. Nichols remained as secretary, taking over Gottron's managerial functions. Harding, Gottron, and Nichols were to report to the Board of Governors. Subsequently, the Board of Governors selected Wasmuth to replace LeFevre and put the Clinic on a new, centrally directed course with true physician leadership.

The Cleveland Clinic's modern era began with Wasmuth's chairmanship of the Board of Governors. He was the Clinic's first genuine physician manager, and the tasks he addressed in this role were similar to those faced by executives in industry, government, or education. In his first year as chairman, he was confronted by a formidable workload, compounded by the fact that there was no one else in the organization to whom he felt comfortable delegating authority. There was no other physician administrator. Wasmuth recalled that he relied heavily on Messrs. James E. Lees, Robert J. Fischer, and Paul E. Widman when he became chairman. However, Wasmuth reserved ultimate administrative control for himself. Lees functioned as an executive assistant, Widman as director of operations, and Fischer as treasurer.

Early in Wasmuth's administration, both Nichols and Harding, the most seasoned professional managers in the administration, resigned. The governors were clinicians with little managerial experience. Wasmuth, therefore, assumed a degree of personal authority unknown since the early days, when the founders themselves had provided day-to-day direction. He considered it essential that he devote full time to his office; therefore, he gave up clinical practice as well as his post as head of the Department of Anesthesiology.

As early as 1968, it was clear that the scope of the chairman's responsibility had become too broad. The Board of Governors was in charge not only of all professional matters but also of operations and could not be conversant with all the necessary details. The key administrative team that kept the Clinic running smoothly and tended to the details in those early years of the Wasmuth era consisted of John A. Auble, general counsel, and Gerald E. Wolf, controller, as well as Fischer, Lees, and Widman. Neither Wasmuth nor any other chairman could have functioned without them. The Board of Trustees required increasing amounts of time and attention, as did a vast array of public interests.

Wasmuth assumed this burden with energy and enthusiasm, but he, the trustees, and the governors realized the need for an "understudy." A search committee identified Dr. William S. Kiser, a urologist who was serving on the Board of Governors, to fill the role of Wasmuth's assistant. Like Wasmuth, Kiser gave up his clinical practice, a decision that was difficult for many staff members to understand. However, the professional staff was determined to have a strong voice in the direction of the institution, and this sacrifice was seen as necessary. Kiser enrolled in the Advanced Management Program at Harvard University, where he became the second physician to complete that course. In due time, he was named vice chairman of the Board of Governors and placed in charge of operations.

During the LeFevre years, the west wing of the hospital had been added. Soon after it opened, however, it became clear that escalating patient demand would require more beds before long. Plans for the south hospital addition and a new research building were developed. It was also necessary to build a hotel and two parking garages. Financing the new development was one of Wasmuth's most important priorities.

The Clinic's traditional "cash on the barrelhead" method of financing capital projects was no longer tenable. The costs were too high, and the Clinic's ongoing operations and routine capital needs required most of the available cash. Therefore, Wasmuth proposed the use of long-term borrowing from local banks to pay the construction costs that could not be supported by current operations. This was the first use of debt financing by The Cleveland Clinic.

Nonetheless, significant commitments of operating funds for these projects in the early 1970s severely restricted cash flow, and money for routine needs was limited. To make matters worse, the federal government imposed price and wage controls at that time. The staff began to grumble. General paranoia was exacerbated by the fact that cost-containment methods were carried to ridiculous lengths, for example, eliminating pens and removing sanitary napkin dispensers from the women's rest rooms. The bitter aftertaste of these ineffective, petty measures dissipated slowly. Yet, throughout the 1970s the Clinic thrived, largely because of the expansion that had increased the capacity to provide patient care. Although the cash squeeze produced by those projects was stressful, the organization's leadership learned important lessons that they would eventually apply to the more grandiose building programs of the 1980s. Few would now deny that Wasmuth deserves plaudits for launching the expansion of the 1970s and for persuading the governors and trustees that all available real estate adjacent to the Clinic should be acquired. He clearly foresaw the Clinic's position as the national and international health resource that it eventually became.

CONFINED EXPANSION AND
COMMUNITY REACTION

As the Clinic purchased land and razed the deteriorated buildings on its new property, its presence became increasingly conspicuous. These activities began to be viewed by some detractors not as neighborhood improvements but rather as evidence of the Clinic's voracious appetite for growth. To put it bluntly, the Clinic was developing a predatory image. As the Clinic became more dependent on public good will to permit new projects and methods of financing growth, the days when it could remain aloof and ignore the public's perceptions and feelings about its actions were over. During the Wasmuth years, there was more adverse public feeling against the Clinic than at any previous time.

During Wasmuth's administration, the Clinic became involved in two public arenas: increased social responsibility and city politics.

The organization gave one million dollars in aid and assistance to the Forest City Hospital, a hospital struggling to survive as a provider of care to many of the urban poor. This hospital later closed its doors. The Collinwood Eldercare Center was partly supported and staffed by the Clinic, and in cooperation with the Cuyahoga County Hospital System the Clinic helped to establish and maintain the Kenneth Clement Family Care Center. A neighborhood revitalization effort, the Fairfax Foundation (now the Fairfax Renaissance Development Corporation), received both financial aid and operational assistance from the Clinic.

The Cleveland Clinic had little or no experience shaping opinions held by such diverse groups as the neighborhood, underserved minorities, the professional community, health care planning agencies, payers, and local politicians. And yet the resolution of issues such as zoning changes and neighborhood use variances, the building of viaducts over city streets, street closures, and the addition of costly technology and hospital beds were all increasingly dependent upon the attitudes and opinions held by these constituencies. For example, a conflict with the local health-planning agency, then called the Metropolitan Health Planning Corporation, took place over the issue of the Clinic's need to add 173 hospital beds in the new South Hospital. Although the Clinic prevailed, it was an unpleasant experience and attracted unfavorable public notice.

In 1976, a committee of governors and trustees chaired by Hughes conducted a confidential inquiry into these matters. The courts eventually had to address some particularly blatant improprieties. The most visible outcome of this inquiry was a change in the Clinic's leadership. The trustees, general counsel's office, and governors worked well together in this effort to preserve the integrity of the Clinic.

While all this was going on, the staff was becoming restless. They felt the Board of Governors had become increasingly estranged from their concerns. This apparent alienation was symbolized by the removal of Wasmuth's office and the boardroom from the first floor of the Main Clinic Building to the new south wing of the hospital in 1974 to an area known informally as "mahogany row." Nearly all the staff had walked by his office door many times a day for several years, and the remoteness of the new, well-furnished location seemed to represent an aloofness. Perhaps a more appropriate symbolism for this move was the shift in emphasis from the outpatient clinic to the hospital, which was, by this time, assuming the financially dominant role

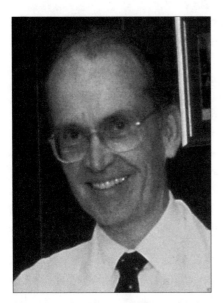

Shattuck W. Hartwell, Jr., M.D.,
Vice Chairman for Professional Affairs,
Founder of the Page Center, Editor of
the second edition of To Act As A Unit

in the Clinic's operations.

The staff was far larger than it had been in the 1950s and early 1960s, and the institutional issues that faced the governing boards took precedence over some of the professional and personal matters that the staff felt should be addressed by the governors. The governors met only once a week, and Wasmuth did not have time for these concerns. Therefore, the Board of Governors appointed Dr. Leonard L. Lovshin, chairman of the Department of Internal Medicine and a former governor, to function as mediator and liaison to the professional staff. He was given the title of Director of Professional Affairs. Lovshin's amiability, popularity, and seniority were assets, but the job was not designed to allow the director to influence policy-making and decisions at the highest level. Recognizing this, the governors eventually took another step to augment the administrative staff that Wasmuth sorely needed by appointing one of their own members to be Vice Chairman for Professional Affairs.

The person they selected to fill this role was Dr. Shattuck W. Hartwell, Jr., a plastic surgeon and member of the Board of Governors and Board of Trustees. Hartwell and Lovshin worked together through the Wasmuth years and into the Kiser era, when Lovshin retired. By that time the Office of Professional Affairs had evolved into a full-time extension of the Board of Governors, assisting the professional divisions in matters of staffing, recruitment, benefits, policy, and dispute resolution. In time, the title of vice chairman of the Board of Governors would be reserved for the chief operating officer, and the title of vice chairman for Professional Affairs would become director, Professional Staff Affairs. Thus, the physician manager continued to evolve toward specialization and assumption of a more important role in the governance of the Clinic during the Wasmuth years. In the Kiser era the position of physician manager was to become even more essential.

8. THE KISER YEARS
1977-1989

By Shattuck Hartwell and John Clough

A decision is an action an executive must
take when he has information so incomplete
that the answer does not suggest itself.
—Arthur William Radford, 1957

A GENTLER STYLE

WILLIAM S. KISER, M.D., OFFICIALLY BECAME THE THIRD CHAIRMAN OF THE
Cleveland Clinic's Board of Governors in January 1977, just before his
49th birthday. A native of West Virginia, Kiser had received his
undergraduate and medical degrees and postgraduate training as a
urologist from the University of Maryland. He had served in the
United States Air Force from 1954 to 1957 with tours of duty in Texas,
Morocco, and Germany, receiving Commendation Medals in 1956
and 1957. After completing his residency in 1961, he had joined the
Surgery Branch of the National Cancer Institute in Bethesda,
Maryland, where he had held the positions of senior investigator and
staff urologist. He had remained at the National Institutes of Health
until he was recruited to join The Cleveland Clinic's Department of
Urology in 1964 by chairman Ralph Straffon, who wished to add a
research dimension to the department.

Kiser's unique background, his bright, enthusiastic personality
and personal warmth, and his clinical skill made him a popular addition to the staff. His election to the Board of Governors in 1972 set him

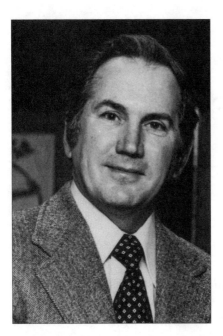

William S. Kiser, M.D., Chairman,
Board of Governors, 1977-1989

on a course that led to his selection by Wasmuth for ultimate succession to the chairmanship, through a search process concluded in 1974 (see chapter 7). Although he was thrust into this role somewhat prematurely and unexpectedly, he rose to the occasion and eventually left his own indelible mark on the Clinic's developmental history.

The Cleveland Clinic's modern period of physician governance had begun with Wasmuth. When Kiser succeeded Wasmuth as chairman, the Board of Governors had been in existence for 20 years. Governance of the Clinic had been evolving over that period of time, and the purview of the board now included a number of new responsibilities, such as policy development, fiscal responsibility, long-range planning, and day-to-day operations. Under Kiser's leadership, these management functions would be increasingly systematized in line with his belief that a corporate model of management should replace the traditional scientific model with which physicians were comfortable.

By 1982, the day-to-day operation of the institution required the cooperative input of the division chairmen whose managerial role was now better defined. This cooperation was formalized by the creation of a committee of the division chairmen called the Management Group. The Management Group reported to the Board of Governors through its chairman, Dr. John J. Eversman. Eversman, an endocrinologist, became the first chief operating officer of the Clinic and a vice chairman of the Board of Governors. He was well suited to these tasks by virtue of his intelligence and additional education, having been the first member of the staff sent by the Clinic to complete an executive M.B.A. program. Kiser, Eversman, and Hartwell were members of the Board of Trustees and its Executive Committee by virtue of their positions.

Differences between Wasmuth and Kiser may be partly due to the way each perceived himself as a chief executive: where Wasmuth had concentrated authority centrally, Kiser encouraged decentralization of operating responsibility among a group of physician managers (the division chairmen) and lay administrators. These managers were accountable, through the chief operating officer, to the Board of Governors (the policy makers). The Board of Trustees held the chairman of the Board of Governors responsible for the operational management of the Clinic.

The distinction between policy making and the implementation of policy has been an important development. It has happened because there has been a conscious effort by institutional leaders to define carefully what the responsibilities are for all groups and individuals and to place accountability appropriately. This has not been easy to do. Doctors are trained in their formative years not only to decide for themselves what is the right thing to do (policy) but also to implement it (operations). Training programs are available for Clinic doctors to enhance their managerial skills. These programs have been very popular.

With the delegation of operational responsibility to the divisions and the departments, decentralization meant that preparation of the annual budget would require input from the department and division chairmen. Inexperience made this problematic at first, but by 1979 budgeting had become a more manageable process for the chairmen, many of whom by then had dedicated administrators. The divisions and departments became responsible for other managerial functions, although there was still a strong egalitarian culture within the staff that made it difficult for the chairmen to be true managers. It seems almost quaint today to review the language of the second edition of this book, which stated, "Large organizations tend naturally to be hierarchical. The titles of department chairman and division chairman indicate responsibilities and influence, but they are not autocratic; this would not be tolerated by the staff."

NEW MANAGERIAL APPROACHES

Beginning in 1975, the relationship of the staff to the Board of Governors was formalized in a process known as the Annual

Professional Review. This relationship was linked to an annual appraisal of the professional departments and of each member within the departments. The reviews, organized by the Office of Professional Staff Affairs, are conducted throughout the year and provide the doctors an opportunity to discuss their accomplishments, plans, career goals, and departmental issues with representatives of the Board of Governors and divisional leaders. More than anything else, the Annual Professional Review keeps the division chairmen and the Board of Governors in touch with the staff and is a potent check on the performance of departmental leadership. The Compensation Committee of the Board of Trustees is apprised of the annual reviews. The reviews, begun in a rudimentary form during Wasmuth's tenure, matured under Kiser and Hartwell and have become a well-established and accepted part of professional life at the Clinic.

The Compensation Committee of the Board of Trustees is regularly informed about the Annual Professional Review of the staff. Since 1975 trustees have been advised by consulting firms that specialize in executive compensation programs. The reviews and the consultants' reports have been key elements in the salary program for the staff and key administrative personnel. Better organized and administered than in the past, the review of salaries and benefits is one of the most important activities of the trustees.

Hartwell, always curious and innovative, left the Office of Professional Staff Affairs in 1986 to form the Page Center for Creative Thinking in Medicine. After an exhaustive search process, he was succeeded as chief in 1987 by Dr. Ralph Straffon, who also received the new title of Chief of Staff. Straffon had been chairman of the Department of Urology and later of the Division of Surgery. He was one of the most highly respected and well-known members of the professional staff. He further strengthened the Annual Professional Review process and computerized the Office of Professional Staff Affairs. In addition, he modernized the staff recruiting process and developed new policies governing the professional staff. Notable among these were redefinition of the category of assistant staff and adoption of the requirement that all members of the full staff be board certified in their (sub)specialties.

One of the important new features of the Clinic's management under Kiser was an attempt to begin an organized long-range planning process in 1979. This was to be a cooperative effort of the Board of Trustees and the Board of Governors. It was necessitated by increasing demand for services, proliferating technology, and staff growth, all leading to crowding of the facilities. The Minneapolis consulting firm Hamilton and Associates worked with the staff and governing groups for two years to develop the Clinic's Master Plan. Although this plan was flawed, and many details were never implemented, it spawned the most ambitious facilities expansion program the Clinic had ever seen—the Century Project—described below.

Concurrent with the planning effort, studies were carried out to determine the best way to finance the growth of the Clinic. Robert Fischer, treasurer of the Foundation, and Gerald E. Wolf, controller, were responsible for financial forecasting, a risky business at best. They correctly predicted that an enormous amount of money would be needed over the next ten years to expand the Clinic. The unfortunate experiences of the mid-1970s, when major capital expansion had been funded from operating revenues, suggested that alternative financing methods should be sought. It was eventually concluded that long-term bonds issued by the county would be the method of choice. The Board of Trustees authorized a bond sale to raise $228,000,000, and in June 1982, all the bonds were quickly sold. This was the largest private financing project in the history of American health care at the time.

Kiser also established offices of public affairs, development, archives, staff benefits, and long-range planning. Wasmuth had been farsighted enough to see the value of a full-time architect, planner, and an internal auditor, and he had filled these positions. Kiser advanced the idea that a support staff of administrative specialists was essential to the continuing development of the Clinic.

CHANGING TIMES

Kiser recognized early on that times were changing for health care and hence for medical practice. Although he initially clung to his modified idea of the Clinic's mission, i.e., "better care of the sick *through specialty care*, research, and education," he knew that an ongoing planning process would be critical and that the institution would have to be prepared to change to meet the new environment.

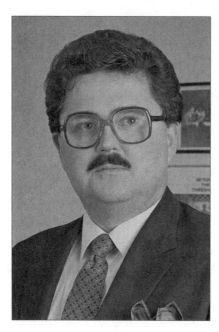

Frank J. Weaver,
Director of Public Affairs, 1980-1989

In 1980, Frank J. Weaver became the Clinic's first director of Public Affairs and Corporate Development, later known as the Divisions of Marketing and Managed Care and of Health Affairs. After Weaver's arrival, the rhetoric changed as well.

Weaver was a professional health care marketer from Texas. Everything about him was big, including his physical size, intellect, capacity for work, and appetites. He cut a natty figure with his boisterous (usually jovial) demeanor, flamboyant clothes, and boutonniere. Weaver had a clearer vision of what lay in store for health care than anyone else at the Clinic, and during his nine-year tenure with the organization, he imprinted many innovative concepts and ideas, which have only recently begun to be appreciated and, in some cases, implemented. He had Kiser's confidence, and for his first years at the Clinic, much of what Kiser said reflected Weaver's thinking.[1]

During the early 1980s, Kiser made some prophetic pronouncements about health care in his "State of the Clinic" addresses, which were traditionally delivered at the second or third staff meeting of each year. In his 1982 speech, for example, he said:

"[N]o single institution can remain an 'island unto itself' in these times. We must seriously consider a departure from the past by developing a strategy for alliance with other groups of physicians and with other health care institutions. We can no longer stand in splendid isolation hoping that patients will come for our attention.

"In the last month Dr. James Krieger [chairman, Division of Surgery], Mr. Dick Taylor [public relations], and Mr. Bill Frazier [head of planning] visited the 15 major group practices in Ohio and Indiana. The observations which they made on location at the various clinics in our region were sobering:

- Referrals of patients more frequently go to other local hospitals because of comparable care and easier access.
- Cleveland Clinic postgraduate courses are no longer a strong attraction to referring physicians due to excessive numbers of CME courses throughout the country—more than 15,000 in 1980!
- Local and university hospitals are actively 'courting' each group for referrals, using incentives the Clinic has used for many years (CME, circuit-riding consultants, timely reporting, etc.)
- Larger groups are developing their own specialty staffs.
- Increasing difficulty communicating with individual Clinic staff members and. . .problems with patient access to our system.

"The conclusions from this survey are that The Cleveland Clinic can no longer count on the reputation of the institution or of its staff to ensure flow of patients in the future. We must formalize relationships with referring doctors or with multi-institutional systems to insure access to patient populations of sufficient size to maintain the economic viability of the Foundation in the future."

BUILDING FOR THE FUTURE

During Kiser's tenure as chairman of the Board of Governors and executive vice president of the Foundation, three major projects that were to change the shape of the organization radically were undertaken. These were (a) the Century Project, (b) the establishment of Cleveland Clinic Florida, and (c) the Economic Improvement Program. Each of these projects warrants some additional discussion.

The Century Project was a building program that grew out of the long-range planning activities referred to previously. Although the Century Project was designed to accommodate the projected growth of the organization through the turn of the century, it was so named because an important feature of it was the construction of a spectacu-

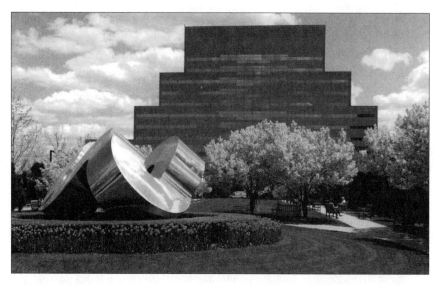

The Crile Building viewed from the mall; in the foreground, Dennis Jones's sculpture "Three for One," a gift from the family of Thomas Vail, Trustee

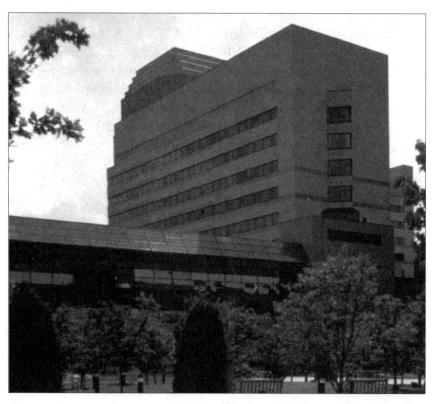

Hospital addition, the "G Wing," 1985

lar new outpatient facility on East 100th Street. The major components of the Century Project as outlined in the Master Plan of 1980 were (a) the East 100th Street outpatient facility (initially called the A Building, but later dedicated as the Crile Building), (b) the enclosed pedestrian walkway from the hospital to the A Building, now known as the Skyway, (c) the southeast wings of the hospital (F and G wings), and (d) the East 100th Street parking garage.

The A Building, designed by award-winning architect Cesar Pelli, opened in September 1985 with an outdoor extravaganza choreographed by Weaver, including speeches by Clinic officials, Speaker of the Ohio State House of Representatives Vernal Riffe, and a congeries of local dignitaries. A high point of the program was the introduction of the newly appointed chairwoman of the Division of Research, Bernadine P. Healy, M.D. Dr. Healy was the first woman appointed to a Cleveland Clinic division chair. Members of the Cleveland Orchestra provided ruffles and flourishes, and they had, fortunately, left by the time a gust of wind blew down their platform. The new building had more than 520,000 square feet of space designed for efficiency by the projected occupants.

The formidable task of moving the outpatient practices of 70% of the staff to the A Building was carried out in just 4 weekends with no interruption of service. The move included the Departments of Allergy, Otolaryngology, Dermatology, Plastic Surgery, Endocrinology, Hypertension and Nephrology, Urology, Internal Medicine, Pediatrics, Pulmonary Disease, Rheumatic Disease, Orthopaedics, Colorectal Surgery, General Surgery, Gynecology, and Ophthalmology. The "stay-behind" departments included Neurology, Neurosurgery, Cardiology, Cardiothoracic Surgery, Vascular Medicine, Vascular Surgery, Primary Care, Gastroenterology, and Infectious Disease. An attempt was made to keep sister services together. Although some shifting of locations has occurred, most departments have remained in their 1985 locations, and the whole design has functioned quite efficiently.

An interesting outgrowth of the work with Pelli on the A building was the creation of a new logo for the organization. Hartwell led this effort, along with architects Pelli, his wife Diana Balmori, and Peter van Dijk, designers Carole Fraenkel and William Ward, and the Burson-Mosteller organization. After 14 months of deliberation, the group proposed the graphic design for the current logo, which was accepted by the Board of Governors and the Board of Trustees.

Hartwell noted that it consists of "four green squares, each showing three rounded corners and overlaid by a perfect golden square," green for medicine and gold for quality. This logo has generated controversy from time to time, on one occasion in a staff meeting having been referred to as a "squashed bug." Nevertheless, it has had remarkable staying power, having survived several efforts at replacement, and according to Mac Ball of the Pelli organization, "it manages to symbolize growth and stability simultaneously . . . [conveying] . . . an optimistic and reassuring feeling."

The Skyway opened at the same time as the A Building. Originally envisioned merely as an environmentally protected, quarter-mile connecting link between the hospital, the new outpatient facilities, and the new garage, it has turned into a meeting ground for all who work at the Clinic. Nearly everyone at the Clinic traverses the Skyway at least once a day, and it is nearly impossible to get from one end to the other without encountering someone with whom some item of business needs to be transacted. Many "curbstone consultations" are conducted on the Skyway, and patient care is the beneficiary. The Skyway has also become the preferred site for numerous events, including the poster sessions for Research Day and many of the events of the annual Martin Luther King, Jr., Celebration of Diversity. It is truly one of the major focal points for life at the Clinic. The comparability of this meeting-place function of the Skyway with that of the "pike" in Boston's old Peter Brent Brigham Hospital was described by Clinic staff member James K. Stoller, M.D., in an article entitled "A Physician's View of Hospital Design" in the December 1988 issue of *Architecture*.

About 3 months after the opening of the A Building, with its associated 1,500-car Carnegie Avenue garage and Skyway, a modern 400-bed addition to the hospital was dedicated. This up-to-date facility included new medical, surgical, and neurological intensive care units, several telemetry units for cardiology patients, a number of regular nursing units and classrooms, and a VIP ward. This allowed closure of some of the oldest areas of the hospital and, thus, represented a net addition of only about 200 beds, bringing the maximum potential bed count to almost 1,200. Given the changes in the health care environment, which were beginning about that time, including a trend to delivering more care in the ambulatory setting, the maximum number of staffed beds peaked at 1,018 during the Kiser era.

A MOVE TO THE SOUTH

While the Century Project was under way, work was beginning on an even more significant undertaking, the establishment of a remote satellite. In 1984, Kiser was approached by physician groups in Florida regarding a possible joint venture with the Clinic. A two-man task force consisting of Robert Fischer, the chief financial officer, and Frank Weaver, the head of public affairs and corporate development, was dispatched to Florida to investigate the possibilities there. At the same time, another task force, pursuant to a 1983 invitation from the Singapore Ministry of Health, was looking into the feasibility of establishing a Cleveland Clinic-like institution in that country. Teams were also created to look at opportunities in Turkey, Sweden, the United Kingdom, Ireland, and Morocco. But eventually attention focused on Florida. Several sites in Florida were evaluated, and, with the help of a 1986 study by the Peat Marwick Mitchell Company, Broward County eventually was selected as the most favorable.

The preliminary work needed to establish a Cleveland Clinic-style group practice in Florida was formidable indeed. In addition to finding the appropriate site, identifying the appropriate physicians, and setting up the necessary hospital affiliations, state legislation allowing The Cleveland Clinic to practice "corporate" medicine had to be passed. All of this was done with some difficulty, but due to the astute work of John Auble, the Clinic's general counsel, James Cuthbertson, Cleveland Clinic Florida's first chief operating officer, and William Hawk, M.D., Cleveland Clinic Florida's first chief executive officer, it was achieved. On February 29, 1988, Cleveland Clinic Florida opened its doors on Cypress Creek Road in Fort Lauderdale with 28 staff physicians and a total of about 100 employees. A month later, Hawk retired, and Carl Gill, M.D., a pediatric cardiac surgeon and medical director of Cleveland Clinic Florida, became chief executive officer.

The Florida physicians had privileges at North Beach Hospital (a for-profit hospital owned and operated by Health Trust, Inc.) located about 10 miles away on the beach. The Cleveland Clinic had leased 50 beds at North Beach and was responsible for filling them or paying for them. Since that 153-bed hospital did not have a certificate of need allowing the performance of cardiac surgery, and because the Clinic was not able to secure one, an arrangement was eventually worked out with Broward General Hospital for the cardiac surgeons to work there. The medical staff of the hospital balked, however, at allowing Cleveland Clinic physicians to have hospital privileges there or even at providing support for the Clinic's cardiac surgeons. This led to a bitter battle and finally to an investigation by the Federal Trade Commission, which found against the Broward General Hospital staff, all of whom were forced to sign a consent decree to avoid prosecution.

During the months before Cleveland Clinic Florida opened, a 320-acre property in Weston, Florida, was acquired. This was to be the ultimate site for the envisioned hospital-clinic-research complex that was to be the fully developed Cleveland Clinic Florida, with initial occupancy of a 200,000-square-foot clinic and a 150-bed hospital at the Weston location by 1992. Although the projected size of the facilities was out of proportion with Peat Marwick Mitchell's estimate that 63 physicians would be needed by 1994, Kiser felt strongly that this institution could grow as large or larger than the Cleveland campus because of (a) the rapid growth of the population in south Florida as compared with the shrinking population in northeast Ohio and (b) the greater accessibility to travelers from Europe, the Middle East, and Latin America, all growing markets for The Cleveland Clinic. This dream sustained the new group through the tough early going. The going remained tough longer than expected, however.

Just as the fledgling clinic was enduring its perinatal angst, the health care environment was changing dramatically. Costs were rising rapidly. Hospital and specialty care, both traditional mainstays of The Cleveland Clinic, were giving way to ambulatory and primary care. Managed care was on the rise. Competition among providers was getting more vicious. All these factors, together with some misreading of the unfamiliar south Florida market by the Clinic's leaders and consultants, led to poor initial financial performance. This was to be one of the major factors necessitating the third big project, the Economic Improvement Program.

Because of reimbursement and practice changes, hospital management was getting more difficult. It was no longer possible to pass cost increases on to the third-party payers; the golden era of cost-based reimbursement had become a thing of the past. In the case of The Cleveland Clinic, in both Cleveland and Florida, this problem was compounded by the relative complexity of the organization, inexperience and lack of training of physician managers to whom authority had been decentralized, and a false sense of permanence created by a period of prosperity that had spanned the entire careers of the majority of the relatively young professional staff.

But the storm clouds were gathering. Although the size of the organization continued to grow unabatedly, growth in new patient activity was slowing, and there were some unexpected cash hemorrhages that began to make the trustees nervous. The Florida project was losing over $1 million per month. A major computer project on the Cleveland campus, which was to have resulted in an electronic medical record and billing system, was floundering, finally failed, and eventually was estimated to have cost the organization millions of dollars. For good measure, it was disclosed that the Florida land had somehow escaped appraisal and was worth less than half of the $55,000 per acre that had been paid for it. Much of this loss was recovered over the next few years by obtaining a land-use change and selling the bulk of the property for residential development. A great deal of the credit for this goes to Mr. Samuel H. Miller, chairman of the board of Forest City Enterprises, Inc., who became one of the Clinic's most active trustees.

The trustees requested Kiser and the Board of Governors to retain McKinsey & Company, a consulting firm with offices in Cleveland noted for masterminding turnarounds for failing companies. Although McKinsey had little health care experience at the time, they took on the project with gusto, and the resulting plan became known within the organization as the Economic Improvement Program. Their initial assessment of the institution's financial status was that if nothing were done, within 18 months the Clinic would have a negative cash flow of $75 million and would begin an economic death spiral from which it could not recover.

On a hot July afternoon in 1989, the Board of Governors held an executive session to consider the situation. During that meeting, Kiser announced his intention to step down as the Clinic's chief executive officer. He agreed to stay on until plans for a smooth transition could be made. The Board of Governors and the Board of Trustees decided to run the institution with a transition team consisting of three of the senior governors, Fawzy G. Estafanous, M.D. (chairman of the Division of Anesthesia), D. Roy Ferguson, M.D. (a member of the Department of Gastroenterology), and Carlos Ferrario,

Ph.D. (chairman of the Department of Brain and Vascular Biology in the Research Institute) along with trustees William MacDonald (chairman of the Board of Trustees), E. Bradley Jones (who became chairman of the Board of Trustees in 1991), and Arthur B. Modell (who became president of The Cleveland Clinic Foundation in 1991). This dedicated team took over the functions of the chief executive officer on July 20, 1989.

The Board of Trustees accepted Kiser's resignation with regret. They approved the hiring of McKinsey in August 1989, and they approved the Economic Improvement Plan the following month.

The Economic Improvement Plan called for implementation of ten projects in two waves. The first five projects included (a) development and implementation of a plan to bring Cleveland Clinic Florida to a cash-flow break-even status by the end of 1991; (b) restriction of capital expenditures to $50 million, freeing $25 million in cash; (c) reduction of costs in Cleveland by $35 million through a combination of difficult measures, including careful control of the employee "head count"; (d) improvement of the budgeting process; and (e) contingency planning. These projects were to start immediately. The second wave of projects, slated to begin during the first quarter of 1990, included (a) the AVA (Activity Value Analysis) project[2]; (b) a "level scheduling" project to improve access; (c) an incentive pay project, euphemistically referred to as "professional staff motivation and rewards"; (d) development of a marketing program that would lead to a 10% increase in patient activity by 1993; and (e) a demonstration project to examine the feasibility of reorganizing into patient-focused activity units rather than traditional specialty departments.

On October 9, 1989, the transition team decreed that the actual first-wave projects would be (a) the Cleveland Clinic Florida project; (b) revenue recapture; (c) AVA; (d) resource utilization; and (e) market strategy. The second-wave activities were to be (a) planning and budgeting; and (b) head count and remuneration. The transition team took on for themselves the tasks of communication and evaluation of information services.

As these projects were getting under way, a search committee composed of the elected members of the Board of Governors and several members of the Trustees' Executive Committee was going about the work of identifying Kiser's successor. Unlike Wasmuth, Kiser had done no succession planning, and there was no one in line to step into the position. Kiser did, however, identify certain promising staff members who were encouraged to obtain further education in management, organizational behavior, or law, who would be candidates for managerial roles in the future. Some have moved into such roles. The search committee reaffirmed the concept that the chief executive should be a physician and interviewed several inside and outside candidates. After deliberating for nearly four months, they chose Floyd D. Loop, M.D., then chairman of the Department of Thoracic and Cardiovascular Surgery and a member of the Board of Governors.

[1] Weaver left the Clinic in 1989 to join Dallas Medical Resource, where he assembled a nine-hospital network to work with self-insured companies in north Texas to provide medical care for their employees. Tragically, he died unexpectedly at the age of 49 on June 16, 1995, in Boston, where he was to have addressed a medical conference.

[2] Activity Value Analysis is a management engineering term that refers to the setting of stretch goals for cost savings followed by the development of ideas for achieving the savings. The ideas are then written up and presented to a leadership team for decisions on which ideas are to be implemented. Many of the ideas involve reductions in personnel.

9. THE LOOP YEARS
(PART I), 1989-1995

By John Clough

It is the bright, the bold, the transparent
who are cleverest among those who are silent:
their ground is down so deep that even
the brightest water does not betray it.
—*Nietzsche, 1892*

TURNAROUND TIME

Floyd D. Loop, M.D., became The Cleveland Clinic's fourth physician chief executive on November 8, 1989, a month before his 53rd birthday. A native of Indiana and son of a country doctor, he was educated in science at Purdue University. He received his medical training at the George Washington University. After he graduated in 1962, he completed a residency in general surgery at George Washington, interrupted by two years in the Air Force. During this residency, his mentor was Brian Blades, M.D., who influenced him to become a thoracic surgeon. Blades was at that time the chief of surgery at George Washington; he was a noted thoracic surgeon, a pioneer in the field of lung cancer surgery, and a friend of the Criles.

Blades arranged for Loop to receive cardiac surgery training at The Cleveland Clinic with the understanding that he would subsequently return to the university to practice cardiovascular surgery. His cardiothoracic surgery training was supervised by Donald B. Effler, M.D., who had been Blades's first chief resident after World

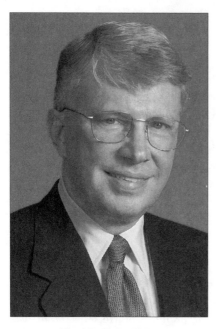

Floyd D. Loop, M.D.,
Chairman of the Board of Governors
and Chief Executive Officer, 1989-2004

War II. Loop's training in Cleveland coincided with the beginning of coronary artery surgery. Effler and his colleagues René Favaloro, M.D., and F. Mason Sones, Jr., M.D., taught him well. When George Washington University was unable to comply with Loop's plans for cardiac surgery there, he joined the Clinic staff in 1970 and, upon Effler's retirement, was appointed department chairman in 1975. Under his leadership the department doubled the volume of cases and became one of the world's great heart centers.

In 1988, Loop was elected to fill the unexpired term of Dr. Carl Gill on the Board of Governors when Gill became a permanent member of the Board by virtue of his executive position with Cleveland Clinic Florida. Loop's unrelenting pursuit of quality led to his appointment with Richard G. Farmer, M.D., then chairman of the Division of Medicine, to co-chair the Quality Assurance Task Force.

At the time Loop succeeded Kiser, shortly after the initiation of the previously mentioned McKinsey "turnaround" projects, the Clinic's future was uncertain. Cash flow had begun a downward spiral in early 1989. Cleveland Clinic Florida had become a symbol of the cash hemorrhage, and there was talk of shutting it down. Loop gave his first *Health of the Clinic* address on February 12, 1990, which he began by citing DaCosta's comment that "[i]t won't help a man much to be a hundred years ahead of his time if he is a month behind in his rent." Though not formally trained in business, Loop became the most visionary and, at the same time, the most fiscally prudent and conservative of the Board of Governors' chairmen. He recognized the opportunity represented by the Florida project, and he knew that the Clinic's future, both in Ohio and Florida, would depend on controlling costs and building market share. The latter could only be accomplished by acknowledging that "[f]or the first time we need to think strategically. We must adapt or we will go the way of the dinosaurs ourselves. We can't rest on our laurels. For a competitive advantage, the choices are clear—we must provide exemplary service of highest quality, increase our patient activity, manage internal systems better, and individually manage our practices better. In other words, if we want to stay the same, things will have to change."

With Loop, the pendulum of leadership had swung back to a more centralized, hierarchical approach, although decentralization of marketing clinical "product lines" was an important feature as well. He reorganized his management team to decrease the number of individuals reporting directly to him. The "professional" divisions (including Medicine, Surgery, Anesthesiology, Pathology and Laboratory Medicine, Radiology, Education, Research, and the "Centers of Excellence") all reported to the Chief of Staff, Ralph Straffon, but the chairpersons of these divisions and centers had direct access to Loop in the Medical Executive Committee, which he also chaired.

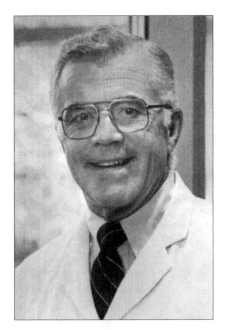

Ralph A. Straffon, M.D., Chief of Staff, 1987-1999

THE NEW TEAM

Perhaps more than any other individual Clinic staff member, Ralph Straffon, whose name appears many times in this book, personified all that is excellent about The Cleveland Clinic's system of medical group practice. A native of Michigan and a graduate of the University of Michigan, he came to the Clinic's Department of Urology in 1959. Just four years later he assumed the department chairmanship and, in 1978, became chairman of the Division of

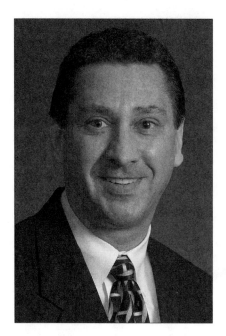
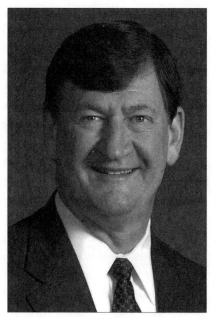

Robert Ivancic, Executive Director,
Human resources

Frank L. Lordeman,
Chief Operating Officer

Surgery. He was appointed Chief of Staff in 1987, and he held that position until his retirement in 1999. He served on the Board of Governors, both as an elected member (1967-1971, 1973-1976) and as a permanent member by virtue of his office (beginning in 1987). He also served on the Medical Executive Committee and the Administrative Council. His professional achievements are too numerous to list completely here, and through all of this he consistently set an enviable example of the group practice ideal of leadership combined with collegiality. A few examples of his national leadership positions include trustee (1973-1979) and president (1979) of the American Board of Urology, member (1974-1980) and chairman (1978) of the Residency Review Committee for Urology, president of the Council of Medical Specialties (1983-1984), and president of the American Association of Genitourinary Surgeons (1986-1987). His crowning achievement was his election as regent (1980-1989) and later to the presidency (1991-1992) of the American College of Surgeons. He has also received the Distinguished Alumnus Award of the University of Michigan (1980), the American Urological Association's Hugh Hampton Young Award (1983), and the National Health Professional Award of the VNA (1989).

On the administrative side, Robert Ivancic was recruited from the Meridia Hospital System to head the Division of Human Resources. John Clough, M.D., relinquished his chairmanship of the Department of Rheumatic and Immunologic Disease to head a new Division of Health Affairs, which encompassed many of the Clinic's external relationships. Daniel J. Harrington, who had been Director of Finance and an officer of the Foundation since 1986, became the Chief Financial Officer. Frank L. Lordeman, formerly the president and chief

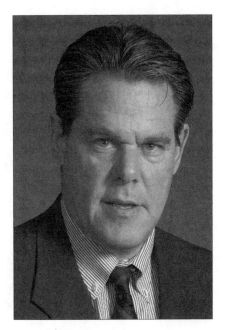

Gene Altus, Executive Administrator, Board of Governors

executive officer of Meridia Hillcrest Hospital, was recruited to the position of Chief Operating Officer to head the Clinic's vast Division of Operations. Along with the rest of the new administrative team, he worked with Loop to engineer the changes that needed to be made in the organization. This team, together with Loop's administrator, Gene Altus, who was also the administrator of the Department of Plastic and Reconstructive Surgery and who had played a vital role in the restructuring of Cleveland Clinic Florida, became the Administrative Council chaired by Loop. After the retirement of John Auble, who had founded the Clinic's legal office two and a half decades before, the office of general counsel was eventually outsourced to Squire, Sanders and Dempsey, a Cleveland firm that appointed David W. Rowan to oversee the Clinic's legal activities. Rowan worked closely with Loop and the Administrative Council on issues requiring his legal input.

In order to strengthen the marketing program in managed care, Peter S. Brumleve was recruited from Group Health Association of Puget Sound in 1994 to become Chief Marketing Officer. Marketing and Managed Care became a separate division under his leadership,

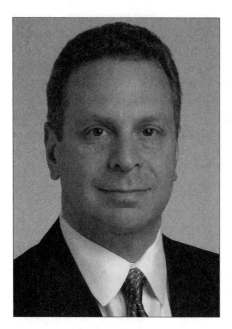

Alan London, M.D.,
Executive Director of Managed Care,
1995-

and he joined the Administrative Council. Two more members were added to the Administrative Council in 1995. Robert Kay, M.D., a pediatric urologist who also held the position of Chief of Medical Operations, and Alan E. London, M.D., Executive Director of Managed Care, formerly medical director of National Medical Enterprises, a California-based corporation that owned a chain of hospitals and managed care organizations, rounded out the Council.

Two more members were added in 1996. C. Martin Harris, M.D., for many years the chief information officer at the Hospital of the University of Pennsylvania, was recruited during the summer of 1996 as the Clinic's first Chief Information Officer and charged with the responsibility of building the ultimate information system to support the Clinic and its network partners. Finally, Melinda Estes, M.D., a neuropathologist and the first woman member of the Board of Governors, was appointed head of a newly created Office of Clinical Effectiveness.

The heart of the Board of Governors continued to be nine elected staff members serving staggered five-year terms. In addition, the Chief of Staff, Chief Financial Officer, Chief Operating Officer, and Chief Executive Officer of Cleveland Clinic Florida, as well as the Chairman, were permanent appointed members. Thus, Loop, Lordeman, and Straffon were members of all three of the major governing bodies.

These administrative changes coincided with the appointment of approximately 30 physician-managers to assume new roles in heading most of the clinical functions. Included among these were Norman S. Abramson, M.D. (emergency medicine), Muzaffar Ahmad, M.D. (Division of Medicine), Jerome L. Belinson, M.D. (gynecology),

David Bronson, M.D. (general internal medicine, later Division of Regional Medical Practice), Delos M.Cosgrove III, M.D. (cardiothoracic surgery), Vincent Dennis, M.D. (nephrology/hypertension), Cynthia Deyling, M.D. (Cleveland Clinic Independence), Charles Faiman, M.D. (endocrinology), William R. Hart, M.D. (pathology and laboratory medicine), J. Michael Henderson, M.B., Ch.B. (general surgery, Transplant Center), Gary Hoffman, M.D. (rheumatic and immunologic disease), Hilel Lewis, M.D. (ophthalmology, Eye Institute), David Longworth, M.D. (infectious disease), Hans Lüders,

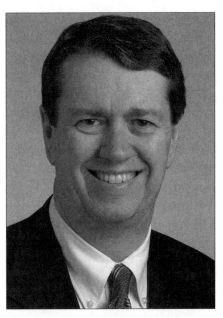

David L. Bronson, M.D., Chairman, Division of Regional Medical Practice, 1995-

M.D., Ph.D. (neurology), Roger Macklis, M.D. (radiation oncology), Maurie Markman, M.D. (hematology/oncology, Cancer Center), Kenneth E. Marks, M.D. (orthopedics), Daniel J. Mazanec, M.D. (Center for the Spine), Harry K. Moon, M.D. (chief of staff, Cleveland Clinic Florida), Thomas J. Morledge, M.D. (Cleveland Clinic Willoughby Hills), Robert Palmer, M.D. (geriatrics), Robert Petras, M.D. (anatomic pathology), Elliot Philipson, M.D. (obstetrics), Joel Richter, M.D. (gastroenterology), Vinod Sahgal, M.D. (physical medicine and rehabilitation, Rehabilitation Institute), Marshall Strome, M.D. (otolaryngology), George Tesar, M.D. (psychiatry), Eric J. Topol, M.D. (cardiology), A. Mary Walborn, M.D. (Cleveland Clinic Westlake), John A. Washington, M.D. (clinical pathology), Herbert P. Wiedemann, M.D. (pulmonary disease), and James Zins, M.D. (plastic and reconstructive surgery).

In the midst of all these changes, George "Barney" Crile, Jr., M.D., the last direct link with the Founders of The Cleveland Clinic, became terminally ill. In a moving ceremony on May 30, 1992, shortly before his death at age 84, the A Building was rechristened the Crile Building in honor of Barney and his father, both of whom had given so much to The Cleveland Clinic throughout its history. More than 40 members of the Crile family attended this Founders Celebration. The building is a living monument to the Criles as well as to the Clinic itself. But within ten years after its grand opening and five years before the turn of the century, it was filled to capacity, and space continued to be an issue for the organization.

FULL STEAM AHEAD

With his team in place, Loop set out to move the Clinic forward into the era of managed care, rapidly accelerating technological development, and growing consumerism. Implementation of the Economic Improvement Plan was the highest priority during the early part of his administration. This included reducing costs through Activity Value Analysis (AVA), revenue recapture, stepping up the marketing effort, making Cleveland Clinic Florida cost effective, and reorganizing the Clinic's management structure. About 135 jobs were eventually eliminated through the AVA process, generating some savings. Among other things, the revenue recapture project led to the first of several revisions of the inpatient and outpatient billing processes, which, according to some, still have plenty of room for improvement. Marketing was initially placed in the Division of Health Affairs, and there emerged a new marketing strategy that emphasized building the Clinic's traditional business while developing managed care capability. In Fort Lauderdale, the Clinic purchased North Beach Hospital from Health Trust, Inc., and started down the difficult path toward converting red ink to black. By early 1990, these measures had produced a $60 million turnaround in cash flow (from −$30 million to +$30 million), and the future seemed brighter.

The Clinic was now poised to tackle several major projects, which would keep the news media, the Ohio Department of Health, and the competition in an unprecedented state of agitation for the next few years. Among these projects were (a) affiliation with Ohio State University; (b) affiliation with Kaiser Permanente; (c) establishment of an inpatient rehabilitation unit; (d) management of the William O. Walker Center for Vocational Rehabilitation; (e) construction of a new state-of-the-art Access Center and emergency facility; (f) formation of the Cleveland Health Network; (g) creation of the Division of Regional Medical Practice; (h) development of the Cleveland Clinic Eye Institute and an eye care network; (i) building of a cancer center; (j) creation of a Division of Pediatrics and a Cleveland Clinic Children's Hospital; (k) reestablishment of obstetrics; and (l) initiation of a major fund-raising campaign to build the Cleveland Clinic Research and Education Institute, the Eye Institute, and the Cancer Center.

Bernadine Healy, M.D., chairperson of the Research Institute from 1985 to 1990, had long recognized the need for the Clinic to develop a strong academic affiliation with a medical school. She and her associates tried hard to work out a satisfactory arrangement with Case Western Reserve University, but for a variety of reasons (mostly related to competition with University Hospitals of Cleveland), this was not possible. So she turned to Ohio State University, where The Cleveland Clinic received a cordial welcome. An affiliation with Ohio State University was consummated and announced in 1991.

This led to an incredible series of events locally, culminating in the appointment of a blue-ribbon panel by the Cleveland Foundation to explore the area's opportunities in medical research and to make recommendations about the advisability of having two separate academic medical centers in the city. After protracted deliberations, the panel finally recognized The Cleveland Clinic as a separate "emerging" academic medical center. Shortly thereafter, officials at Case Western Reserve University arranged an affiliation with the Henry Ford Hospital in Detroit. The Clinic's Ohio State affiliation, though beneficial, did not progress to the establishment of a medical school on the Cleveland Clinic's campus. As it became clear that this would be necessary, the Clinic and the University parted amicably over a three-year period beginning in 2001.

The Clinic's exposure to managed care was greatly enhanced by the completion of a contract with Kaiser Permanente in 1992 under which Cleveland Clinic Hospital became the major inpatient care site for Kaiser members in northern Ohio. The earliest discussions about possible affiliation had taken place in the late 1980s between the Clinic's Dr. Shattuck W. Hartwell, Jr., and the Ohio Permanente Medical Group's Dr. Ronald Potts. Loop resurrected the concept after he assumed the role of chairman of the Board of Governors. Dr.

Robert Kay played a key role in bringing about the affiliation. This dramatic and, in the eyes of some, unlikely linkage was made possible through the strong leadership and vision of Loop along with Ronald Potts, M.D., Medical Director of the Ohio Permanente Medical Group, and Kathryn Paul, Regional Manager of the Kaiser Health Plan. Hospitals that had previously provided inpatient facilities for Kaiser Permanente (St. Luke's on the east side and MetroHealth[1] on the west side, which had recently merged) waged media campaigns and filed lawsuits in an attempt to derail the affiliation, but to no avail. As a result of this agreement, many physicians in the Ohio Permanente Medical Group were granted staff privileges to admit and care for their patients in Cleveland Clinic Hospital, and Kaiser, which had at one time operated three hospitals in the Cleveland area, closed its last remaining hospital. This was the first time that physicians other than those employed by The Cleveland Clinic had been admitted to the Clinic's medical staff, an arrangement that was problematic for some Clinic physicians in their quest to continue to act as a unit. However, the affiliation has greatly benefited both organizations since full consolidation occurred in January 1994, and the Clinic doctors have had an enlightening look at HMO-style primary care as delivered by the experts.

Clinic leaders saw the necessity to develop satellites to deliver geographically distributed primary care services. This became the responsibility of the new Division of Regional Medical Practice under the direction of David L. Bronson, M.D. Five satellite Family Health Centers were planned, each to be 30-45 minutes' driving time from the main campus. This was the "ring concept," first proposed by Frank Weaver, director of marketing in the early 1980s. In Weaver's proposed strategy, there was to have been an "inner ring" of primary care facilities within 45 minutes of the main campus and a more distant "outer ring" of such facilities, to provide easier access to the Cleveland Clinic for patients from surrounding areas. The first of these facilities to open was in Independence, located in the Crown Centre Building at Interstate 77 and Rockside Road. The second was in Willoughby Hills on Ohio Route 91 (S.O.M. Center Road) and Interstate 90. The third was in Westlake at Interstate 90 and Crocker-Bassett Road. The further development of the satellites, called Family Health Centers, is described more fully in the next chapter.

Vinod Sahgal, M.D., an internationally known physiatrist from the Chicago Institute of Rehabilitation, joined the staff in 1992 to build a Rehabilitation Institute. As a necessary first step in this process, the Clinic applied for a certificate of need to operate a 34-bed rehabilitation unit. The Cleveland Clinic had never had a problem obtaining state approval for new programs or technology, but times had changed. Nonetheless, despite opposition from the competition, Loop negotiated a settlement with the Director of the Ohio Department of Health, which allowed the Clinic to open a 20-bed unit. Legal appeals went on for another two years before finally being laid to rest.

Because of an increasing need for an improved emergency medicine facility, both on the part of the Clinic's established patients as well as residents of the inner city, Clinic leaders decided to build a new Emergency Medicine and Access Center. It was located on the south side of Carnegie Avenue between East 93rd and East 90th Streets and was designed to house four separate units on its first floor: (a) The Cleveland Clinic's Emergency Medicine Department, which was about six times the size of the old facility, (b) Kaiser Permanente's Emergency Department, which enabled them to close their old east-side emergency room, (c) a shared Clinical Decision Unit with 20 observation beds, and (d) The Cleveland Clinic's Access Department, intended to provide same-day service for outpatients. These departments opened in the spring of 1994 and were formally dedicated in October of that year. The second floor of the Access Center Building, which opened in 1996, housed 24 new operating rooms, replacing the same number of outmoded operating rooms that had served the Clinic's needs for some four decades. The third floor contained the offices of the Divisions of Surgery and Anesthesia as well as a high-tech training facility for minimally invasive surgery.

After many months of intricate negotiations led by Frank Lordeman, Loop hosted a press conference on May 13, 1994, to announce the formation of the Cleveland Health Network. Flanked by Robert Shakno, chief executive officer of Mt. Sinai Hospital, and Thomas LaMotte, chief executive officer of Fairview General Hospital, representing the charter members of the network, Loop announced the association of ten hospital systems (Cleveland Clinic, Mt. Sinai/Laurelwood, Fairview Health System [Fairview/Lutheran], Parma, MetroHealth, Elyria Memorial, Summa [St. Thomas/Akron

City], Akron Children's, and Aultman [Canton]; Marymount joined later) and their affiliated physician hospital organizations (PHOs) for the purpose of contracting to provide managed care.

The Cleveland Health Network was unlike the other local hospital systems (Meridia and University Hospitals Health System) in that it did not involve single ownership of all the participating hospitals. It was also considerably bigger and geographically more far flung, with participating hospitals in five counties. It encompassed three preexisting two-hospital networks: Summa (Akron City and St. Thomas Hospitals), Fairview Health System (formerly Health Cleveland, including Fairview and Lutheran Hospitals), and the Mt. Sinai Health System (Mt. Sinai and Laurelwood Hospitals). Marymount Hospital merged with The Cleveland Clinic and joined the network in 1995, and ties with MetroHealth became stronger. Development of a Cleveland Health Network managed care organization, composed of the above-named hospitals and hundreds of their affiliated physicians, was the major focus of the network, and the development of this was considered crucial to the overall success of the network. Dr. Alan London had the responsibility of organizing this important component of the Cleveland Health Network.

To outsiders, the most surprising member of the network was MetroHealth, the Cuyahoga County hospital, which had recently been at odds with the Clinic over the Clinic's reestablishment of rehabilitation services and had a long history of close affiliation with Case Western Reserve University, the parent organization of University Hospitals. MetroHealth and The Cleveland Clinic had complementary strengths, however, and the association was beneficial for both.

The acquisition of Marymount Hospital was more significant than most people realized at the time. It turned out to be the first step in formation of the Cleveland Clinic Health System (see the next chapter), initiating another quantum leap in the size and complexity of the organization and signaling the beginning of the institution's third era, that of system and consolidation.

Meanwhile, on the main campus, in preparation for the formation of The Cleveland Clinic Eye Institute, Hilel Lewis, M.D., was recruited from the Jules Stein Eye Institute of Los Angeles to head it. The Department of Ophthalmology was removed from the Division of Surgery and accorded divisional status. Plans were developed for a new building to house both clinical and research activities related to the eye. Lewis expanded the already excellent ophthalmologic services available at the Clinic by adding new talent to the group, and he set about forming a network of community ophthalmologists and optometrists to offer eye services on a contractual basis.

Pediatrics, which had existed as a department since the early 1950s, was also granted divisional status and removed from the Division of Medicine. Under the chairmanship of Douglas Moodie, M.D., the new Division of Pediatrics, together with The Children's Hospital at The Cleveland Clinic, newly remodeled and containing a state-of-the-art pediatric intensive care unit as well as new pediatric cardiac surgery suites, assumed a leadership role in the care of diseases of children. The Cleveland Clinic Children's Hospital had been accepted as an associate member of the National Association of Children's Hospitals and Related Institutions (NACHRI) in 1987. In 1989, the Ohio Children's Hospitals Association successfully lobbied the state to add a definition of the term "children's hospital" to the certificate-of-need law that specifically excluded The Cleveland Clinic Children's Hospital on the grounds that it did not have 150 beds! No other state has such a law, and NACHRI does not have this requirement. Fortunately, it was (and is) not necessary to have a certificate of need for designation as a children's hospital.

In Chapter 6, we noted that the Clinic's obstetrical program had closed down in 1966 to make room for the growing cardiac surgery program. On June 1, 1995, the program was reopened under the direction of Elliot Philipson, M.D. Its location on the sixth floor of the hospital is just around the corner from its original site, and the delivery suites, which had in the interim sequentially served cardiac surgery, orthopedic surgery, and ambulatory surgery, were returned to their original function. Outpatient obstetrical services became available both on the main campus and in the satellites.

After several fits and starts at fund raising, and one successful, but relatively small, campaign that raised $30 million for phase 1 of the Research and Education Institute (the Sherwin Building), the Board of Trustees approved a full-scale five-year campaign, designated "Securing the 21st Century." This campaign had a $225-million goal to build the remainder of the Research and Education Institute, the Cancer Center, and the Eye Institute. William Grimberg was recruited from Cleveland Tomorrow to head the Department of Institutional Advancement, which had the responsibility for organizing the campaign. Grimberg had cut his teeth on the campaign that revitalized Cleveland's Playhouse Square a few years earlier, and he had become interested in health research and technology through his association with the Technology Leadership Council of Cleveland Tomorrow. He was no stranger to The Cleveland Clinic, having labored mightily to develop collaborative arrangements between the Clinic and Case Western Reserve University to attract state money to support research at both institutions. This campaign was completed two years early, having raised some $236 million, up to that time the most successful campaign ever conducted at The Cleveland Clinic.

By the end of 1994, The Cleveland Clinic's prospects had never been brighter. National and international recognition of the Clinic as a provider of extremely high-quality medical care was at an all-time high. In the *U.S. News and World Report's* annual evaluation of hospitals, The Cleveland Clinic had been recognized among the top 10 hospitals in the country every year the survey had been done. Singled out for special recognition were cardiology (tops in the nation each year from 1995 through 2003), urology, gastroenterology, neurology, otolaryngology, rheumatology, gynecology, and orthopedics. No other hospital in the state or the region had been so recognized. Moreover, many of the staff had received similar recognition in lists of "best doctors" assembled by various organizations. Although the health care scene was undergoing fundamental change, characterized by a shift to managed care and increasing emphasis on primary care and prevention, the Clinic's new initiatives were designed to allow the organization to continue as a major player in the health care of the future while maintaining the institution's underlying values. But now the organization was entering a new era, and the formation of the Cleveland Clinic Health System had quietly begun.

---

[1] MetroHealth is the reincarnation of the old Cleveland Metropolitan General Hospital. It was set up to provide an umbrella organization for the merger of that hospital and St. Luke's into a "system." Shortly after the completion of the agreement between The Cleveland Clinic and Kaiser Permanente, the merger was dissolved, and the name "MetroHealth" subsequently referred only to the county hospital.

SYSTEM AND CONSOLIDATION

10. THE LOOP YEARS
(PART II), 1995-2004

By JOHN CLOUGH

Leadership is action, not position.
—Donald H. MacGannon

BEGINNING IN THE MID-1990S, THE PACE OF GROWTH IN SIZE AND complexity of the organization accelerated dramatically. These developments, though they occurred simultaneously, followed pathways that are best understood when considered separately. They included (a) acquisition of nine hospitals in the northeast Ohio region, the assembly of the Cleveland Clinic Health System, and the formation of the Physician Organization (PO); (b) building integrated clinics and hospitals in Naples and Fort Lauderdale, Florida (see Chapter 21); (c) creation of fourteen family health centers; (d) construction of a research and education institute, an eye institute, and a cancer center on the Cleveland campus; (e) establishing new and expanded emergency services at a site that included twenty-four new operating rooms (see Chapter 9); (f) establishment of The Cleveland Clinic Lerner College of Medicine of Case Western Reserve University; (g) strengthening of information technology and implementation of the ambulatory electronic medical record; (h) reorganization and strengthening of clinical and administrative management; (i) initiating a comprehensive leadership program called World Class Service; and (j) reorganization of the academic enterprise toward programmatic research, i.e., "investigation of their problems."

ASSEMBLY OF THE CLEVELAND CLINIC HEALTH SYSTEM

Over a three-year period beginning in 1995, nine hospitals in Cleveland and the surrounding suburbs came together and merged with The Cleveland Clinic Hospital to form the core of the Cleveland Clinic Health System. These hospitals included Marymount, Lakewood, Fairview, Lutheran, Meridia Hillcrest, Meridia Huron, Meridia Euclid, Meridia South Pointe, and Health Hill. In the process, the Meridia name was dropped in favor of the original individual hospital names, and Health Hill became the Cleveland Clinic Children's Hospital for Rehabilitation.

At the same time, two additional systems formed in Cleveland, the University Hospitals Health System, and the ill-fated Mt. Sinai Health System. By the time the dust died down, only a handful of Cleveland's hospitals remained independent: Deaconess, Parma Community Hospital, MetroHealth Hospital, and the Veteran's Administration hospitals. With the exception of Deaconess, these facilities were governmentally owned.

In 1996, Mt. Sinai's economic problems led that organization to sell their system, which included Mt. Sinai Hospital, Mt. Sinai Hospital East (the former Richmond General Osteopathic Hospital), and the Integrated Medical Campus in Beachwood to the for-profit Primary Health System, creating at the same time the Mt. Sinai Foundation, another conversion foundation. They also sold Laurelwood Hospital to the University Hospitals Health System. In separate transactions, Primary Health System also acquired St. Alexis Hospital and Deaconess Hospital, converting them to for-profit entities. The former deal also resulted in a name change of St. Alexis Hospital to St. Michael Hospital.

During these years, Mt. Sinai and St. Luke's Hospitals closed.

Several factors led to the sudden emergence of hospital merger activity. These included (a) the aggressive rise of the for-profit hospital systems (especially Columbia-HCA, which was at the height of its strength) and their targeting of the Cleveland market at that time, (b) the repeal of Ohio's certificate-of-need law in 1995, (c) the failure of the Clinton health care reform initiative in 1994, (d) the concentration of market power in the insurance companies and their dominance in the health care marketplace, and (e) the threat of a merger between

Blue Cross of Ohio and Columbia-HCA.

Columbia-HCA entered the market by acquiring a half-interest in several area hospitals, the other half held by the Sisters of Charity. The hospitals were St. Luke's (having just been cast loose by MetroHealth after a brief merger), St. Vincent Charity, St. John West Shore, and Timken Mercy (Canton, Ohio). The resulting organization was called Caritas, and its formation generated the St. Luke's Foundation, a so-called conversion foundation, resulting from the conversion of a nonprofit to a for-profit entity. The conversion foundations had the purpose of making sure that the endowments were used for community benefit.

Jack Burry, then president of Blue Cross of Ohio, concluded a deal with Rick Scott, chief executive of Columbia-HCA, which would have made the insurance company a part of Columbia-HCA. The Ohio Attorney General struck this deal down, and in the process the Blue Cross-Blue Shield Association canceled the membership of Blue Cross of Ohio, which since then has been known by its original name, Medical Mutual of Ohio. All of these factors combined to convince the community hospitals' executives and boards to seek refuge under the protective wings of the better managed and economically strong Cleveland Clinic.

For The Cleveland Clinic, the process began when, during discussions between Cleveland Clinic leadership and Marymount Hospital's CEO Thomas Trudell in 1995 about Marymount's joining the Cleveland Health Network (see Chapter 9), Trudell suggested consideration of a merger instead. Convinced that merger was the relationship they wanted, they quickly concluded a handshake agreement with The Cleveland Clinic, which was formalized in December 1995. Among other things, the agreement recognized and supported Marymount's Catholic mission and protected the interests of the retired nuns who had staffed Marymount for many years. At the time, no one recognized the importance of this event or predicted what was to follow over the next two years. Although Trudell lived to see the formation of the Cleveland Clinic Health System, initiated by the merger of Marymount with The Cleveland Clinic, he died suddenly in 2002, while at the peak of his career.

In May 1996, Lakewood Hospital, with 295 beds and a level-2 trauma center, became part of the emerging Cleveland Clinic Health System through a three-way agreement of The Cleveland Clinic with the City of Lakewood and the non-profit Lakewood Hospital Association. Lakewood, previously affiliated with University Hospitals, had been looking for a new partner and had explored joining the Columbia-HCA system, but their board ultimately preferred to remain nonprofit. It is the only municipal hospital in the system. The City of Lakewood owns the building and leases it to the Lakewood Hospital Association, which is now part of the Cleveland Clinic Health System.

A few months later, in the fall of 1996, Fairview Health System and The Cleveland Clinic agreed to merge, bringing Fairview General Hospital (469 beds) and Lutheran General Hospital (204 beds) into the fold. Fairview Health System and Meridia had been engaged in merger discussions, but Fairview decided to join The Cleveland Clinic. Fairview Health System, previously known as Health Cleveland, was a two-hospital system consisting of Fairview General and Lutheran General Hospitals. Together with Lakewood Hospital, these hospitals became the Western Region of the Cleveland Clinic Health System. A search committee selected Louis Caravella, M.D., a prominent and widely respected ophthalmologist, to lead the region. When Caravella stepped down in 2003, the Clinic selected Fred DeGrandis, then the chief executive officer of St. John West Shore Hospital, to succeed him.

Meridia had continued to look for a partner, weighing the pros and cons of joining The Cleveland Clinic vs. University Hospitals. For Meridia this was a prolonged process, involving the use of a national consultant (Goldman Sachs Group) to evaluate the opportunities that remained. One important factor in the ultimate choice was support for the Clinic from the Meridia trustees.

In March 1997, the Meridia Hospital System, having failed to conclude its merger with Fairview, agreed to merge with The Cleveland Clinic. This merger brought Hillcrest (347 beds and a level-2 trauma center), Huron Road (387 beds and a level-2 trauma center), Euclid General (371 beds, including a 48-bed rehabilitation unit), and South Pointe (166 beds, formed from the 1994 merger of Suburban and Brentwood Osteopathic) Hospitals into the Cleveland Clinic Health System. The former Meridia Health System became the Eastern Region of the Cleveland Clinic Health System, under the leadership of Charles Miner. When Miner announced his intention to leave the Cleveland Clinic Health System in 2003, the Clinic chose Tom Selden, long-time chief executive officer of Parma Community

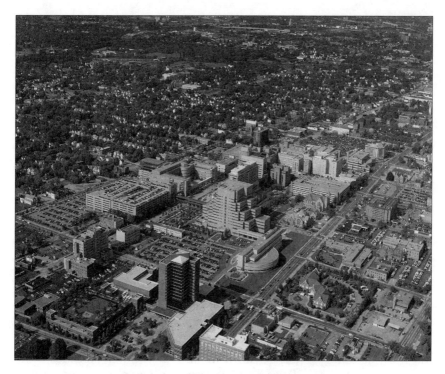

Aerial view of The Cleveland Clinic, 2003

Hospital, to replace him.

In July 1998, the Cleveland Clinic Health System admitted Health Hill, a 52-bed children's rehabilitation hospital, and shortly thereafter, the name was changed to the Cleveland Clinic Children's Hospital for Rehabilitation. It became a part of Children's Hospital at The Cleveland Clinic for administrative purposes.

Along with Loop, the key Cleveland Clinic executive most intimately involved in assembling the Cleveland Clinic Health System was Frank Lordeman, the Clinic's chief operating officer. Originally from California, Lordeman had come to Cleveland to serve as president and chief operating officer of Meridia Hillcrest Hospital. Lordeman was no stranger to hospital consolidation, having served as president of Health Ventures, Inc., a for-profit hospital system based in Oakland, California. The Meridia system, led at that time by Richard McCann, had formed from the merger of five hospitals (Hillcrest, Euclid General, Huron Road, Suburban, and Brentwood) in the mid-1980s. The latter two hospitals, located adjacent to each other on Warrensville Center Road, soon merged all their operations to form

South Pointe Hospital. Brentwood was an osteopathic hospital with strong academic ties to Ohio's only osteopathic medical school at Ohio University in Athens, Ohio.

Shortly after Lordeman left Hillcrest to join The Cleveland Clinic in 1992, Blue Cross of Ohio attempted a merger with the Meridia system, which was looking for a partner. Charles Miner, formerly an executive with Figgie International, succeeded Lordeman at Hillcrest. This merger went forward, and McCann became an employee of Blue Cross, but the union dissolved soon thereafter because of the Meridia board's cultural differences with Burry, president of Blue Cross of Ohio. When McCann moved to Blue Cross, Miner became the chief executive of the Meridia System.

Blue Cross then went on to an ill-fated attempt to merge with Columbia-HCA, which was hungrily eyeing the Cleveland marketplace. However, about that time, Columbia-HCA ran afoul of the Justice Department and began to downsize, eventually giving up on the idea of entering the Cleveland marketplace. Almost no one thought this merger was a good idea, anyway. Ohio Attorney General Betty Montgomery refused to allow it, and the Blue Cross-Blue Shield Association dismissed Blue Cross of Ohio from membership. Since then the company has been known as Medical Mutual. It is still one of the strongest health insurers in the region.

Several other organizations have affiliated with the Cleveland Clinic Health System, although they are not formally merged with The Cleveland Clinic. These include the Ashtabula Medical Center, with its 226-bed hospital, the Ashtabula Clinic, and seven satellite locations in Ashtabula, Ohio; the Summa Health System, comprising Akron City Hospital and St. Thomas Hospital in Akron, Ohio; and Grace Hospital, an 87-bed, long-term acute care hospital in Cleveland.

While all this was going on, University Hospitals also assembled a system that included the following hospitals: University Hospitals, Bedford Medical Center, Geauga Regional Hospital, Memorial Hospital of Geneva, and Brown Memorial Hospital (in Conneaut, Ohio). When Columbia-HCA abandoned Northeast Ohio, University Hospitals bought their half interest in Caritas, a group of Catholic hospitals including St. Vincent Charity, St. John West Shore, St. Luke's, and Timken Mercy in Canton, Ohio. University Hospitals ultimately closed St. Luke's Hospital, long a Cleveland icon, after a brief attempt to make it succeed as a psychiatric hospital. After Primary Health System

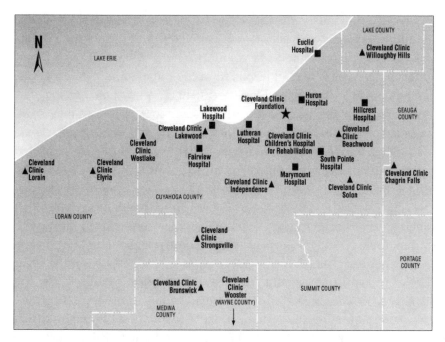

*The Cleveland Clinic Health System, showing locations of Cleveland Clinic Hospital
(star), system hospitals (squares), and Family Health Centers (triangles)*

closed Mt. Sinai in 1999 and went bankrupt the following year, University Hospitals acquired St. Michael Hospital and Mt. Sinai Hospital East (the former Richmond General Hospital) to round out their system. In a related negotiation, the Cleveland Clinic bought the Mt. Sinai ambulatory building, which became the Cleveland Clinic Beachwood Family Health and Ambulatory Surgery Center.

The formation of the Cleveland Clinic Health System presented an opportunity to consolidate some administrative functions and gain some economies of scale. The Administrative Council defined six systemic functions for centralization: (a) finance, (b) marketing, (c) human resources, (d) information technology, (e) managed care, and (f) medical operations. Local operations, community relations, media relations, fund raising, volunteer services, and government relations were left to the devices of the individual hospitals or to the regions. The System did not undertake rationalization of medical services among the hospitals. Each of the six functions was to be led by the appropriate member of the Administrative Council. An Executive Council, consisting of the heads of the various entities in the System, was established to direct the affairs of the Cleveland Clinic Health System. As referred to previously, the Cleveland Clinic Health System was divided into three regions: Eastern, Western, and Central (the latter including the main campus and Marymount). The Cleveland Clinic's Board of Trustees, with a few additions from the member hospitals' boards, functioned also as the board for the system. There was no organization comparable to the Clinic's Board of Governors at the system level, because physicians had a much more limited role in the System hospitals than on the Clinic's main campus. However, under the managed care arm of system management, a system-wide Physicians' Organization was established to deal with physician-specific issues.

The establishment of the Cleveland Clinic Health System also had another significant result. It made The Cleveland Clinic, now with approximately 25,000 employees, the fourth largest employer in the state, behind General Motors, Delphi Automotive, and Kroger Company, and one of only two health care organizations in the top twenty-five. The other health care organization in the top 25 private-sector employers in Ohio was University Hospitals of Cleveland, which ranked ninth based on the *2000 Harris Ohio Industrial Directory*. The Cleveland Clinic had truly joined the ranks of big business.

THE CLEVELAND CLINIC HEALTH SYSTEM'S PHYSICIANS' ORGANIZATION

Associated with the hospitals that joined the Cleveland Clinic Health System were four physician hospital organizations (PHOs). On the east side of Cleveland were the Meridia PHO (the largest of the four), which was linked to the four Meridia hospitals (Hillcrest, Euclid, Huron, and South Pointe), and the Marymount Hospital PHO. On the west side of the city were the PHOs of Lakewood Hospital and the Fairview Hospital System (Fairview and Lutheran Hospitals). The purpose of these PHOs was to allow the hospitals and their associated physicians to act as combined entities in contracting with payers for the delivery of managed care. Altogether, approximately 2,000 physicians were members of these PHOs. As the Cleveland Clinic Health System came together, it became necessary to decide the direction in which the relationship of the new hospital system to the physicians in the PHOs would evolve.

The need to contract with payers for managed care still existed, and the PHO physicians were used to the idea of working with their respective hospitals. There was, nevertheless, some unease among the physicians about having the same sort of relationship with a large hospital system anchored by The Cleveland Clinic. Many were concerned that The Cleveland Clinic would force them into an employed, salaried relationship, like that in The Cleveland Clinic's staff model. Some, on the other hand, had actively campaigned against their hospitals' joining The Cleveland Clinic, because they wanted a relationship with a system that would buy their practices. There was also fear that The Cleveland Clinic would impose controls on their freedom to practice as they chose. It fell to Dr. Alan London, The Cleveland Clinic's dynamic, young Executive Director of Managed Care, to resolve these issues and work out a satisfactory working relationship with the PHO physicians.

As noted in the previous chapter, London had come to the Clinic in 1995 from Tenet Healthcare Corporation in California. He grew up in Cleveland and got his medical degree from the Medical College of Ohio in Toledo. He received his training in family practice at the University of California, Irvine. At Tenet, then known as National Medical Enterprises, he was executive vice president and national medical director. He had developed and directed a broad spectrum of managed care and healthcare delivery programs within the Tenet network both in the United States and abroad. Thus, he was well suited to the difficult task that now confronted the institution.

The first assignment was to develop a strategic plan to bring the groups together. All this work was completed by November 1998, and the Physician Organization (PO) Board, chaired by London, began to meet then to hammer out a physician participation agreement. The PO Board's 15 members consisted of four physician-elected trustees, six regional hospital-nominated trustees, and five member (CCF) trustees. The physician members were half specialists and half primary care physicians. Elected Board members served for terms of two years. Although for all intents and purposes, the agreement was finished by May 1999, it was not agreed to until September of that year. The Board also established the following committees: risk pool, medical management, finance and contracting, and membership and credentialing. All but about 200 of the original PHO members chose to stay in the merged organization, and the size of the PO has remained constant at about 2,000 (22% primary care).

DEPLOYMENT OF FAMILY HEALTH CENTERS AND AMBULATORY SURGERY CENTERS

The Cleveland Clinic established its first off-site medical practice in the nearby community of Independence, just south of Cleveland. The original idea for this arose in the sports medicine section of the Department of Orthopaedic Surgery, and orthopedists Dr. John Bergfeld, team physician of the Cleveland Browns, and Dr. Ken Marks, head of the department, pushed hard for its establishment. Bergfeld and Marks saw an opportunity to take the Clinic's elite sports medicine program out into the community where it could be more accessible to scholastic sports participants. They were anxious to more fully develop the concept in a Clinic-owned facility.

Thus, the first Cleveland Clinic Family Health Center opened in leased space in Crown Centre, a large new office building near the intersection of I-77 and Rockside Road in Independence, under the direction of internist Cynthia Deyling in September 1993. It was an immediate success. The original sports medicine concept was successfully implemented there as well. Within a couple of years, the practice had outgrown its original quarters, and The Cleveland Clinic constructed a new building, Crown Centre II, adjacent to the first site. The physicians working in this facility were all employees of The Cleveland Clinic and were included in a new Division of Regional Medical Practice headed by David L. Bronson, M.D.

Bronson had been recruited from the University of Vermont to head the Clinic's department of general internal medicine in 1992. Originally from Maine, Bronson received his M.D. degree from the University of Maine and trained in internal medicine at the University of Wisconsin. After finishing his training, he returned to New England and joined the faculty of the University of Vermont. While in Vermont, as a faculty member and later as associate chairman of the department of internal medicine at the University of Vermont, he had become interested in innovative delivery of medical care. Subsequent to his arrival in Cleveland, it quickly became apparent that he would make an outstanding leader for the formation and management of a group of strategically placed, primary care-oriented practices that could function as access points to the main campus's subspecialty-oriented physicians. Bronson assumed the leadership of the new division in 1995.

In the early 1990s, the time was clearly right for this initiative, and several factors were important in creating a favorable setting for establishment of satellites. Managed care appeared to be replacing traditional fee-for-service indemnity health care insurance coverage, and for physicians this favored banding together "to act as a unit" in contracting with the payers. Furthermore, it appeared then that primary care physicians would finally assume their long sought-after role as gatekeepers and that Cleveland Clinic-style specialists would have a less central role in care management.

The Clinton administration was pushing for a modified version of the "managed competition" care delivery model envisioned by the Jackson Hole Group, led by Alain Enthoven and his colleagues. This model encouraged the formation of groups of primary care physicians with strong administrative capabilities ("Accountable Health Plans") that could contract directly with employers and other payers and manage the health of "populations" of patients through careful attention to prevention. Capitated payment was the order of the day. This, so the story went, would keep the patients out of the hospitals and away from the expensive subspecialists, save money, and result in great outcomes. Although capitated HMO-type managed care never really caught on in Cleveland, the primary care satellite concept worked very well for The Cleveland Clinic and its widely distributed patient population.

Dr. Cynthia Deyling continued to lead the first family health center at Independence, which moved to the new adjacent building in 2000. The three other original family health centers opened in Willoughby Hills to the east, Westlake to the west, and Solon to the southeast. Primary care physicians led all of them. Dr. Thomas Morledge (internist) was the director of the Willoughby Hills facility, Dr. Mary Walborn (internist) led the Westlake center, and Dr. Ruth Imrie (pediatrician) was in charge of the Solon location. As had occurred in Independence, these practices also grew rapidly. An "inner ring" strategy began to take shape.

Over the next five years, several additional Family Health Centers came into being. In 1998, The Cleveland Clinic acquired the Wooster Clinic, a highly-regarded group practice in Wooster, Ohio, headed by Dr. James Murphy. Many of The Cleveland Clinic's physicians had close referral relationships with the doctors at the Wooster Clinic, so the association was natural. In fact, this relationship brought the

Clinic back to its roots, in a sense, because George Crile, Sr., had graduated from Wooster College's long defunct medical school in the nineteenth century. This acquisition also turned out to be the first of the "outer ring" facilities.

Also in 1998, the Lorain Ambulatory Surgery Center was added. John Costin, M.D., an irrepressible and entrepreneurial Cleveland Clinic-trained ophthalmologist, and Michael Kolczun, M.D., a prominent alumnus of The Cleveland Clinic's orthopedic surgery program, played important roles in getting the project started. A number of successful Lorain County physicians joined in this endeavor, and it has become one of the leading medical facilities in the region.

The following year, The Cleveland Clinic opened its Strongsville facility, under the leadership of internist Dr. Howard Graman. This was the first of the Family Health Centers built using the pyramid-like Crile Building as its architectural model. Subsequent newly constructed Family Health Centers follow the same design. In addition to primary care, the Strongsville Family Health Center has an ambulatory surgery component.

In 2000, The Cleveland Clinic opened its Beachwood facility in the same building that had housed Mt. Sinai's Integrated Medical Campus. The Clinic purchased this building from the bankrupt Primary Health System. Interestingly, the original plan was for The Cleveland Clinic to purchase the Integrated Medical Campus along with two hospital buildings (St. Michael and Mt. Sinai East) that were to have been closed by Primary Health Systems. However, the proposed closure of these two hospitals, though they were both losing money and suffered from chronic low occupancy (less than 30% in both cases), precipitated community protests that were fanned by local politicians. Ultimately, University Hospitals bought the hospitals for $12 million and promised to keep them open as full-service hospitals. Since Mt. Sinai East had the same Medicaid provider number as the already closed Mt. Sinai Hospital in University Circle, University Hospitals reaped the federal and state monies that Mt. Sinai, if it had remained open, would have received through Ohio's Hospital Care Assurance Program (HCAP) for indigent care in 1998 and 1999. It is probably not coincidental that the amount of these payments was approximately $12 million. In September 2003, University Hospitals Health System announced the impending closure of St. Michael Hospital after having lost $33 million trying to keep it running, and it closed at the end of the year. Like Strongsville, the Beachwood Family Health Center also had ambulatory surgery and a fairly broad range of subspecialists.

In addition to the eight major facilities described above, several smaller centers (Brunswick, Lakewood, Chagrin Falls [formerly Curtis Clinic], Elyria, Chardon Road/Willoughby Hills, and Creston, as well as a sports health center at the Jewish Community Center in Beachwood) also opened. In all, by 2002 the Family Health Centers, some with ambulatory surgery centers, employed over 250 physicians and accounted for about half of the outpatient visits to The Cleveland Clinic. Eighty-nine primary care residents and 99 medical students received part of their training at the Family Health Centers in 2001. The Family Health and Ambulatory Surgery Centers filled an extremely important role for The Cleveland Clinic's delivery system.

NEW BUILDINGS: ACQUISITIONS AND NEW CONSTRUCTION

After the Century Project was completed in 1986, there was a brief lull in new building construction and expansion. Nevertheless, the staff continued to grow at its exponential rate (see Epilogue) and, by the early 1990s, it was clear that this could not continue without the addition of space for clinical and research activities. Some of the existing facilities, moreover, were showing the effects of age and changes in design requirements for the Clinic's growing and increasingly complex needs. For example, all the organization's computing facilities were at that time located in a basement under the East 90th Street employee garage. With the institution's increasing dependence on technology to support its voracious appetite for information, this was clearly a vulnerable point in the system.

Lack of adequate laboratory space had become an obstacle to recruiting first-class scientists to the Research Institute. Besides the research facilities in the FF Building, which had been constructed in 1974, there was some very old space in a loading dock area abutting the south side of the L Building, which at that time housed the artificial organs program. The Sherwin Building, which had opened in 1991, funded by a $30 million campaign led by Bernadine Healy, M.D., chairwoman of the Research Institute, and Arthur B. Modell, president (1991-1996) of The Cleveland Clinic Foundation, relieved the pressure temporarily. The Sherwin Building represented the first phase in a grander design (see Chapter 9).

Lerner Research Institute

The realization of this grand design was the Lerner Research Institute, funding for the construction of which was the major purpose of the campaign called "Securing the 21st Century." This campaign, led by trustee Joseph Callahan and managed by William Grimberg, the director of Institutional Advancement, provided about $190 million toward the building of the Lerner Research Institute, of which $16 million was a gift from Mr. and Mrs. Alfred Lerner. Lerner was, at the time, president (1996-2002) of The Cleveland Clinic Foundation.

The Lerner Research Institute is a five-story, U-shaped building designed by Cesar Pelli and located on the south side of Carnegie Avenue between East 97th and 100th Streets. The western limb of the U houses the Department of Biomedical Engineering. It contains a fully equipped machine shop as well as an array of laboratories, supporting, among other things, The Cleveland Clinic's artificial heart development program.

The base of the U contains traditional laboratories for biomedical research, housing the Clinic's extensive programs in molecular biology as well as other basic research programs. On the first floor of this part of the building is the Reinberger Commons, a rotunda area designed to promote collaborative interaction among the scientists and named for the philanthropic Reinberger brothers, distinguished fellows of The Cleveland Clinic Foundation.

The eastern limb of the U provides a home for the Division of Education and the Cleveland Clinic Educational Foundation. A prominent feature of this part of the building is the Alumni Library, which occupies most of the third and fourth floors of the east wing. The north ends of the limbs of the U are connected by a skyway at the third-floor level, and short bridges connect the west end of the Lerner Research Institute to the laboratory medicine building at the second level and the east end to the East 100th Street garage and the skyway to the Crile Building at the third level.

Occupancy of the Lerner Research Institute began early in 1999, and the building was formally opened and dedicated in May of that year, with a week-long series of celebrations. Although the original intent was to occupy floors one through four initially and later build out and open the top floor, by the end of 1999 the building was full, and the Research Institute was already looking for additional space.

Cole Eye Institute

The establishment of the Cleveland Clinic Eye Institute and recruitment of Hilel Lewis, M.D., in 1992 had signaled the Clinic's intent to support this activity with the construction of new facilities for ophthalmology and eye research. An important part of this process was the success of the previously mentioned Securing the 21st Century campaign in raising $30 million, anchored by a $10-million gift from Jeffrey Cole, needed to fund the construction of the building to house the Institute. The Cole Eye Institute, which opened in 1999, is located on the south side of Euclid Avenue between East 100th and 105th Streets, just east of the Crile Building and connected to it by a skyway. An important feature of this building, designed by Lewis, is the radial design of the examining rooms, which are long and narrow, and arrayed in a semicircle. This design permits the examining-room entrances to be closer together than they would be with traditional design, thus facilitating access and promoting efficiency. It is also responsible for the distinctive curved appearance of the north face of the building.

Taussig Cancer Center

Although not part of the original program for Securing the 21st Century, a significant gift from the Taussig family enabled the Clinic to accelerate plans for a new building to house the Cancer Center. Once again, Cesar Pelli's considerable talents were employed to develop the dramatic S-curved appearance of the $49-million Taussig Cancer Center, which opened in 2000. It occupies the south side of Euclid Avenue between East 89th and 90th Streets. It houses clinical examining and treatment rooms on the first and second floors and research laboratories on the upper floors. It is connected to the radiation oncology department of the Cancer Center (in the T Building) through a second-level bridge across East 90th Street.

W.O. Walker Center

In the mid-1980s, the State of Ohio began construction of a $72-million, 15-story building occupying the land bounded on the west by East 105th Street, on the north by Euclid Avenue, on the east by Stokes Boulevard, and on the south by the Ohio School of Podiatry. This building, named after William O. Walker, the founder and longtime publisher of the *Call and Post* newspaper, was intended to house a state-of-the-art residential rehabilitation center to be operated by the Ohio Bureau of Workers' Compensation. It was similar to, but bigger than, a similar facility in Columbus, the Leonard Camera Center. Despite valiant attempts, neither of these operations was successful. In Columbus, Ohio State University took over operation of the Camera Center, using it primarily for sports medicine services. In Cleveland, after a prolonged negotiation, the state sold the Walker Center to The Cleveland Clinic and University Hospitals late in 1996 for $44 million. The two organizations each paid half of the purchase price, occupied alternating floors, and shared certain common facilities.

The Cleveland Clinic had several clinical services in the Walker Center, including the Spine Institute, Pain Management, outpatient rehabilitation facilities, and the histocompatibility laboratory. Management of the facility required ongoing cooperation between The Cleveland Clinic and University Hospitals, something that few would have predicted possible. Nonetheless, the project went forward smoothly.

Parker Hannifin Building

In September 1997, the Parker Hannifin Company, a well-established Cleveland equipment manufacturer, moved its corporate headquarters to a new building in suburban Mayfield Heights, Ohio.

They donated their old corporate headquarters building at 17325 Euclid Avenue (between Ivanhoe and London Streets) to The Cleveland Clinic. This structure, with more than 500,000 square feet of usable space, housed the Cleveland Clinic Health System's Information Technology Division, as well as several other administrative functions.

TRW Building

Following its acquisition by Northrop Grumman, TRW's aerospace division was moved to California and its automotive division to Livonia, Michigan. Thus, in December 2002, TRW donated its corporate headquarters in suburban Lyndhurst, Ohio, to The Cleveland Clinic. This 300,000-square-foot facility is situated on a 58-acre wooded parcel of land on the west side of Richmond Road between Legacy Village Mall on the south and Hawken Lower School on the north. This is a portion of the old Bolton Estate. Besides the land and office complex, which contains a large auditorium and a spectacular atrium, TRW's gift included a 300,000-square-foot garage that accommodates 577 cars, a 5,000 square-foot repair facility, and the Bolton House. The latter is a 21,836-square-foot mansion built in 1917 and completely renovated by TRW in the mid-1980s to provide housing for corporate visitors and conferences. The house has 12 bedrooms, each with a private bath.

Heart Center

Plans for a new Heart Center, to be funded mostly by philanthropy, had been incubating since the successful completion of the Securing the 21st Century campaign. As these plans took shape, the concept emerged of a nearly one million square-foot building to house the new center, including 288 hospital beds, laboratories, and outpatient facilities. Replacement of the parking garage on the south side of Euclid Avenue at East 93rd Street with a new parking and office structure on the north side of Euclid made space for the new building. A tunnel under Euclid Avenue eased access to the new facility.

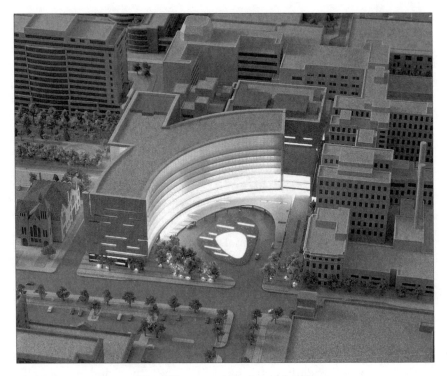

Heart Center, architect's model, 2003

THE ACADEMIC ENTERPRISE AND
THE MEDICAL SCHOOL

In March 2001, Loop announced the reorganization of The Cleveland Clinic's academic enterprise. The Board of Governors appointed Dr. Eric Topol, a distinguished clinical investigator and head of the Clinic's cardiology department, as Chief Academic Officer. His team consisted of Dr. Andrew Fishleder, who would continue to head the Clinic's postgraduate education programs, Dr. Richard Rudick, head of the newly created Office of Clinical Research, and Dr. Paul DiCorleto, head of the Lerner Research Institute, the Clinic's basic research program. Brian Williams, Ph.D., Edward Plow, Ph.D., Andrew Novick, M.D., and Joseph Iannotti, M.D., Ph.D. filled the remaining seats on the Academic Council.

Just over a year later, in May 2002, through a formal agreement with Case Western Reserve University supported by the University's new president, Dr. Edward Hundert, and a generous gift from Alfred

Lerner, the president of The Cleveland Clinic Foundation, The Cleveland Clinic Lerner College of Medicine of Case Western Reserve University was born. This event greatly pleased many of Cleveland's traditional leaders, who had long sought to bring The Cleveland Clinic and Case Western Reserve University together. This process was difficult because of competition between The Cleveland Clinic and University Hospitals, but it was greatly eased by changes in leadership at University Hospitals and the resolution of conflict between University Hospitals and the University itself. The purpose of the new medical

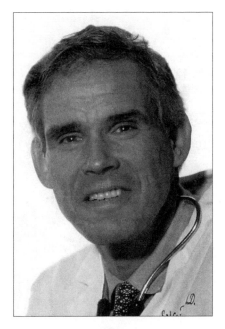

Eric J. Topol, M.D.,
Chief Academic Officer, 2001-

school was to produce physician investigators, an increasingly rare breed of medical graduates. The first class of 32 students was scheduled to enroll in July 2004.

INFORMATION TECHNOLOGY AND THE ELECTRONIC MEDICAL RECORD

Computers had appeared at The Cleveland Clinic in a big way during the early 1980s. The idea of managing as many functions as possible, including patient care, with the help of computers led to several ill-fated, institution-wide projects, but the technology then simply wasn't up to the task. Instead, many different systems and networks serving various functions (billing, scheduling, laboratory management and reporting, radiology, pathology, and a proliferating gaggle of clinical registries) sprang up, Babel-like in their inability to communicate with each other. The ideal of an institution-wide electronic medical record seemed as though it should be achievable but had always been just out of reach. Commercially available prod-

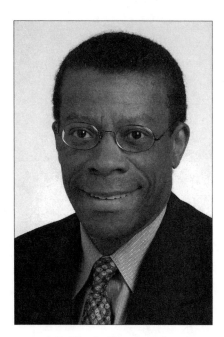

C. Martin Harris, M.D.,
Chief Information Officer, 1999-

ucts were unable to cope with the sheer size and complexity of The Cleveland Clinic, although they were capable of serving small medical offices. Some institutions developed home-grown electronic medical records (e.g., Harvard Community Health Plan, Kaiser Permanente, and others), but attempts to do this at The Cleveland Clinic were unsuccessful and costly. Part of the problem was that the Clinic's early computer experts did not understand the needs of medicine, and the Clinic's medical experts were unsophisticated in the realm of digital technology.

In 1996, Dr. C. Martin Harris was recruited from the University of Pennsylvania to fill the role of the Clinic's first Chief Information Officer. Harris is a nearly unique individual in that he is a highly skilled internist as well as a computer expert with a degree from the Wharton School of Business. Thus, he understands the needs of medicine, but he also clearly understands the capabilities of the technology and its cost implications. His communication skills are such that he can talk the languages of the key players and bring all the pieces together in a way that none of his predecessors had been able to do. He has a methodical business approach that enables him accurately to evaluate existing products and make choices that do not lead to unpleasant surprises after implementation begins.

Harris's first task, however, was to develop a plan that would get the Clinic through a looming problem that few people could accurately evaluate, i.e., "Y2K." In 1998, concern began to grow about what would happen on January 1, 2000, to the computer-based infrastructure upon which U.S. business (including hospitals) and government had become increasingly reliant. This concern stemmed from the fact that much of the software serving major date-sensitive functions, written over the previous 25 years, recognized only the last two digits of the year, assuming "19" for the first two digits. Nobody knew what would happen to scheduling systems or equipment programmed to require service on certain dates (such as pacemakers, etc.) when "99" flipped over to "00" at the turn of the century. Articles predicted that airplanes would fall out of the sky, that the world monetary system would collapse, and that disastrous events killing many patients would occur in hospitals. Lawyers were salivating at the prospect.

Harris devised a plan in which all computer-based functions at the Clinic would be classified into (a) those that had to be fixed because they were likely to fail with significant bad results, (b) those that were likely to fail but could be discarded and replaced, and (c) those that would not be affected by the arrival of Y2K—the year 2000. Millions of lines of code in the scheduling, admission, and billing systems had to be examined and corrected. Every computer in the Clinic had to be checked for date-sensitive software, and every piece of equipment with a microprocessor in it also had to be tested. Then each piece of equipment and software had to be classified into one of the three categories listed above and certified as Y2K-ready or discarded and replaced. Amazingly, despite a certain level of hysteria that prevailed both inside and outside the institution, Harris and his team accomplished all this six months ahead of schedule, and Y2K came and went uneventfully at the Clinic.

For his next task, Harris and his colleagues in the Information Technology Division (ITD) addressed the previously unsolved issue of the electronic medical record. By this time, several departments had begun experimenting with one or another of the commercial products that were becoming available. Harris organized the evaluation scheme, piloted several of the products, and concluded that the Epic system, with EpiCare as the front end, had the capacity, flexibility, and user-friendliness required to meet the needs of patient care at The Cleveland Clinic. Introduction of this system to clinical practice began in 2001 and was essentially complete in the outpatient clinics by the end of 2002. The next hurdle will be implementation of an electronic medical record in the hospital, including computerized physician order entry (CPOE).

While all this was taking place, the Internet had developed from a curiosity, mainly frequented by computer "nerds," into a potentially important tool for dissemination of information and for marketing. The Cleveland Clinic's presence on the World Wide Web began, somewhat primitively, in 1994. By 1996, there was an organized web site (www.ccf.org) providing much information about the Clinic and its departments (including the entire third edition of *To Act As a Unit*), but very limited capability for interaction. This was solved in 2002 with the introduction of *e-ClevelandClinic.com*, the commercial arm of the Clinic's web site. *e-ClevelandClinic.com* grew out of an idea conceived by Dr. Eric Topol, head of the Clinic's cardiology department. The purpose was to make on-line, second-opinion consultation with Cleveland Clinic specialists available to the public in a secure, protected web environment. The Clinic's partnership with WebMD, a popular health care portal to the Internet, provided greater ease of access to the Clinic's web site.

The ITD division, under Harris's leadership, has truly brought the organization into the 21st century by providing the nervous system for the widely disseminated components of the Cleveland Clinic Health System. With the sophisticated connectivity that now exists, the Clinic is poised for whatever the future may bring.

STRENGTHENING OF MANAGEMENT

While all of this was going on, several significant changes took place in the executive management of The Cleveland Clinic.

After 18 years of dedicated service, Daniel Harrington, the Clinic's Chief Financial Officer, retired in 1999. Michael O'Boyle was eventually recruited to fill the role of Chief Financial Officer for the Cleveland Clinic Health System. He came to the Clinic from his position as Executive Vice President and Chief Financial Officer of MedStar Health, Inc., of Columbia, Maryland. MedStar was the largest healthcare network in the Baltimore-Washington metropolitan area. He had 18 years experience as chief financial officer for medical organizations.

Also in 1999, Ralph Straffon, M.D., the Clinic's Chief of Staff, retired and was replaced by Robert Kay, M.D., a pediatric urologist. Straffon died after a prolonged illness on January 22, 2004. Kay had most recently served, as previously mentioned, in the role of Director of Medical Operations. He was a lifelong Californian prior

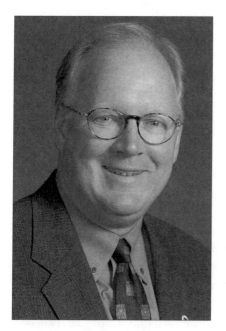

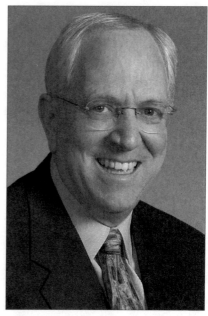

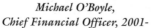

Michael O'Boyle,
Chief Financial Officer, 2001-

Robert Kay, M.D.,
Chief of Staff, 1999-

to his recruitment by Straffon to join the Clinic's staff in 1980 as head of the Section of Pediatric Urology. He obtained his M.D. from the University of California Los Angeles in 1971. Since joining the Clinic, he has had a distinguished medical career, including his service as chairman of the Section on Urology of the American Academy of Pediatrics. He has held numerous administrative positions at the Clinic, including service on the Board of Governors and the Board of Trustees. He has received much recognition for excellence as a physician and is consistently listed among America's best doctors. He also obtained an M.B.A. degree from Case Western Reserve University in 1990.

Melinda Estes, M.D., returned to The Cleveland Clinic in 2000 after a three-year stint as Executive Vice President and Chief of Staff at MetroHealth Medical Center to serve as Executive Director of a newly created Division of Business Development. Loop soon prevailed on her to assume the reins at Cleveland Clinic Florida, where she became CEO in 2001, replacing Dr. Harry Moon. Estes received her M.D. degree from the University of Texas, Galveston. After joining the medical staff at The Cleveland Clinic in 1982, she

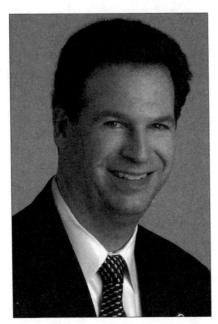

James Blazar,
Chief Marketing Officer, 1999-

was appointed head of the section of neuropathology, a position she held until moving to MetroHealth in 1997. In addition, she served on the Clinic's Board of Governors from 1990 to 1995 and as Associate Chief of Staff from 1990 to 1997. Estes resigned in 2003 to accept a hospital CEO position in Vermont.

Following the departure of Chief Marketing Officer Peter Brumleve, James Blazar was recruited from the Henry Ford Health System to fill this position in 1999. Blazar had 24 years of experience in marketing, mostly in health care. He had received his undergraduate education at the University of Cincinnati and an M.B.A. degree from the University of Chicago. He worked at Henry Ford Health System for eight years, where he began as Vice President of Marketing and Product Development, later moving to the Vice Presidency of Primary Care and Clinical Services for Henry Ford's medical group.

Finally, when William Grimberg, head of Institutional Advancement, left the Clinic in 2001, Bruce Loessin moved over from Case Western Reserve University, where he had served as Vice President for Development and Alumni Affairs, to take the helm of the fund-raising department, now known as Institutional Relations and Development. Since completing his education at the University of Michigan in 1972, Loessin had gained experience at several institutions, encompassing teaching and research, fund-raising, capital support, broadcasting, special events, continuing education, international studies, and federal relations. His successes at Case Western Reserve University made him the ideal candidate to succeed Grimberg.

By 2003, the Administrative Council had expanded to 12 members, but dropped back to 11 members with Estes's departure.

Chaired by Loop, the group now included Altus, O'Boyle, Kay, Lordeman, Blazar, Harris, London, Ivancic, Bronson, and Clough. The Board of Governors and the Medical Executive Committee remained constituted as before, although the personnel changed from time to time.

Professional divisional and especially departmental management also underwent some significant changes during this period.

At the divisional level, Paul DiCorleto, Ph.D., replaced George Stark, Ph.D., as chairman of the Lerner Research Institute in 2002. DiCorleto, also a molecular biologist, has worked extensively with cytokines. He has served on the Board of Governors, the Medical Executive Committee, and the Academic Council and is an able successor to Stark, who remains active in research. In 2003, Michael Levine, M.D., a pediatric endocrinologist from Johns Hopkins University, replaced Moodie as chairman of the Division of Pediatrics and head of The Children's Hospital at The Cleveland Clinic. In October 2003, three other significant divisional leadership changes occurred. Claire Young, R.N., replaced Shawn Ulreich as Chief Nursing Officer. Kenneth Ouriel, M.D., head of the Department of Vascular Surgery, replaced Hahn as chairman of the Division of Surgery, and James B. Young, M.D., co-chair of the Heart Failure Center, replaced Ahmad as chairman of the Division of Medicine.

At the departmental level, numerous changes have taken place since the last edition of this book. In 2003, Dr. Charles Emerman headed the Clinic's Emergency Department, which operates jointly with the emergency department at MetroHealth Medical Center. Tommaso Falcone, M.D., became the chairman of Obstetrics and Gynecology, having succeeded Jerome Belinson, M.D. After Bronson moved to the Division of Regional Medical Practice, Joseph Cash, M.D., briefly headed the Department of General Internal Medicine until his untimely death in 1999. Dr. Richard Lang replaced him. Sethu Reddy, M.D., succeeded Charles Faiman, M.D., as the head of Endocrinology. Joseph Iannotti, M.D., Ph.D., became chair of Orthopaedics, following Kenneth Marks, M.D. Both Anatomic Pathology and Clinical Pathology received new chairmen, with John Goldblum, M.D., now in charge of the former and Raymond Tubbs, D.O., the latter. The Department of Vascular Medicine was merged into Cardiovascular Medicine and no longer has a department chair. As the result of the departure of David Longworth, M.D., a search for his successor in Infectious Disease is under way. Finally, in November 2003, Derek Raghavan, M.D., Ph.D., from the University of Southern California, was appointed the new chairman of the Taussig Cancer Center, succeeding Maurie Markman, M.D.

TAKING STOCK: A PROGRESS REPORT

As Loop prepares to retire after nearly 15 years as chief executive officer, it is instructive to consider how far the organization has advanced during that time. We have been looking at the trees in the last two chapters; now it is time to look at the forest.

In 1990, the organization had annual revenues of $572 million and equity of $301 million with debt of $365 million. In 2003 the debt had approximately tripled to $1 billion, but the annual revenues had risen sixfold to $3.5 billion, and equity had grown to $1.3 billion, a fourfold increase. In Cleveland, there were 650 thousand outpatient visits to the main campus in 1990, but by 2003 this total had increased to 2.1 million visits to the Clinic's facilities, now supplemented by 14 family health centers and four ambulatory surgery centers. On the hospital side, the organization has grown from one hospital in Cleveland and one in Florida in 1990 to 10 hospitals in Cleveland and two new hospitals on two new unified campuses in Florida (Weston and Naples) in 2003.

Accompanying these physical and financial changes, the Clinic's culture has changed as well. A sense of proactive urgency has replaced the relaxed camaraderie of past years. Although there is still a marked emphasis on leadership, teamwork, active practice, and academic achievement, we now require excellence in more than one endeavor, and we recognize a stronger need for intellectual growth, practice building, communication, and service excellence. This is Loop's "New Professionalism," and it is reflected further in the shift of the Clinic's university affiliation from Ohio State University to Case Western Reserve University. Research has metamorphosed from a small and unfocused sideline to a highly sophisticated, programmatic enterprise. Fund raising, which was negligible in the past, is now well organized and productive, and the endowment has increased from $150 million to $800 million. The Annual Professional Review has progressed from a predominantly subjective to a more objective exercise, and this progression continues.

Finally, on June 2, 2004, Board of Trustees Chairman A. Malachi Mixon III announced the election of Delos M. "Toby" Cosgrove as the Clinic's next chief executive officer. Cosgrove had succeeded Loop as chairman of cardiovascular surgery, and would now succeed him again as CEO. This would be the Clinic's smoothest succession at the top leadership position, and the staff enthusiastically welcomed the transition.

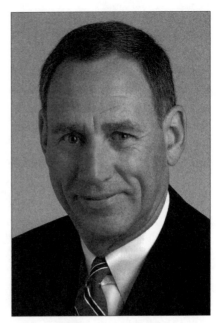

Delos M. Cosgrove, M.D., Chairman of the Board of Governors and Chief Executive Officer, 2004-

The combination of new divisional and departmental leadership as well as dynamic leadership at the top has kept the organization's energy level at high intensity. Coupled with the World Class Service leadership development initiative that began in 2003, these changes promise to catapult The Cleveland Clinic and the Cleveland Clinic Health System to new heights of accomplishment in the decades to come.

DIVISIONS, DEPARTMENTS, INSTITUTES, AND CENTERS

11. DIVISION OF MEDICINE

By Muzaffar Ahmad, Claudia D'Arcangelo, and John Clough

A good physician knows his patient through and through,
and his knowledge is bought dearly. Time, sympathy,
and understanding must be lavishly dispensed, but
the reward is to be found in that personal bond, which
forms the greatest satisfaction of medical practice.
—A.C. Ernstene

BEGINNINGS

The Division of Medicine has played an important role in the development of medical practice at The Cleveland Clinic since its opening in 1921. Dr. John Phillips, the only internist among the four founders, was the first chief of the Division of Medicine, then called the Medical Department. He was a true family physician who saw medicine begin to move away from house calls and toward an office-based practice during the eight years between 1921 and his untimely death in 1929 at age 50. Nevertheless, he continued to treat patients with diverse disorders and make house calls, often spending his entire weekend visiting patients in their homes.

Despite his own inclination and experience, Phillips recognized the value of specialization. In 1921, he assigned Henry J. John, M.D., the field of diabetes and supervision of the clinical laboratories. In 1923, he appointed Earl W. Netherton, M.D., head of the Department of Dermatology, and in 1929, E. Perry McCullagh, M.D., head of the Department of Endocrinology. The rest of the staff, like Phillips, practiced general medicine.

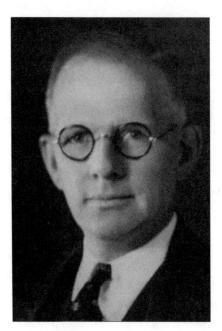

Russell L. Haden, M.D.,
Chief of Medicine, 1930-1949

In September 1930, one and a half years after Phillips's death (see Chapter 3), Russell L. Haden, M.D., was appointed chief of the Division of Medicine. Formerly a professor of experimental medicine at the University of Kansas School of Medicine, he approached medicine in a significantly different way. Whereas Phillips had been interested primarily in the clinical aspects of disease, Haden was a modern, laboratory-oriented medical scientist. During his eight years at the Clinic, Phillips published 26 papers, 23 of which were concerned with unusual cases or the diagnosis or treatment of diseases. In contrast, Haden's first five years at the Clinic saw publication of 26 papers, 23 of which were descriptions of laboratory innovations or attempts to define the causes or interrelationships of various diseases. Although his interests spanned the entire field of internal medicine, he was a hematologist, and he made many important contributions to the field of blood diseases, most notably the discovery of spherohemolytic anemia. However, his enthusiasm for physical therapy combined with the reluctance of most physicians to tackle the problems of arthritic patients resulted in a large referral practice in rheumatic diseases. Dynamic, brilliant, and possessing impeccable manners, Haden treated everyone with equal respect. Renowned as a superb clinician, he impressed patients and physicians alike by the speed at which he arrived at correct conclusions.

Residents coming to Haden's service did so with apprehension because "the chief" demanded high performance. This challenge usually brought out the best in the young physicians. Haden never seemed to forget small mistakes and frequently reminded the offender much later. However, he rarely mentioned major errors again because he knew how miserable the trainee felt and that the lesson had been learned. Although he never complimented residents for a job well done, they knew when Haden was pleased by the twinkle in his eye and slight smile.

Haden's first appointment to the Clinic staff was A. Carlton Ernstene, M.D., as head of the Department of Cardiorespiratory Disease in 1932. Ernstene had been trained in internal medicine and cardiology on the Harvard services of Boston City Hospital and served on the Harvard faculty. His interest in laboratory and clinical research made him an excellent choice to direct the new department. In 1939, H.S. Van Ordstrand, M.D., who had been appointed head of the Section of Pulmonary Disease, joined Ernstene.

Gastroenterology, allergy, and physical medicine were added between 1932 and 1937. Then economic restrictions imposed by the Great Depression required the staff to devote most of their energy to providing the highest volume of patient care at the lowest cost. The Clinic experienced almost no further growth until World War II.

A gradually improving economy brought visions of expansion that were dimmed by the war. Young physician candidates for the staff were drafted into military service, along with several members of the Division of Medicine and many residents. The entire Cardiorespiratory Department was depleted when Ernstene and Van Ordstrand departed for military service. Fortunately, Fay A. LeFevre, M.D., a former fellow, was able to return to the Clinic to replace them.

Immediately after the war, the Clinic experienced a rapid increase in staff as well as further specialization. As a result of military training, many young physicians recognized the value of group practice and applied to the Clinic for training. Haden preferred to accept those who had served their country and actually took more than his residency program needed.

When Haden retired in 1949, the chairmanship fell on Ernstene. Aside from his love of work and clinical abilities, he had little in common with Haden. Meticulous order was his hallmark. He started his hospital rounds at 8 A.M. and finished in one hour. He would rapidly complete any brief, unscheduled activities before he returned to his office, by which time he expected his first patient of the day to have been examined by his resident. He would question the patient closely, recheck much of the physical examination, and make careful and concise notes in a tight, angular, small script. Residents were occasionally heard to comment that Ernstene's hand-

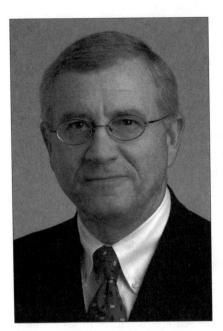

James Young, M.D.,
Chairman, Division of Medicine, 2003-

writing was reminiscent of 60-cycle interference commonly seen on the electrocardiograms of the time. Although he had a good background in internal medicine, cardiology was his field and he had all the attributes of an outstanding clinical cardiologist. Ernstene was a model of uncluttered, perfectly logical judgment, although he was not a good teacher in the traditional sense. His lectures were excellent because of their superb organization and precise delivery.

Seven new departments were established during Ernstene's tenure as division chairman, and the Department of Cardiorespiratory Disease was divided into Clinical Cardiology and Pulmonary Disease. The new departments were Internal Medicine (1949), Pediatrics (1951), Peripheral Vascular Disease (1952), Rheumatic Disease (1952), Hematology (1953), Hypertension (1959), and Pediatric Cardiology (1960). However, Ernstene discovered that as a physician with a large practice who also served as an officer of several national medical societies, administrative duties were burdensome. He formed a committee to advise and assist him, and this was the beginning of democratic governance in the Division of Medicine.

At the time of Ernstene's retirement as chairman in 1965, the Division of Medicine had 28 staff physicians. Expansion continued under the successive chairmanships of Van Ordstrand, Ray A. Van Ommen, M.D., Richard G. Farmer, M.D., and Muzaffar Ahmad, M.D. They were, respectively, specialists in pulmonary disease, infectious disease, gastroenterology, and pulmonary disease, but each sought a balanced development in the division, and each brought a unique character and style to the job. By 2003, there were 304 staff members in the division, excluding the pediatricians who had become part of a separate Division of Pediatrics in 1994. As this book was nearing completion in October 2003, cardiologist Dr. James B. Young replaced Ahmad as Division Chairman.

NEPHROLOGY AND HYPERTENSION

The senior Crile was interested in blood pressure his whole life, and early in his career he made notable contributions to the understanding of blood pressure maintenance under certain conditions. Through a considerable amount of experimental and clinical work, he became convinced that hypertension was mediated through the sympathetic nervous system, and that denervation of the celiac ganglion would be beneficial to the hypertensive patient. Although the therapeutic results of his surgical endeavors did not meet his expectations, he remained interested in hypertension and tried, with mixed success, to interest others on staff.

For many years, hypertensive patients at the Clinic were treated by general internists and cardiologists. After 1945, those with severe problems were studied in the hospital and then followed in the clinic by Robert D. Taylor, M.D., from the Division of Research. It was natural that with the large number of patients referred for the treatment of hypertension, drugs for its treatment were often tested at the Clinic. Soon, the need for specialized services to supplement those provided by Taylor became evident. In 1959, the Clinic formed a new Department of Hypertension and appointed David C. Humphrey, M.D., to head it.

In 1967, Ray W. Gifford, Jr., M.D., succeeded Humphrey. Gifford forged a strong alliance between the clinical and research programs in hypertension. Innovative and accomplished investigators, such as Irvine Page, Merlin Bumpus, Robert Tarazi, and Harriet Dustan, and their successors, Fetnat Fouad and Emmanuel Bravo, pioneered research programs in the humoral, hemodynamic, and neurologic aspects of hypertension. These activities were linked to clinical programs that focused on treatment options and their benefits as well as the education of physicians and their patients, leading to a national standard of excellence for departments of hypertension.

The Division of Research also addressed the development and application of dialysis. Willem J. Kolff, M.D., head of the Department of Artificial Organs, had developed an artificial kidney in Holland in 1940 and demonstrated its value in the treatment of reversible kidney disease. At the Clinic, it was discovered that regular dialysis could prolong life and relative comfort even when kidney function was seriously impaired.

Kolff was one of a trio of physicians who profoundly influenced the development of cardiology at the Clinic. The other two were cardiologist F. Mason Sones, Jr., M.D., and Donald B. Effler, M.D., a cardiovascular surgeon. Their contributions were monumental and received international acclaim. There were times, however, when these men did not get along. Their effect upon one another became so stressful to them and others around them that the Board of Governors decided that something had to be done and formed a committee to address the issue in 1956. It was headed by William L. Proudfit, M.D., a cardiologist on speaking terms with each of the dissident colleagues. The four men met daily at 8 A.M. and often would talk to each other only through the chairman. Much of the dissension surrounded the death of several high risk-patients who were operated on and had been expected to live. At one point, Effler decided to stop operating. However, Dr. John W. Kirklin, then at the Mayo Clinic, said he felt there was nothing wrong with the approach or selection of patients and that the operations should be resumed. His judgment proved correct, and with improved results, bad tempers eased. Nevertheless, Kolff left the Clinic in 1967 to continue his work with artificial organs at the University of Utah.

This activity was officially merged with hypertension in 1967 to form the Department of Hypertension and Nephrology. Members of the department led the development of standard hemodialysis techniques and newer approaches to prolong life in end-stage renal disease, including slow continuous ultrafiltration, continuous ambulatory peritoneal dialysis, and special interventions for critically ill patients in intensive care units.

Donald G. Vidt, M.D., an investigator and practitioner of pharmacologic approaches to hypertension, became chairman of the combined department in 1985. He consolidated programs in hypertension and expanded those in nephrology to include all aspects of dialysis. Gifford remained on Vidt's staff until his retirement in 1994, at which time the department established the Ray W. Gifford, Jr., Chair in Hypertension and Nephrology, and honored him as Distinguished Alumnus.

The succession of department chairmen with roots in The Cleveland Clinic changed in 1992 with the appointment of Vincent W. Dennis, M.D., from Duke University. By this time, the department was heavily engaged in research and patient care in kidney diseases, and so it was renamed Nephrology and Hypertension. In 2003, the department was composed of nine members with research and practice specialties in renovascular hypertension, immunologic aspects of transplantation, endocrine causes of hypertension, treatment for acute renal failure, and metabolic disturbances in kidney disease and stone disease. They were also closely involved in the selection and treatment of patients in the kidney and kidney-pancreas transplant program. Although the first cadaver kidney transplant was done elsewhere, the Clinic was one of the first institutions to apply this technique, in 1963. The Clinic's program was the first long-term successful series. Dennis stepped down from the chairmanship in 2003, and a search for his successor was under way at the time of this writing.

CARDIOVASCULAR MEDICINE

The Department of Cardiology has its roots in the Department of Cardiorespiratory Disease, which was established in 1932. In the late 1950s, when image-amplifying radiographic equipment first became available, Sones became interested in photographing the coronary arteries. Some incidental photographs showing portions of the coronary arteries already had been made in Sweden, but Sones attempted to photograph the vessels by injecting contrast material near their openings. One day he accidentally injected a large amount of dye directly into a coronary artery. When no dire consequences were noted, he deliberately injected small doses directly into the coronary arteries. The result was a clear x-ray picture of the coronary arteries. Thus, selective coronary arteriography began, and Sones was soon able to use his technique to verify the location of blockages in the arteries as well as the effectiveness of a coronary bypass operation.

In 1960, an offshoot of the department was formed to reflect the diagnostic laboratory studies developed under Sones. Named the Department of Pediatric Cardiology, it was renamed the Department of Cardiovascular Disease and Cardiac Laboratory in 1967, and

Sones was appointed chairman. Two years earlier, Ernstene had retired as chairman of Clinical Cardiology and had been replaced by William L. Proudfit, M.D. Although the two cardiology departments overlapped in many areas, their relationship remained harmonious.

Upon Proudfit's retirement in 1974, the two departments were merged into one Department of Cardiology, and William C. Sheldon, M.D., was named chairman. After 16 years of excellent leadership, in 1991, Sheldon was replaced by Eric J. Topol, M.D., a pioneer researcher in the field of ischemic heart disease and leader in interventional cardiology.

Over the next decade, the department grew from 33 to more than 72 physicians. Beyond its primary mission of delivering outstanding patient care, the department has gained a reputation for international leadership in education and research through its exceptional contributions to the specialty. These include the orchestration and successful completion of a 41,000-patient heart attack trial in 15 countries (with the acronym GUSTO), the development of new antiplatelet drugs used in millions of patients each year (IIb/IIIa blockers and clopidogrel), and becoming the leading center in the world for ablation of atrial fibrillation and carotid stenting, as well as one of the foremost centers for heart failure and transplantation.

In 2001, the department of Vascular Medicine merged with the department of Cardiology to form a new department of Cardiovascular Medicine, bringing the total membership of the department to 73 as of this writing in 2003.

PULMONARY AND CRITICAL CARE MEDICINE

The Department of Pulmonary Disease separated from the Department of Cardiorespiratory Disease in 1958. Howard S. Van Ordstrand, M.D., who subsequently became chairman of the Division of Medicine, was appointed its first head. Van Ordstrand also served a one-year term as president of the American College of Chest Physicians. He was known for his original description of acute berylliosis, a potentially lethal inflammatory disorder of the lungs that occurred in workers exposed to high concentrations of beryllium. Van Ordstrand worked on this problem with Sharad D. Deodhar, M.D., Ph.D., of the Department of Immunopathology.

Deodhar demonstrated the immunological nature of berylliosis, an outstanding example of the interdivisional collaboration that typifies the Clinic's approach to clinical investigation.

In 1973, Joseph F. Tomashefski, M.D., succeeded Van Ordstrand as department chairman. Under Tomashefski, the department successfully navigated the changes that were rapidly transforming the specialty of pulmonary medicine. During this time, fiberoptic bronchoscopy and the activities of the Pulmonary Function Laboratory were formally organized. The department also was given responsibility for the medical intensive care unit.

Following "Dr. Tom's" retirement in 1983, Muzaffar Ahmad, M.D., was appointed chairman. During his eight years of leadership, effective recruiting practices doubled the number of staff members to 10 and established a productive blend of individuals who contributed to the department's growing national reputation for clinical expertise and research. In 1985, the department became the first in the Division of Medicine to appoint a full-time laboratory scientist, Mary Jane Thomassen, Ph.D., to its primary staff, thus providing an important model for collaborative research. The addition of a Section of Respiratory Therapy laid the groundwork for subsequent growth in clinical activity and academic accomplishment.

After Ahmad's appointment as chairman of the Division of Medicine in 1991, Herbert P. Wiedemann, M.D., was designated chairman of the department, and its name was changed to Pulmonary and Critical Care Medicine. Under Wiedemann's direction, clinical and research activity continued to increase. In conjunction with the Department of Thoracic and Cardiovascular Surgery, the department developed one of the leading programs of lung transplantation in the country which is, at this time, the only one in Ohio (see Chapter 15). Seventeen physicians were on the staff in 2003, including two adult allergists.

In 1991, the Department of Pulmonary and Critical Care Medicine absorbed the Department of Allergy, which became the Section of Adult Allergy and Immunology. It had been created in 1934 with I. M. Hinnant, M.D., as head. Subsequent heads were J. Warrick Thomas, M.D. (1939-44); C. R. K. Johnston, M.D. (1944-66); Richard R. Evans, M.D. (1966-76), co-discoverer of the enzymatic defect responsible for hereditary angioneurotic edema; Joseph F. Kelley, M.D. (1976-86); and Sami Bahna, M.D. (1987-90). Today, the section concentrates on rhinitis and sinusitis, asthma, and latex allergy.

The National Institutes of Health supports five separate research projects in the department: a clinical center for research in adult respiratory distress syndrome (ARDS); a data-coordinating center for the registry of patients with severe deficiency of alpha-1 antitrypsin; a study of alveolar macrophage function in lung disorders; the development of inducible vectors for gene therapy; and the assessment of pulmonary function in pediatric AIDS patients. Other research projects, such as the investigation of innovative therapies for sepsis, ARDS, and asthma, and new bronchoscopy techniques for detecting or palliating lung cancer, are supported by private donations. As a link to the past, the department recently rekindled its research into beryllium-induced lung disease.

ENDOCRINOLOGY

Although the treatment of hypertension and coronary artery disease greatly influenced the Clinic's growth and development, significant advances were made in many other specialties. The first medical specialty at the Clinic was endocrinology, which was established in 1921 as a "diabetic service" under Henry J. John, M.D. A formal Department of Endocrinology was formed in 1928 with E. Perry McCullagh, M.D., as chairman. McCullagh had started his training in surgery, but he gradually shifted his interest to endocrinology, which was a new specialty at that time. Like John, he started with diabetes, but soon expanded to encompass the entire field of endocrinology. He was a walking encyclopedia, a colorful and friendly person with an inexhaustible supply of poems, jokes, and stories.

Sometimes McCullagh gave orders that were clear only to him. Once his resident misinterpreted an order and requested that a radiological examination of the colon be done on a woman with no gastrointestinal symptoms. The patient was undergoing the study when McCullagh was making rounds, and he became visibly annoyed. However, the x-ray film showed a large cancer of the colon, so McCullagh accepted the report in good grace and complimented the resident.

In the early days, McCullagh was engaged in laboratory and clinical research on a wide variety of endocrinologic topics. His work with testosterone and intermedin received wide recognition. His belief in rigid control of blood glucose levels for diabetics was later discounted, but is now being revived. With McCullagh's support, John and his wife founded Camp Ho Mita Koda, the world's first summer camp for diabetic children.

Diabetes has remained a driving interest of the department, which, following McCullagh, was headed successively by Penn G. Skillern, M.D., O. Peter Schumacher, M.D., Byron J. Hoogwerf, M.D., Charles Faiman, M.D., and, most recently, Sethu Reddy, M.D. Over the years, the department's interests have included lipid disorders, bone and mineral metabolism, and general endocrinology. The areas of reproductive medicine and pituitary disorders, which fascinated McCullagh, have recently again become centers of attention. The Clinic's research and education in endocrinology and metabolism have earned widespread respect. As of 2003, the department had five staff members.

DERMATOLOGY

The second specialist appointed to the Clinic staff was Earl Netherton, M.D., who served as chairman of the Department of Dermatology from 1923 to 1958. Although dermatology was generally disliked and even omitted from most training programs at that time, it was a treasured rotation among the Clinic's internal medicine residents. Netherton was a kindly teacher, respectful of students' opinions and intent on sharpening their observational skills. His charts vividly describe patients' skin lesions along with their diagnoses and treatments and include prescriptions and directions for use. A true "hands-on" physician, Netherton could tell whether or not an ointment had been prepared properly by merely rubbing it between his fingers. He was a pioneer in dermatopathology and safe radiation therapy for skin diseases and was an expert in the tedious investigation of patients with contact dermatitis.

John R. Haserick, M.D., succeeded Netherton as chairman of dermatology in 1958. He is best known for his contributions to the diagnosis and treatment of disseminated lupus erythematosus, a disease sometimes affecting only the skin but which often attacks other organs and leads to death if untreated. Haserick discovered the L. E. cell phenomenon, which for years was the mainstay diagnostic test for this disease. He never really got credit for this, however, because his publication was a few months behind that of Hargreaves at Mayo Clinic, who had simultaneously observed the same phenomenon. Haserick was the first to describe the fact that the phenomenon was due to a circulating "factor," which later turned out to be one of the antinuclear antibodies.

Henry H. Roenigk, M.D., who led the department into several new areas of endeavor, followed Haserick. Among these were hair transplantation and dermabrasion surgery, photochemotherapy for psoriasis, and topical and systemic chemotherapy for cutaneous lymphomas. He also began the department's long and highly recognized efforts in pharmaceutical research.

The current chairman is Philip L. Bailin, M.D., M.B.A., who assumed that role in 1977. Under Bailin's guidance, the department has grown from four to eleven staff physicians at the main campus, making it one of the nation's largest academic dermatology programs. Bailin also expanded the residency program to include a basic research track. In addition, he developed post-residency fellowships in dermatologic surgery, dermatopathology, and environmental dermatology.

With the establishment of The Cleveland Clinic's Family Health Centers, the department added a Section of Community Dermatology, now with eleven dermatologists in several of these regional offices. Cleveland Clinic Florida also added dermatology services with multi-physician sites at both Weston and Naples. In 2000, the department appointed Edward Maytin, M.D., Ph.D., to head the newly created Section of Molecular Dermatology, with dedicated basic laboratory facilities in the Lerner Research Institute. This NIH-funded effort examines the role of transcription factors and other molecular pathways in skin growth and development in both normal and disease states. The department has achieved expertise in cutaneous oncology (Mohs' surgery and malignant melanoma), cutaneous laser therapy, pediatric dermatology, oral medicine and cutaneous immunology, contact dermatitis, psoriasis and related disorders, and cosmetic dermatology.

Dermatology has also been active in organized medicine. One of the best known members of the department, Wilma Bergfeld, M.D., holds the distinction of having been the first woman president of the Academy of Medicine of Cleveland. She was also elected president of the American Academy of Dermatology. Bailin has served as president of the American Society for Dermatologic Surgery, the American College of Mohs' Micrographic Surgery and Cutaneous Oncology, and the Association of Academic Dermatologic Surgeons. James Taylor, M.D., has been president of the American Contact Dermatitis Society. Several members have served as president of the state and local dermatologic societies, and on the boards of many national organizations.

The department has 13 members. In 2003, Bailin stepped down from the department chair, and at the time of this writing, a search was under way for his successor.

GASTROENTEROLOGY

E. N. Collins, M.D., came to the Clinic in 1931 as a radiologist with a special interest in disorders of the digestive tract. By 1934, his reputation as a "stomach specialist" was firmly established, and he was asked to set up a Department of Gastroenterology. Thus, he became a practicing internist. His background in radiology, extensive knowledge, and aptitude for teaching made him popular with residents. R. J. F. Renshaw, M.D., an early member of the department, helped lay the groundwork for the emerging field of endoscopy in the late 1930s and early 1940s.

Upon Collins' death in 1959, Charles H. Brown, M.D., was named head of the department. During his tenure, he added two important physicians to the staff: Benjamin H. Sullivan, Jr., M.D., and Richard G. Farmer, M.D. Sullivan, picking up the baton from Renshaw, was a pioneer in the development and popularization of fiberoptic endoscopy, which greatly affected the practice of that subspecialty worldwide. Farmer, who was destined to succeed Brown as chairman of the department, shared his interest in inflammatory bowel disease. By working with his colleagues in pediatrics, surgery, and pathology, Farmer led the Clinic to international prominence in the management of this affliction.

When Farmer became chairman of the Division of Medicine, Bertram Fleshler, M.D., was named his successor in the Department of Gastroenterology. Fleshler continued to strengthen the department, particularly in the areas of motility and diseases of the esophagus.

The next chairman was Michael Sivak, M.D., who established an outstanding training program in innovative endoscopic technology and procedures, including endoscopic ultrasound and sclerosis of bleeding varices.

Joel Richter, M.D., has chaired the Department of Gastroenterology since 1994. Richter divided the 20-member group into six academic centers of excellence: colon cancer, endoscopy, hepatology, gastrointestinal motility (with a swallowing center), inflammatory bowel disease, and nutrition. Their goal is to expand clinical and research activities while working with colleagues in Colorectal Surgery, General Surgery, Liver Transplant Surgery, Thoracic Surgery, Radiology, and Pathology to make the Clinic's Digestive Disease Center one of the best in the country.

The Department of Gastroenterology, with 23 members as of 2003, now provides care in the new facilities of the Digestive Disease Center in the Crile Building. On one floor, all the clinical activities and research of both the Departments of Gastroenterology and Hepatology and Colorectal Surgery are housed together. This is the only combined center of its kind in the United States, and it significantly enhances the ability to give excellent clinical care in an environment of teaching and patient-related research.

NEUROLOGY

The need for a Department of Neuropsychiatry brought Professor Louis J. Karnosh from City Hospital (now called MetroHealth Medical Center) to the Clinic in 1946. His stature lent immediate prestige to the new department. According to his colleagues, what Karnosh did not know about neuropsychiatry was either unimportant or false.

Karnosh was a master neuropsychologist who inspired the confidence of patients, residents, and colleagues. His clinical approach was characterized by insightful questioning and therapeutic recommendations. His clinical notes were so complete and exquisitely phrased and executed that he never dictated reports to physicians; his secretaries merely copied his notes. Underneath his sharp features and stern countenance lay a good sense of humor, which was intensified by his deadpan delivery. Karnosh found time to write books and illustrate them with superb woodcuts of his own making. He also built a model railroad system and cultivated an encyclopedic knowledge of railroading.

When Karnosh retired in 1957, Guy H. "Red" Williams, M.D., succeeded him. He was a gentle, good-natured man and an accomplished physician who was popular with his staff. He gradually expanded the department and developed an outstanding Section of Electroencephalography. Due to increasing specialization in both areas, Williams advised that Neuropsychiatry be divided into two departments. This was accomplished in 1960. Williams became chairman of the new Department of Neurology, and A. Dixon Weatherhead, M.D., was appointed chairman of the Department of Psychiatry (see next section).

In 1976, John P. Conomy, M.D., became chairman of the Department of Neurology, succeeding the brief and tumultuous but productive chairmanship of Arnold H. Greenhouse, M.D. Greenhouse had recruited several young, highly talented neurologists, including Conomy, who eventually came to occupy leadership positions within the department. As chairman, Conomy expanded the department by adding experts in all major neurological subspecialties. Today, the effort continues under Hans O. Lüders, M.D., who joined the Clinic in 1978 as head of the Section of Electroencephalography and was appointed department chairman in 1991.

Since Lüders' appointment, Asa Wilbourn, M.D., established an electromyographic laboratory of national repute, and Hiroshi Mitsumoto, M.D., developed a Section of Neuromuscular Disease and a laboratory for amyotrophic lateral sclerosis (ALS) research. Conomy was instrumental in establishing the Mellen Center for Multiple Sclerosis, which has become a model of integrated clinical and research efforts (see Chapter 15).

Under Lüders' direction, the Section of Epilepsy and Sleep Disorders became an international leader, with a four-bed adult monitoring unit and specialized four-bed pediatric unit. The section was taken over by Harold "Holly" Morris, M.D., in 1991.

The department, with 43 members as of 2003, established subspecialty programs of national visibility and clinical research efforts in the fields of pediatric neurology, neuro-oncology, and movement disorders. The creation of the Department of Neuroscience within the Lerner Research Institute under the direction of Bruce Trapp, Ph.D., provided the necessary infrastructure to help the Neurology Department make essential contributions in the quest to conquer neurologic diseases.

PSYCHIATRY AND PSYCHOLOGY

The Department of Psychiatry developed more gradually during Weatherhead's tenure as chairman, which began in 1960. The department's emergence at that time paralleled the introduction in this country of a new and expanding pharmacopoeia of antipsychotic, antidepressant, and non-barbiturate sedative-hypnotic (benzodiazepine) drugs. Weatherhead was among the first U.S. psychiatrists to use the then-novel mood stabilizer, lithium, developed in Scandinavia. Under his leadership, the department grew into an interdisciplinary group of psychiatrists, psychologists, and social workers, providing services to adults as well as children. David A. Rodgers, Ph.D., the department's first clinical psychologist, was hired in 1966, followed shortly by Michael McKee, Ph.D., and Gary DeNelsky, Ph.D.

Clare Robinson, M.S., had been hired as a child psychologist by the Department of Pediatrics in 1953. However, lack of a Ph.D. degree prevented her from being promoted to full membership on the professional staff. When the "Associate Staff" category was created in 1968, she was immediately promoted to that position.

When Richard M. Steinhilber, M.D., was named chairman in 1977, a five-year growth spurt brought the number of staff members to a total of 13 psychiatrists and three psychologists. Steinhilber was dynamic and energetic in a way that belies the stereotype of the quiet, thoughtful, contemplative psychiatrist. Farmer used to say, "Within his chest beats the heart of an orthopedic surgeon." He added special Sections of Child and Adolescent Psychiatry, Consultation-Liaison Psychiatry, Alcohol and Drug Recovery, Chronic Pain Management, and Psychology. Ricky Huerta, M.D., A. Dale Gulledge, M.D., Gregory B. Collins, M.D., and Edward C. Covington, M.D., were recruited to lead the new sections of Child and Adolescent Psychiatry, Consultation-Liaison Psychiatry, Chemical Dependency, and Chronic Pain Management, respectively.

Neal Krupp, M.D., who succeeded Steinhilber in 1982, recognized the broader membership by changing the name to the Department of Psychiatry and Psychology. Krupp added the Section of Neuropsychology in 1985 and expanded the psychiatry residency and post-doctoral training in psychology.

George E. Tesar, M.D., assumed the chairmanship in 1993. During his first 10 years of leadership, he guided his staff through the turbulent waters of managed care. Important programmatic developments included the Anxiety and Mood Disorders Subspecialty Unit, the Child and Adolescent Fellowship, and extension of mental health services to the regional medical practices. As of 2003, the department had 19 members.

RHEUMATIC AND IMMUNOLOGIC DISEASE

Despite Russell Haden's interests in arthritis in the 1930s and 1940s, the Department of Rheumatology was not established until 1953. Arthur L. Scherbel, M.D., was named the first chairman and held the post for 27 years.

In Scherbel's time, most practitioners were discouraged by the problems of joint disease. Yet his optimistic attitude helped to create a great demand for this service. During his tenure, the department conducted important studies in cytotoxic drugs, especially mechlorethamine and methotrexate, for rheumatoid arthritis, systemic lupus erythematosus, vasculitis, and allied disorders. Scherbel also had a strong interest in scleroderma and was one of the first to recognize the importance of vascular lability and ischemia in this disease.

In 1981, John D. Clough, M.D., succeeded Scherbel as department chairman. Within a few years, he increased the department to 11 physicians in order to handle the growing patient load as well as increased interest in the specialty by young physicians. He also changed the name to the Department of Rheumatic and Immunologic Disease to recognize the staff's involvement in the care of patients with immunologic abnormalities and in immunologic research. Beginning in 1974, the department also operated the Special Immunology Laboratory in the Department of Immunopathology, where modern testing for autoantibodies and immune complexes was developed and research projects on immunocyte interaction were conducted. This laboratory was another model of interdivisional collaboration, but it fell victim to the reorganization of the Division of Laboratory Medicine that occurred subsequent to Deodhar's retirement.

Leonard H. Calabrese, D.O., the first osteopath appointed to the staff, became the head of Clinical Immunology. Calabrese has achieved national prominence for his work with rheumatological manifestations of AIDS, central nervous system vasculitis, and inclusion-body myopathy. William S. Wilke, M.D., has played a prominent role in the popularization of methotrexate for the treatment of severe rheumatoid arthritis and some forms of systemic lupus erythematosus. Daniel J. Mazanec, M.D., led the department's efforts in metabolic bone disease, and Anna P. Koo, M.D., ran the therapeutic apheresis program.

In 1992, Gary S. Hoffman, M.D., became the third chairman of the department, filling the vacancy created when Clough was named Director of Health Affairs for The Cleveland Clinic. During his years at the National Institutes of Health, Hoffman had founded the International Network for the Study of Systemic Vasculitides, of which he is chairman. The organization is now based at the Clinic and serves to coordinate large, multicenter studies for a variety of rare disorders. Hoffman is an internationally known expert in Wegener granulomatosis, giant-cell arteritis, and Takayasu arteritis.

The department has established a commitment to basic science in the area of immunogenetics. Starting in the year 2000, efforts have focused on identifying variations in candidate immunoregulatory genes in patients with vasculitis. Thomas Hamilton, Ph.D., chairman of the Department of Immunology, has facilitated linkage of his department with the Department of Rheumatic and Immunologic Diseases, providing expertise and space for Dr. Yihua Zhou and visiting scientists working in this area. In 2000, Hoffman and Calabrese were honored with the creation of the Harold C. Schott Chair in Rheumatic and Immunologic Diseases and the Richard Fasenmyer Chair in Clinical Immunology, respectively.

Chad Deal, M.D. joined the department in 1998 and developed a multidisciplinary Center for Osteoporosis and Metabolic Bone Disease, active at both the main campus and the Family Health Centers.

The department has formed a Section of Pediatric Rheumatology, headed by Philip Hashkes, M.D., and continues to support a variety of research activities aimed at enhancing the understanding and quality of care in rheumatoid arthritis, fibromyalgia, chronic fatigue syndrome, systemic lupus erythematosus, and vasculitis. As of 2003, the department had nine members.

HEMATOLOGY AND MEDICAL ONCOLOGY

Although Haden was primarily a hematologist, the Department of Hematology was not established until 1953. John D. Battle, M.D., was its first chairman. Over time, the medical treatment of cancer was recognized as a separate specialty, and the name was changed to the Department of Hematology and Medical Oncology.

James S. Hewlett, M.D., succeeded Battle in 1971. One of Hewlett's most important contributions to the field was his use of exchange transfusion for the effective treatment of thrombotic thrombocytopenic purpura, which previously had almost always been fatal. This treatment became the standard therapy until it was replaced by the much simpler technique of plasmapheresis, which was also pioneered at the Clinic.

When Hewlett retired, Robert B. Livingston, M.D., led the department until 1982. Livingston established the Predictive Assay Laboratory, where tumor cells from patients are grown and their reactions to various chemotherapeutic agents are determined.

James K. Weick, M.D., assumed the chairmanship in 1983 and held the post until he left to become chairman of the Department of Hematology and Medical Oncology as well as chairman of the Division of Medicine at Cleveland Clinic Florida in 1991 (see Chapter 21).

Maurie Markman, M.D., recruited from Memorial Sloan-Kettering Cancer Center in 1992, chaired the department until he left the institution in 2004. Under Markman and subsequent to his departure, the staff was active in testing the effectiveness of experimental drugs and drug combinations in the treatment of malignant disease. This commitment required a great deal of time, accurate record-keeping, careful analysis, and persistent optimism, despite frequently discouraging responses. The staff treated benign hematological conditions as well.

Beginning in the mid-1980s, the Department of Hematology and Medical Oncology demonstrated significant growth in patient numbers as well as the size and scope of clinical research programs. Bone marrow transplantation, chemotherapy, and immunotherapy were among the treatments widely used by the staff. The bone marrow transplant program, which performed 50 percent of all transplants in Ohio, became nationally recognized. The department's palliative care and hospice program was designated a pilot program of the World Health Organization, and the Horvitz Center, which opened in 1994, provided a unique focus on symptom management of patients hospitalized with cancer.

The Hematology/Oncology's 25 staff members have played a major role in the Clinic's multidisciplinary cancer efforts, including its highly regarded program in experimental therapeutics, headed by Ronald Bukowski, M.D., which examined innovative treatments for malignant disease. The search for effective treatments continues, often drawing upon the cooperation of other medical and surgical departments at the Clinic.

In the fall of 2000, the Department of Hematology and Medical Oncology moved into the new Taussig Cancer Center (see also Chapter 15). This wonderful new facility permitted significant growth in patient numbers, dramatically enhanced the department's ability to conduct innovative clinical research in hematologic and solid malignancies, and enabled recruitment of outstanding laboratory and clinical scientists.

GENERAL INTERNAL MEDICINE

Notwithstanding the rapid growth of specialty medicine at the Clinic, the institution recognized the value of general internal medicine by formally establishing the Department of Internal Medicine in 1949. John Tucker, M.D., the first chairman, had been a member of the Division of Medicine since 1921. He was succeeded in 1960 by Leonard L. Lovshin, M.D., who founded the Section of Headache Medicine. The growth of this subspecialty continued under the stewardship of Robert Kunkel, M.D., an internationally recognized headache specialist. Glen Solomon, M.D., joined him in 1986 and became section head in 1994. All three physicians have held national leadership roles in the study of headache, bringing the Clinic wide recognition in experimental therapeutics and medical outcomes in this field. The section was transferred to the Department of Neurology in 1998.

Ray A. Van Ommen, M.D., became the third chairman of the Department of Internal Medicine in 1970, and he also served as chairman of the Division of Medicine as well as founder of the Department of Infectious Disease. William H. Shafer, M.D., served ably as department chairman from 1972 until 1989. In 1971, the Clinic responded to corporations seeking periodic health evaluation for their executives by establishing a Section of Health Services under the direction of Alfred M. Taylor, M.D. Richard N. Matzen, M.D., succeeded him, and the section eventually became a department (Department of Preventive Medicine).

Beginning in 1986, Dennis Jahnigen, M.D., who was recruited from the University of Colorado, formed and headed a Section of Geriatric Medicine. Under his direction, the program became one of the top ten geriatric medicine programs in the United States. When Jahnigen left the Clinic in 1994, Robert M. Palmer, M.D., was appointed as section head.

In 1989, Stephen Ockner, M.D., restructured the Department of Internal Medicine. The Department of Preventive Medicine became a section in the Department of General Internal Medicine with Richard S. Lang, M.D., as section head. At the same time, the Department of Primary Health Care, which had been established in 1974 for the care of employees and their families and headed by Gilbert Lowenthal, M.D., also joined General Internal Medicine. Geoffrey Lefferts, M.D., was appointed head of the new Section of Primary Care. To reflect the wider scope of activities encompassed by the internists, the department was renamed General Internal Medicine.

After this consolidation, the Clinic recruited David L. Bronson, M.D., from the University of Vermont to serve as department chairman. Tremendous growth in the number of new staff members, patient visits, and residents occurred between 1992 and 1995. By the end of 1994, the department was logging more than 97,000 patient visits annually, making it the busiest in the Clinic. The residency program had grown to include 110 internal medicine residents, most of whom were receiving a large portion of their training in the Department of General Internal Medicine.

In the early 1990s, Clinic leaders recognized that the organization could provide more convenient service to patients in the surrounding communities through satellite facilities. The first satellite opened in Independence, Ohio, in 1993, with a group of orthopedic surgeons and one internist, Cynthia Deyling, M.D. Additional satellites were established, a new Division of Regional Medical Practice was created, and Dr. Bronson was appointed Division Chairman. Joseph M. Cash, M.D., originally a member of the Department of Rheumatic and Immunologic Disease, succeeded Bronson as department chairman in 1996. Following Cash's untimely death in 1998, Richard S. Lang, M.D., became acting chairman of the department and was appointed chairman in 2000.

From 1997 through 2003, the department formed new sections and explored fresh directions. The Section of Women's Health was established in 1997, headed by Holly L. Thacker, M.D. Clinical activity for this enterprise grew steadily, leading ultimately to establishment of the multidisciplinary Flo and Stanley Gault Avon Women's Health Center on the first floor of the Crile Building in 2002.

To address the facilitation of preoperative medical evaluation of surgical patients, the department created the Internal Medicine Preoperative Assessment Consultation and Treatment (IMPACT) Center in 1997 under the direction of David Litaker, M.D. This center handled almost 11,000 consultations in 2002, among the largest such operations in the United States.

To care better for hospitalized medical patients, the department established the Section of Hospital Medicine, which began as the hospitalist program in 1997 and formally became a section in 1999. Franklin A. Michota, Jr., M.D., who had directed the program from its outset, served as section head. Hospital admissions to the department increased dramatically in the following years, reflecting growth in main campus Emergency Department activity, maturing of the Regional Medical Practice Family Health Centers, and a trend toward shifting of admissions from subspecialty services to the Department of General Internal Medicine. The availability of internal medicine residents for coverage of inpatients on the internal medicine services considerably reinforced this trend. Admissions to the department increased from 1,226 in 1992 to 4,466 in 2002.

By 2003, the Department of General Internal Medicine had 45

professional staff members and, in addition to carrying out the varied clinical duties and activities outlined, also covered the Subacute Care Unit; performed a major role in education of students, residents, and fellows; participated significantly in the implementation of the electronic medical record; established fellowship training in geriatric medicine, women's health, medical informatics, and hospital medicine; and provided leadership in the establishment and planning of The Cleveland Clinic Lerner College of Medicine of Case Western Reserve University with Alan L. Hull, M.D., Ph.D., serving as Associate Dean of Curricular Affairs and J. Harry (Bud) Isaacson, M.D., as Director of Clinical Education. The department is among the largest and most diverse clinical entities in the institution.

INFECTIOUS DISEASE

The Department of Infectious Disease originated as a section of the Department of Internal Medicine under Van Ommen. In 1972, a separate department emerged, and Martin C. McHenry, M.D., was named chairman.

The department flourished under McHenry's guidance, and was soon recognized for excellence in both clinical medicine and education. McHenry epitomized the consummate scholar, combining excellence at the bedside with compassionate care, superlative teaching, and active clinical research. For these reasons, he was the first recipient of the Bruce Hubbard Stewart Award for humanism in the practice of medicine.

During McHenry's chairmanship, the department grew to five physicians and conducted clinical trials and outcomes research in many areas, including new antimicrobials, heart and bloodstream infections, and osteomyelitis.

McHenry stepped down in 1991, and David L. Longworth, M.D., was appointed chairman in 1992. Three new staff physicians were recruited, and the department intensified its commitment to research. Programs in transplantation, infectious disease, outcomes research related to hospital epidemiology, and laboratory-based investigation regarding antiviral susceptibility testing were initiated. Numerous clinical trials of newer antimicrobial agents were begun, along with studies to determine the optimal therapy for difficult infectious diseases.

The department's close relationship with the Section of Microbiology in the Department of Clinical Pathology has proven to be fruitful. Many collaborative studies have resulted from this, as well as a combined fellowship program leading to certification in both disciplines. Clinical activity has grown steadily, with routine evaluations performed on difficult infectious disease problems in the areas of nosocomial and postoperative infections, endocarditis, bone and joint infections, HIV disease, fever of unknown origin, tropical disease, and community-acquired infections. Under Longworth's leadership, research productivity increased, and the department has achieved national stature commensurate with its recognized excellence in clinical medicine and education.

Longworth left the Clinic in June 2002. As of this writing in 2004, a search for his successor was still under way.

EMERGENCY MEDICINE

In May 1994, The Cleveland Clinic strengthened its emergency medicine program with the opening of an 18,000-square-foot facility on the southwest corner of E. 93rd St. and Carnegie Avenue, the E Building. The new facility, which was a far cry from a standard emergency room, included a 19-bed emergency treatment area and a 12-bed minor illness area. It was adjacent to a 20-bed Clinical Decision Unit—an advanced concept in emergency medicine shared with Kaiser Permanente. In this unit, patients who do not require immediate hospitalization can be observed and treated for up to 24 hours after their initial evaluation. This unit has become a national model for the evaluation of chest pain and the treatment of heart failure.

Kaiser Permanente of Ohio, a branch of the giant health maintenance organization, which formed a partnership with the Clinic in 1992, shared space in the Clinical Decision Unit and had a separate emergency department within the same building. Patients of both organizations benefited from on-site radiology facilities, operating rooms directly overhead, efficient access to the clinical laboratories, and a rooftop helipad.

Responsibility for providing care in this new facility belonged to the Department of Emergency Medicine, which the Board of Governors created in 1993 in anticipation of the new enterprise. Norman S. Abramson, M.D., became its first chairman. In the first year, he assembled a board-certified emergency medicine staff and, working with Sharon Coulter (Director of Nursing), expanded the nursing staff to accommodate the patient volume. The department instituted education and training programs for Ohio State University medical students and Cleveland Clinic internal medicine residents and laid plans for an emergency medicine residency program. The Department of Emergency Medicine became the home base for establishing centers for the evaluation and treatment of patients with chest pain, stroke, and asthma, as well as pediatric emergencies.

Charles L. Emerman, M.D., assumed the chairmanship in 1996. He expanded the staff to 17 members by 2003 to meet the increasing patient volume and educational needs. The department affiliated with the MetroHealth Medical Center Emergency Medicine residency program in 1996 and currently trains 33 emergency medicine residents.

CONCLUSION

Although practice methods have become more scientific since 1921, the Clinic's approach to patient care has remained unchanged: one physician is responsible for each patient's care and orders any consultations with other physicians that may be required. With drastic changes in health care under way, the Clinic agrees that the role of the primary physician is more important than ever to ensure appropriate care and the timely, judicious use of resources.

12. DIVISION OF PEDIATRICS

By John Lampe

Children are poor men's riches.
—English Proverb

PEDIATRICS BEGINS

CHILDREN WITH RARE AND COMPLICATED DISEASES HAVE BEEN CARED FOR AT The Cleveland Clinic since its inception. When co-founder John Phillips, M.D., moved his practice to the Clinic from Western Reserve University, he brought with him the tradition of caring for children, a skill for which he was widely known in those days. At that time, the care was disease-oriented rather than child-centered. That changed in 1951 when Robert D. Mercer, M.D., arrived from Western Reserve University, as Phillips had done some three decades before, to start a Department of Pediatrics.

Mercer was already well known in the community before he arrived at The Cleveland Clinic. He and his wife, Ann, had helped to found the Cleveland chapter of United Cerebral Palsy, now located on the Clinic's main campus. He was a gifted teacher, and he had a massive slide collection, the envy of his colleagues, which he continued to expand throughout his career. His willingness to share this asset with anyone who had need of it was legendary. Long after he retired, Mercer was honored for his contributions to medicine and to The Cleveland Clinic during the dedication ceremony for the Alumni Library in the educational wing of the newly opened Lerner Research Institute in 2000. United Cerebral Palsy also dedicated a room in his honor in their new building at that time. He died in 2002.

The Clinic's first pediatric outpatient department was located in two rooms "loaned" by the Department of Urology. They were just around the corner from Sones's original cardiac catheterization laboratory. A pediatric cardiologist, Sones was using his new cardiac visualization technique to help Clinic surgeons perform heart operations on children, with excellent results. At that time there, was no pediatric cardiologist or pediatric cardiac surgeon at Western Reserve University, and patients from that institution were sent to the Mayo Clinic. With the formal establishment of the pediatrics department, the Clinic reserved 30 of its 357 hospital beds for a pediatric ward.

The first pediatrician Mercer recruited was Viola Startzman, M.D., a superb clinician admired and respected throughout the community. Startzman had been trained as a laboratory technician before going to medical school, and her understanding of blood chemistry proved invaluable.

Nineteen fifty-three was a landmark year in which the Department of Pediatrics started a residency program, paying the residents the princely salary of $150 per month, and gave its first postgraduate education course. It was also the year Clare Robinson, M.S., became the department's third staff member. Considered to be one of the best pediatric and adolescent psychologists in the profession, she nevertheless lacked the doctoral degree necessary for full staff status. When the "Associate Staff" category was created in 1968, she was appointed to that position, as noted in the previous chapter.

In 1954, the department initiated a program with St. John School of Nursing for training student nurses in pediatrics. This was the first student nurse program at The Cleveland Clinic. A few years later, the department developed a curriculum for training third-year medical students, and this became the Clinic's first medical school program.

RELATIONSHIP WITH OBSTETRICS

During those years, the Clinic had an excellent Department of Obstetrics under the supervision of Howard P. Taylor, M.D. It was among the first in the country (a) to make use of amniocentesis, (b) to invite fathers into the delivery room, and (c) to permit newborns to stay in their mothers' hospital rooms. Clinic obstetricians even carried out intrauterine transfusions. Their newborn nursery was open to all pediatricians in the community. Yet despite all these successes, the Clinic closed the Department of Obstetrics in 1966 to make room for expansion of cardiac surgery, which was on the brink of explosive progress. This was, nevertheless, a severe blow to the pediatricians, whose patient base in large part was composed of babies born at the Clinic. In any case, pediatrics survived and ultimately separated from the Division of Medicine, becoming a division in its own right. After a 29-year absence, obstetrics reopened at the Clinic in 1995 (see Chapter 13).

PEDIATRIC SPECIALIZATION

Mercer recognized the value of specialization and began the process around the same time it was going on throughout the Division of Medicine, in which pediatrics was then still a department. In 1956, Mercer invited Mary Harmon, M.D., to join the staff. A specialist in metabolic abnormalities in babies, she established a unit that was designated by the State of Ohio as a center for the treatment of phenylketonuria.

The department next added gastroenterology with the appointment of William M. Michener, M.D., in 1961. He left to accept an academic position in New Mexico in 1968 but returned five years later to become Director of Education for The Cleveland Clinic (see Chapter 19). He then resumed his pediatric practice on a part-time basis. His colleagues greatly valued his ability to distinguish chronic ulcerative colitis from Crohn's disease. It was not until the early 1980s that the department recruited a second gastroenterologist, Robert Wyllie, M.D. Thereafter, the section rapidly grew into one of the largest groups of pediatric gastroenterologists in the country, gaining additional national recognition in the treatment of inflammatory bowel disease as well as hepatitis, gastrointestinal bleeding, and the procedures of endoscopy and liver transplantation. Wyllie set the national standards for pediatric endoscopy and was the senior editor of a major textbook in pediatric gastroenterology. Drs. Rita Steffen and Marsha Kay received staff positions in 1996 and 1997, respectively, after completing their pediatric gastroenterology fellowships at the Clinic. Barbara Kaplan, M.D., joined the department in 1998 from Mt. Sinai Hospital in Cleveland, and Vera Hupertz, M.D., arrived the next year from Rainbow Babies and Children's Hospital, a pediatric hospital-within-a-hospital at University Hospitals of Cleveland.

Mercer had helped conduct the first successful chemotherapy during his pathology residency at Boston Children's Hospital. The study in which he participated included a large number of patients, and its success gave birth to the subspecialty of pediatric oncology. At the Clinic, Mercer continued to care for cancer patients himself until his other pediatric patients and administrative duties necessitated looking for help. In 1962, he recruited Derrick Lonsdale, M.D., a pediatrician with a special interest in childhood cancer, to assume the care of the Clinic's young patients with leukemia and other childhood cancers. Paul Dyment, M.D., arrived and assumed leadership of the pediatric hematology/oncology section in 1971, and was later joined by Donald Norris, M.D. (1981), Michael Levien, M.D. (1989), and Karen Bringelsen, M.D. (1991).

In 1960, Mercer started one of the first laboratories in the state for the culture of cells and study of chromosomes and their role in genetics. He very early recognized the need for these studies to aid in diagnosis of certain congenital disorders. Once the procedures were well established, he turned the laboratory over to the Department of Laboratory Medicine.

In 1971, residency programs began to graduate a new wave of physicians and surgeons with training in pediatric specialties, and the Clinic recruited two: Dyment, as mentioned above, and Ronald L. Price, M.D., a pediatric ophthalmologist. Price joined the Department of Ophthalmology and received a joint appointment in Pediatrics. Dyment became a well-known pediatric specialist and was appointed department chairman upon Mercer's retirement in 1980. These and other additions allowed the Clinic to begin offering the specialty care in pediatrics that has distinguished it in adult medicine.

In 1973, the appointment of A. David Rothner, M.D., enabled the Clinic to establish a section devoted to pediatric neurology. Over the years, the section has grown and has developed particular expertise in the treatment of headaches, neurofibromatosis, learning disabilities, brain tumors, and metabolic and neuromuscular disorders. Gerald Erenberg, M.D., joined Rothner in 1976, later becoming nationally known for his treatment of patients with Tourette's syndrome.

Bruce Cohen, M.D., in 1991, brought to pediatric neurology new expertise in neuro-oncology, and Neil Friedman, M.D. (1998), provided additional abilities in the care of neuromuscular diseases. By the mid-1980s, so many children with epilepsy were being evaluated at the Clinic that a special childhood epilepsy service was established, headed by Elaine Wyllie, M.D., soon joined by Prakash Kotagal, M.D. The pediatric neurologists offered a 24-hour, fully computerized epilepsy and sleep studies unit, and with their neurosurgical colleagues (including William Bingaman, M.D., 1997) they developed an international reputation in epilepsy surgery for children.

In 1977, Carl C. Gill, M.D., joined the staff to organize a pediatric cardiac surgery program. A year later, Douglas S. Moodie, M.D., a pediatric cardiologist who had worked with Gill at the Mayo Clinic, rejoined him as the first head of the section of pediatric cardiology. Pediatric cardiologists with expertise in pediatric electrophysiology (Richard Sterba, M.D.), echocardiography (Daniel Murphy, M.D.), cardiac catheterization (Lourdes Prieto, M.D.), and cardiac transplantation (Maryanne Kichuk-Chrisant, M.D.), were subsequently added. The section developed a unique program that provided continuity of care for patients with congenital heart defects from birth through old age. Today, the Clinic's pediatric cardiologists and cardiac surgeons care for the largest number of adult congenital heart disease patients in the country. Capitalizing on this expertise, they developed fellowships in adult congenital heart disease (1993) and pediatric interventional cardiology (1994)—both unusual training programs in this country. Larry Latson, M.D., was recruited in 1993 to become chairman of a rapidly expanding and diversifying department of pediatric cardiology.

In 1986, Dyment left the Clinic to become chairman of pediatrics at the Eastern Maine Medical Center in Portland and was succeeded as department chairman by Moodie. Moodie oversaw a period of unprecedented growth in pediatrics, including successful recruitment of pediatric staff members representing the full complement of pediatric specialty services as well as a children's hospital at The Cleveland Clinic.

After Gill left Cleveland in 1987 to become chief of staff and then chief executive officer of Cleveland Clinic Florida, Eliot Rosenkranz, M.D., was named the new head of the Section of Congenital Heart Surgery. Renowned Australian pediatric cardiothoracic surgeon Roger B. Mee, M.B., Ch.B., succeeded him, bringing with him an international reputation for excellence and innovation. A second congenital heart surgeon was added in 1993. Together, they doubled the number of pediatric open-heart cases and at the same time achieved one of the lowest mortality and morbidity rates in the world.

Robert Kay, M.D., started the section of pediatric urology in 1980, and quickly became known as an outstanding urologist. However, he became so busy with his responsibilities as Director of Medical Operations (and later Chief of Staff) for the Clinic that a second surgeon, Jonathan H. Ross, M.D., had to be added to the staff in 1992.

The first full-time practitioner of pediatric general surgery at the Clinic was Hugh V. Firor, M.D., who arrived in 1981 and operated primarily on children with abdominal and bowel disease. He left the Clinic in 1991 and was replaced by Fred Alexander, M.D. By 2002, Alexander was performing more than 800 operations annually and investigating the feasibility of doing small-bowel transplantation in children. John DiFiore, M.D., was recruited to join the pediatric surgery department in 1998 after completing his training at Boston Children's Hospital. Anthony Stallion, M.D., joined them in 2002, following his residency at the University of Cincinnati.

By the 1980s, the Clinic was becoming well known worldwide for pediatric specialty care but was not known in the community for general pediatrics. A section of general pediatrics had existed since the appointment of Dr. Ruth Imrie in 1978, but it was part of the Department of Primary Care and existed to provide care for the children of staff and employees. In 1982, Moodie recruited Michael L. Macknin, M.D., a highly regarded academic pediatrician. Two well-known community pediatricians, Daniel Shapiro, M.D., and Richard Garcia, M.D., were added to the growing general pediatric department in the mid 1980s. In 1991, Moodie brought the section into the Department of Pediatrics to give it a higher profile in the community.

Robert J. Cunningham, M.D., became head of pediatric nephrology in 1981 and assumed directorship of the pediatric residency program in 1985. He built the largest pediatric nephrology service in northeastern Ohio, was named vice-chairman of Pediatrics, and became associate director of The Children's Hospital at The Cleveland Clinic. Accordingly, the need arose for a second nephrologist. When Ben Brouhard, M.D., joined the staff in 1988, he brought expertise in pediatric hypertension and renal transplantation. Deepa Chand, M.D., joined them in 2002.

Because of Brouhard's strong research background, he subsequently became director of pediatric research and developed an excellent program for both staff and residents. Johanna Goldfarb, M.D., a well-known pediatric infectious disease specialist, subsequently assumed the directorship of pediatric research. While only a quarter of the pediatric programs in the country require their residents to do research, The Cleveland Clinic requires pediatric residents to present the results of a research project each year. Brouhard also encouraged staff members to publish, speak, and spread their expertise as visiting professors.

Although neurosurgery chairman Donald F. Dohn, M.D., regularly performed surgery on children, the first designated pediatric neurosurgeon was Joseph F. Hahn, M.D., who eventually succeeded Dohn as department chairman. In 1987, Hahn's patient-care capacity was reduced when he was appointed chief of the Division of Surgery while maintaining his departmental leadership. The growing need for a full-time pediatric neurosurgeon led Moodie to recruit the Clinic's first pediatric-trained neurosurgeon, Mark S. Luciano, M.D., in 1993.

A similar situation existed in endocrinology. Department chairman O. Peter Schumacher, M.D. Ph.D., had developed a solid reputation in pediatric diabetes, but he had been trained in adult endocrinology. The Clinic's first pediatric endocrinologist, Geoffrey Redmond, M.D., arrived in 1982. When he left for private practice in 1991, he was replaced by Douglas G. Rogers, M.D., a specialist in pediatric diabetes. Rogers also became the first quality assurance officer for Pediatrics, a post he held until 1995 when it was assumed by gastroenterologist Marsha Kay, M.D. Ajuah Davis, M.D., joined Rogers in 2000 in the busy endocrinology section.

Michael J. McHugh, M.D., was recruited to head pediatric intensive care in 1979 and became director of the new Pediatric Intensive Care Unit (PICU) in 1992. Competition with University Hospitals was intense at that time, and the issue of pediatrics, particularly pediatric intensive care, was a hot-button issue with them. University Hospitals used the certificate-of-need process to try to block the establishment of this unit. In the end, they failed to make their case, and the state granted the certificate of need.

McHugh also took over directorship of the residency program from Cunningham in 1992. Under his leadership, the number of residents has more than doubled to 33. In addition, up to 60 medical students now rotate through pediatrics every year, and fellowships have been developed in the pediatric subspecialties of neurology, gastroenterology, allergy and immunology, critical care, interventional cardiology, psychology, and adult congenital heart disease. Gary Williams, M.D., who had joined the Department of General Pediatrics in 1991, became the director of the pediatric residency program in 1996. During his tenure, the pediatric residency program continued to flourish, increasing the number of residents to 13 in each of the three years of pediatric residency training. Ronald Holtzman, M.D., was appointed chairman of the Department of Neonatology in 2000 and oversaw the opening of the Clinic's first level III Neonatal Intensive Care Unit (NICU) a year later.

Gita P. Gidwani, M.D., came to the Clinic in 1976 from Kaiser Permanente to establish the pediatric and adolescent gynecology practice. She was the institution's only gynecologist with special training in the problems of adolescence until the arrival of Dr. Marjan Attaran in 1996. Both physicians worked closely with Ellen Rome, M.D., a specialist in adolescent pediatrics who joined the staff in 1994, Ruth Imrie, M.D., who had developed an interest and expertise in the problems of teenagers over the years, and Karen Vargo, M.D., who had brought her adolescent medicine specialty experience to the Clinic from the Children's Hospital of Pittsburgh in 1999.

Under Moodie's direction, the Department of Pediatric and Adolescent Medicine took a quantum leap from a small but respected group of pediatric specialists to a large and comprehensive pediatric program. He expanded existing sections, and he added the first pediatric specialists in many fields to care for the growing number of children. These included allergy (Alton L. Melton, M.D., 1988, and Velma Paschall, M.D., 1988), infectious disease (Barbara Baetz-Greenwald, M.D., 1988, Johanna Goldfarb, M.D., 1992, and Camille Sabella, M.D., 1995), dermatology (Teri A. Kahn, M.D., in 1992), plastic surgery (Frank A. Papay, M.D., 1992), orthopedics (Alan Gurd, M.D., 1976, and Jack Andrish, M.D., 1977, joined by Thomas Kuivila, M.D., in 1995), ophthalmology (Elias Traboulsi, M.D., 1997) pulmonary disease (Paul C. Stillwell, M.D., 1992, who was succeeded by Karen McDowell, M.D., in 1998), rheumatology

(Bernhard Singsen, M.D., 1993, replaced by Philip Hashkes, M.D., 2003), otolaryngology (Diana Traquina, M.D., 1993, followed by Peter Koltai, M.D., in 1998), and neonatology (Jeffrey Schwersenski, M.D., 1994). John B. Lampe, M.D., a general pediatrician recruited in 1991, had a special interest in pediatric dermatology and provided new expertise in this area. Kahn was the first trained pediatric dermatologist at the Clinic, and she had established the largest practice of its kind in northern Ohio.

The PICU, which had opened in 1992 under the leadership of Michael McHugh, M.D., soon needed dramatic expansion to accommodate the burgeoning pediatric surgical practices. McHugh was joined at this time by Stephen Davis, M.D., and Demetrious Bourdakos, M.D., in 1996; Kathryn Weise, M.D., in 1997; and A. Marc Harrison, M.D., and Elumalai Appachi, M.D., in 1999. Their 24-hour in-house attending physician level of care yielded one of the lowest mortality rates in the nation. The Clinic opened a pediatric cardiac surgery operating room adjacent to the intensive care unit and moved all pediatric cardiology and cardiac surgery services into The Children's Hospital at The Cleveland Clinic toward the end of 1994.

THE CHILDREN'S HOSPITAL AT THE CLEVELAND CLINIC

In 1987, the Clinic opened its Children's Hospital and became an associate member of the National Association of Children's Hospitals and Related Institutions. This hospital-within-a-hospital occupied the third and fourth floors of the old hospital. In one unit, children under age 10 are cared for in single rooms. Each room provides space for the patient's own toys as well as a convertible chair bed to accommodate a parent.

A rooftop play deck provides a safe outdoor play area for patients right off the hospital wing. The Jennifer Ferchill Play Deck is a highly valued component of The Cleveland Clinic Children's Hospital. Located right off the pediatric hospital wing, its wide doors, flat surface, and oxygen hook-ups ensure that even wheelchair-bound and intravenous-tethered children can enjoy fresh air. A glass house between the outdoor portion and the hospital provides an outdoor-type setting where children can play during the winter. The play deck was donated by John Ferchill, a corporate developer, in gratitude for the care his young daughter had received at the Clinic during her battle with a brain tumor. Ferchill persuaded Cleveland's construction community to donate almost $700,000 worth of labor to construct the deck.

A separate unit, designed for adolescent patients, is staffed with nurses specially trained in treating teenagers. To make hospitalization as pleasant an experience as possible, the unit included a recreation room with appropriate furniture, stereo equipment, and games. A four-bed special-care unit, originally placed on this unit to treat patients needing more intensive nursing care, has evolved into an epilepsy-monitoring unit.

Vanessa Jensen, Psy.D., reinvigorated the Department of Pediatric Psychology when she joined the Clinic in 1992. Her expertise in autistic spectrum disorders was widely sought, and the increasing demand for psychology services soon mandated the addition of pediatric psychologists Beth Anne Martin, Ph.D., and Amy Lee, Ph.D. Michael Manos, Ph.D., joined the department in 1999, bringing his expertise in attention-deficit hyperactivity disorder, as did Gerard Banez, Ph.D., whose particular interest was childhood functional disorders.

Pediatric radiology expertise was essential to The Children's Hospital at The Cleveland Clinic. Marilyn Goske, M.D., became head of this section in 1993 and quickly recruited outstanding colleagues to provide the full range of imaging and interventional services, including David Frankel, M.D., in 1997; Janet Reid, M.D., and Stuart Morrison, M.D., in 1999; and Sunny Chung, M.D., in 2001.

In 1998, as The Cleveland Clinic was establishing the Cleveland Clinic Health System, Health Hill Hospital added its 52 beds to The Children's Hospital at The Cleveland Clinic, in the process changing its name to the Cleveland Clinic Children's Hospital for Rehabilitation.

THE DIVISION OF PEDIATRICS

In 1994, the Department of Pediatrics, with a staff of 79 physicians, achieved division status in recognition of its increased importance in the institution and to help coordinate and administer all pediatric activity at The Cleveland Clinic.

In 2002, Moodie left The Cleveland Clinic to take on the challenge of developing a strong pediatrics program at the Ochsner Clinic in New Orleans. After a national search, his successor was identified as Michael Levine, M.D., who was recruited from Johns Hopkins University. Levine arrived in March 2003.

The future of pediatrics at The Cleveland Clinic promises to be exciting. The staff anticipates rapid growth in the general pediatrics programs as well as the specialty programs, The Children's Hospital facilities, satellite pediatric programs, and obstetrics. A common focus on providing the best possible care of sick children unifies these activities. Active research programs in many areas, including the study and treatment of genetic and immunologic diseases, will constantly reaffirm and support this goal.

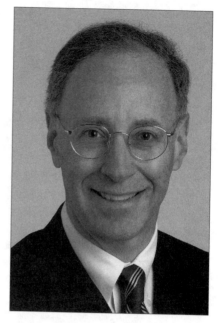

Michael Levine, M.D.,
Chairman, Division of Pediatrics, 2002-

13. DIVISION OF SURGERY

By Joseph Hahn

*A surgeon must have a hand as light as
floating perfume, an eye as quick as a
darting sunbeam, a heart as compassionate
as all humanity, and a soul as pure as
the water of Lebanon.*
—*John Chalmers DaCosta*

WHEN THE CLINIC OPENED IN 1921, UROLOGY AND OTOLARYNGOLOGY (THEN called ear-nose-throat) were the only surgical specialties represented. General surgeons did all other operations. Urology had not, however, formally separated from general surgery, and Lower performed almost as many thyroidectomies, cholecystectomies, and general surgical procedures as urologic procedures.

The first otolaryngologist, and later, orthopedic, neurological, and ophthalmic surgeons, strictly limited their practices to their specialties. Eventually, specialists in plastic surgery, gynecology, thoracic surgery, vascular surgery, and colorectal surgery were added to the staff. General surgery gradually became one of the smaller services, limited in scope to the treatment of diseases of the upper abdomen, thyroid, and breast, and to hernia repair.

Nevertheless, many of the physicians who helped shape The Cleveland Clinic Foundation in its early days were general surgeons. For this reason, the development of the Division of Surgery has been closely intertwined with the history of the Department of General Surgery and the practice of surgery as a whole in the 20th century.

GENERAL SURGERY

Thyroidectomies provided the bulk of the financial support for the original Clinic and Hospital. In 1921, following the discovery that iodine made thyroidectomy possible for patients with Graves' disease, surgeons suddenly were confronted with a backlog of previously inoperable patients. Nontoxic goiters that were endemic in the Great Lakes region increased this backlog. Improvements in surgical techniques introduced by Crile and the Mayo brothers made thyroidectomy safe, and, in 1927, Clinic surgeons were performing an average of ten a day. Their mortality rate for this procedure was the lowest ever reported.

The greatest danger at that time was thyroid crisis, a dramatic chain of events that was likely to occur when a patient with Graves' disease and severe hyperthyroidism was subjected to general anesthesia, surgery, infection, or even a bad fright. The patient's pulse rate would soar, the heart often fibrillated, and the body temperature rose to 105° or 106°F. The patient literally was consumed in the fire of his own metabolism. Ice bags and oxygen tents sometimes helped; transfusions did not. The crisis tended to run its course, peaking on the second night after surgery, and then, if the patient survived, subsiding.

Crile believed that fear could trigger such a crisis. To avoid it, he developed a system called "stealing the thyroid." The patient would not be told when the operation was to take place. Every morning, breakfast was withheld and the nurse anesthetist would go to the patient's bedside and administer just enough nitrous oxide to make the patient a bit giddy and confused. On the morning of surgery, the routine was the same except that the analgesia was a little deeper, so the patient took no notice when the team moved in. The neck was prepared with ether, iodine, and alcohol, and then draped. A floor nurse or the patient's private nurse stood on a chair behind the head of the bed and illuminated the operative field with a shaded light held on the end of a pole.

With a single stroke, Crile would make a gracefully curved incision and then dissect the skin flap. He never stopped to clamp bleeders; that was the function of the first assistant. The second assistant, hanging uncomfortably over the head of the bed, would retract the skin and cut the thread after the knots were tied. These 10-minute operations were bloody and unanatomic, but in the days before intravenous anesthesia, speed was necessary. A transfusion team was always available to give blood when there was excessive loss. The same team stood ready to do tracheotomies when necessary, since the incidence of injury to the recurrent laryngeal nerves was high. Postoperative hemorrhage was fairly common, too, because the main vessels were not tied.

Better surgical training and technique and improved anesthesia gradually enabled increasing numbers of these operations to be done in community hospitals. The introduction of iodized

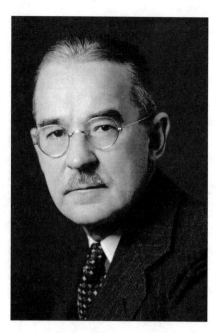

Thomas E. Jones, M.D.,
Chief of Surgery, 1943-1949

salt, better food transportation, antithyroid drugs, and radioactive iodine eventually obviated the need to operate on patients for Graves' disease. After 1927, the frequency of thyroidectomy at The Cleveland Clinic declined steadily.

Despite the large number of thyroidectomies performed in 1927, not one patient was diagnosed as having hyperparathyroidism. In 1969 Clinic surgeons performed 32 operations on the parathyroid. By the 1990s, as the result of better diagnostic techniques and the reputation of Caldwell B. Esselstyn, Jr., M.D., over 100 operations for hyperparathyroidism were performed annually.

At the same time, the number of operations for cancer of the colon and rectum grew. Thomas E. Jones, M.D., an accomplished abdominal surgeon, returned from a trip to London having learned a one-stage combined abdominoperineal resection procedure, which he proceeded to perfect into a fine art. He could perform three or four of these complex operations in a morning when it took most surgeons three or four hours to do one.

Jones was operating in the days before sulfonamides or antibiotics, and mortality from colon resection with anastomosis was

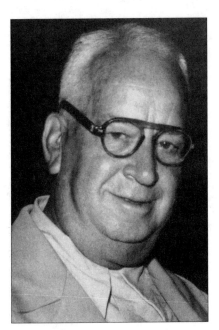

Robert S. Dinsmore, M.D.,
Chief of Surgery, 1949-1957

high everywhere. The fatal problem was peritonitis, which Jones avoided by not opening the bowel or anastomosing it. Cancers located well above the rectum were treated by abdominoperineal resection with end colostomy. After a resection of the left colon or transverse colon, he usually exteriorized the tumor over a Rankin clamp and performed an obstructive resection. There were no anastomoses except after resections of the right colon, which had few complications. The result was an astonishingly low mortality rate for surgery of the colon and rectum, but the price was a high incidence of colostomy.

Jones was a true general surgeon whose versatility encompassed not only abdominal surgery, but also gynecology, varicose veins, radical dissections of the neck, and some thoracic surgery. A pioneer in implanting radium and gold radon seeds into cancers, Jones mastered the techniques of surgical irradiation and was considered a leading authority on the treatment of cancer. He performed a successful local resection of a lung cancer several years before the first reported successful pneumonectomy for this disease, and he pioneered the use of electrocoagulation with implantation of radon seeds in selected low-lying rectal cancers. Although his results were excellent, he never reported them.

In 1949, Jones was 57 years old and at the peak of his career when he collapsed in the surgeons' locker room from a ruptured left ventricle. Efforts to resuscitate him failed. At the time of his death, he was the principal surgeon in the Department of General Surgery and chairman of the Division of Surgery. After Jones's sudden death, he was replaced by Robert S. Dinsmore, M.D., one of the two remaining general surgeons in the department. He held the titles of principal surgeon and chairman of the Division of Surgery until his own death in 1957. During that eight-year period, the hospital expanded. Dinsmore, wisely looking ahead, planned a 23-room operating pavilion. Many members of the staff felt that this was far too big, since antibiotics, antithyroid drugs, and radioactive iodine were rapidly drying up the source of thyroid operations. But by the time the building was finished, the operating rooms were fully used. Ten years later, after closure of the obstetrics department, six more rooms had to be opened to accommodate the growing number of cardiac cases.

Upon Dinsmore's death, Stanley O. Hoerr, M.D., was appointed chairman of the Division of Surgery, and George Crile Jr., M.D., became chairman of the

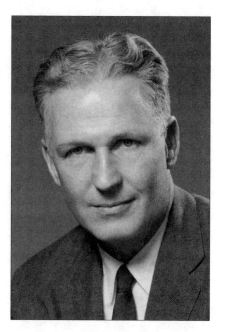

George "Barney" Crile, Jr., M.D., son of Founder Crile, General Surgeon, Co-Editor of the first edition of To Act As A Unit

Department of General Surgery. They had been colleagues in the Department of General Surgery under Dinsmore. Thus arose a unique situation in which Hoerr was Crile's chairman in the division and Crile was Hoerr's chairman in the department. The arrangement worked, undoubtedly because the men respected each other and had no cause for conflict.

James S. Krieger, M.D., succeeded Hoerr as chairman of the Division of Surgery in 1971 and served until his retirement. Bruce H. Stewart, M.D., a urologist, held the position from 1980 until his untimely death from cancer in 1983. Ralph A. Straffon, M.D., Stewart's colleague and chairman of the Department of Urology, was then appointed chairman of the Division of Surgery. When Straffon was tapped to become Chief of Staff in 1986, Joseph F. Hahn, M.D., former chairman of the Department of Neurological Surgery, took over the position. In 2003 Hahn stepped down to assume leadership of Cleveland Clinic Foundation Innovations, and Kenneth Ouriel, M.D., ascended to the division chair.

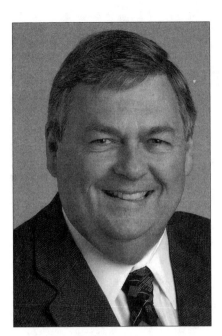

Joseph F. Hahn, M.D., Chairman,
Division of Surgery, 1987-2003

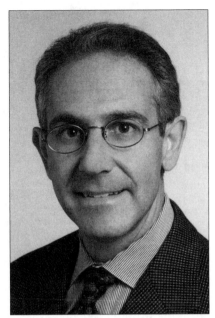

Kenneth Ouriel, M.D., Chairman,
Division of Surgery, 2003-

For more than six decades, Clinic surgeons have tried to find ways to avoid the morbidities associated with radical operations for cancer. In 1955, when the worldwide trend was towards more radical and, therefore, extensive and deforming operations, Crile, Jr., began to treat selected patients with small breast cancers by wide local excision or partial mastectomy, usually combined with axillary dissection. He abandoned radical mastectomy, setting a national trend. In 1980, Caldwell B. Esselstyn, Jr., M.D., began to combine local excision of small breast cancers with specialized radiation. The Breast Center, opened in 1995, builds on this philosophy as it provides a multidisciplinary approach to treating breast cancer.

In 1968, Crile, Jr., who had always planned to retire at age 60, resigned as head of the Department of General Surgery and became a senior consultant. Hoerr served as head for one year before following in Crile's footsteps. Robert E. Hermann, M.D., a member of the staff with a special interest in teaching, was chosen to head the department. An exuberant man and an excellent surgeon, Hermann made friends for the Clinic all over the world. The department, with six other surgeons, continued to see and treat breast disease, upper

abdominal problems, and hernias. In addition, Hermann also started a successful liver transplantation program that complemented
the department's previous experience with liver surgery, major bile
duct surgery, and portal hypertension (see chapter 15).

With the cooperation of their colleagues in the Department of
Gastroenterology, the general surgeons developed a Section of
Surgical Endoscopy.

Hermann resigned as chairman in 1989, but remained on the
active staff for five more years. After a lengthy search, Scottish-
trained liver surgeon J. Michael Henderson, M.B., Ch.B., was chosen
in 1992 to head the department as well as the Transplant Center. The
department grew to a staff of fifteen by 2002. While most staff members maintained their general surgery roots, there was a growing
emphasis on specialization, particularly in breast diseases, hepato-
biliary-pancreatic surgery, minimally invasive surgery, endocrine
surgery, and surgical endoscopy. The practice also extended to the
Clinic's Ambulatory Surgery Centers and Family Health Centers for
routine general surgery and some resident teaching.

The Breast Center opened in 1995 on the ground floor of the Crile
Building under the leadership of Dr. Joseph Crowe. This center emphasized a multidisciplinary approach to the evaluation and management
of patients, integrating radiology, medical breast specialty, oncology,
radiation therapy, and plastic surgery with the general surgery.

The department expanded hepato-biliary-pancreatic surgery. As
this specialty matured, the Clinic's higher volume and multidisciplinary approach resulted in superior outcomes. Living-related partial
adult liver transplantation became an option for some patients in 1999.

Laparoscopic and endoscopic expertise expanded significantly
through the 1990s under Dr. Jeffrey Ponsky's leadership, placing the
Clinic at the cutting edge, as it were, of innovation in these fields.
Development of education programs for residents and fellows was a
highlight of these new approaches in surgery.

Surgery of the thyroid and parathyroid glands (endocrine surgery) was an early mainstay of the surgical practice at The Cleveland
Clinic. Both of the Criles did extensive work in this area, which was
carried on by Esselstyn until his retirement in 2000. The baton was
then passed to Dr. Allan Siperstein, who had been trained in San
Francisco, and who capably assumed the responsibility of maintaining the tradition of excellence established by his predecessors.

COLORECTAL SURGERY

After Jones's death, Rupert B. Turnbull, Jr., M.D., performed most of the colon operations. Before long he became so expert in diagnosis and management that the Clinic established a Department of Colonic and Rectal Surgery in 1968 and named him chairman. Later that same year, the Board of Governors simplified the name to "Colon and Rectal Surgery." Turnbull introduced many innovations and operations that circumvented the need for permanent colostomy and reduced morbidity.

Turnbull carried an extremely large hospital service, sometimes with as many as 50 or 60 patients at various stages of preparation for or recovery from surgery. Considering the complex nature of what he was doing and the potential frequency of unexpected (mostly bad) sequelae, the pressures on him were enormous. Nonetheless, he always exuded calmness and confidence, even in the operating room, where the norm for many of his contemporaries was considerably different. With his tall stature and flowing white hair, he seemed to float serenely above the fray.

Turnbull was succeeded by Victor W. Fazio, M.B., M.S., F.R.A.C.S., under whose direction the department has developed an international reputation. They were the first to use stapled ileal pouch anastomoses, and with 150 cases per year they have the greatest experience in the world with this procedure. The pouch database exceeded 2,400 cases by the year 2001.

The department maintained its preeminence in surgery for inflammatory bowel disease and performed more operations for Crohn's disease, especially the bowel-conserving strictureplasty, than any other institution. The staff developed the world's most extensive experience with the advancement rectal flap operation for Crohn's anal and anovaginal fistulas, as well as with the stapled valve-pouch and T-pouch operation for continent ileostomy. They were the first to use the advancement pelvic pouch anal anastomosis for fistula-stricture complications and the advancement rectal sleeve operation for Crohn's anal and anovaginal fistulas. The group also devised the combination strictureplasty technique for Crohn's stricture and restorative colo-anal anastomosis for rectal Crohn's disease. In addition, they perfected many new laparoscopic bowel surgery techniques that greatly shorten hospital stay and recovery time.

Much of the department's success stems from basic research on colorectal cancer and inflammatory bowel disease. A major program for research and clinical application of laparoscopic bowel surgery began in 1992 with a $1.7 million grant awarded to Dr. Scott Strong. Endowments also funded personnel for the familial polyposis and Crohn's disease registries, ulcerative colitis research, and laboratory technicians. By 2001, research nurses and managers had oversight of twelve disease and treatment-specific databases, supervised by Feza Remzi, M.D.

Election of many of these surgeons to positions in prestigious national and international subspecialty organizations demonstrated the esteem in which their peers held them. Fazio himself served as president of the American Board of Colon and Rectal Surgery in 1992 and was president of the American Society of Colon and Rectal Surgery in 1995. Dr. Ian Lavery also served as President of the American Board of Colon and Rectal Surgery beginning in 2002. Dr. James Church, founder of the Collaborative Group of the Americas and head of the David Jagelman Registries, was honored by his colleagues through his appointment as president of the Leeds Castle Group and also the International Hereditary Non Polyposis Colorectal Cancer Group (HNPCC)—the first person to be thus doubly honored—thereby bringing together the two leading societies in this field.

The David Jagelman Registries, which contain information on patients with familial polyposis and colorectal cancer, were posthumously named for David Jagelman, M.D., a staff member who was instrumental in setting them up. When Cleveland Clinic Florida began in 1988, Jagelman was one of the original "Pioneers" there, and he started the colorectal surgery service in Ft. Lauderdale. Tragically, he died of cancer at a young age a few years later, and the registries, among the largest of their kind worldwide, were named in his memory.

Jeffrey Milsom, M.D., started the department's program in laparoscopic bowel surgery in 1990, and Anthony Senagore, M.D., brought the department to leadership in the field with the assistance of Conor Delaney, M.D. Dr. Tracy Hull did seminal work in anorectal functional disorders, especially fecal incontinence, and developed the artificial anal sphincter program. In the fall of 2000, James Wu, M.D., became the first department member to provide service at the Clinic's satellite outpatient facilities and regional hospitals.

OTOLARYNGOLOGY

In 1921, ear, nose, and throat (ENT) surgeons were preoccupied with tonsils and adenoids. The concept of chronic infection as a cause of many illnesses was gaining popularity, and the tonsils bore the brunt of the surgeon's assault. In those days before sulfanilamide and antibiotics, the treatment of mastoid infections was a great challenge. The correction of deviated nasal septa, an easier procedure, was also in vogue.

Justin M. Waugh, M.D., was the Clinic's first ENT surgeon. After his retirement, William V. Mullin, M.D., took over and did much to develop the technique of operating on the mastoid. After Mullin's untimely death from an overwhelming bacterial infection, Paul M. Moore, M.D., headed the department. He was succeeded by Harold E. Harris, M.D., a young surgeon with superb technical skill and clinical judgment.

By the 1940s, cancer of the larynx was becoming increasingly common. Pediatricians and internists were beginning to take a second look at tonsillectomy and to wonder whether the tonsils might be serving some useful function. Most importantly, an operation for otosclerosis, a disease that fused together the tiny bones of the inner ear, causing progressive deafness, was developed. When the surgeon who developed the procedure organized a course to teach other otolaryngologists how to do it, Harris was among the first to apply.

As a result of learning this new technique, he was swamped with patients. By 1955, the need for operations in which he had been trained (i.e., tonsillectomy, adenoidectomy, mastoidectomy, and correction of a deviated septum) had all but disappeared. In their place were new operations for cancers of the larynx, tongue, and mouth. Competition for the care of patients with these cancers caused conflict with the newly formed Department of Plastic Surgery. Bronchoscopic operations, historically performed by the otolaryngologists who had developed the technique, were rapidly shifting into the domain of the thoracic surgeons, who could then operate on whatever pulmonary disease was visualized. Thus, a struggle developed, and resolution of this conflict seemed insoluble without casualties.

Fortunately, the Clinic's Surgical Committee, composed of the contestants' peers, acted discreetly and with tact. They took no action on bronchoscopy, believing that there would be enough to provide training for residents in both departments. They charged a subcommittee to review the results of neck dissections in the presence of the surgeons who had done them. It soon became clear that the plastic surgeons, who had been trained to do radical surgery, performed the operations in about one-third the time and with fewer complications. Soon, the plastic surgeons and otolaryngologists were cooperating, the latter doing the laryngeal part of the operations and the former doing the neck dissections assisted by ENT residents.

After Harris' death in 1975, Harvey M. Tucker, M.D., was named chairman of the Department of Otolaryngology and Communicative Disorders. By 1985, the department had six members who were specializing in head and neck cancers, nerve reconstruction, cosmetic surgery of the face, and hearing problems. Newer diagnostic tests for dizziness and hearing loss were implemented. The addition of otolaryngologists with special expertise in head and neck cancer ensured a steady flow of patients formerly referred to plastic surgeons.

Under the chairmanship of Marshall Strome, M.D., who assumed the post in 1993, the department's residency program was lengthened one year to accommodate a full year of research. Graduates can now receive a Master of Science degree for their work during that year. Each year since the initiation of the research program, residents have won one or more of the Academy of Otolaryngology's prestigious research awards. Further, the department added a Section of Pediatric Otolaryngology and the Center for the Professional Voice, as well as Sections of Rhinologic Disorders, Medical Otolaryngology, and Regional Medical Practice.

Under Dr. Donald Lanza's direction, the Section of Rhinology, with three staff physicians, became the largest nationally and the only one with two fellowship-trained rhinologists.

New programs attracting local and national recognition included laser palatal surgery for snoring, phonosurgery for the larynx, cochlear implantation, endoscopic sinus surgery alone and in conjunction with laser surgery, and innovative techniques for managing skull base tumors.

Strome performed the first total human larynx transplant in 1998, and the patient was still doing well in 2004. Also associated with that operative procedure were human thyroid and parathyroid transplantation. Ongoing research in the otolaryngology transplantation laboratory holds the promise for frequent transplantation of all three organs.

Research flourished in all sections. Clinical studies improved the understanding of autoimmune inner ear disease. Rhinology explored the importance of the eosinophil in the genesis of chronic sinusitis and polyposis. Further, with its new basic science laboratory, otology investigated cellular involvement in noise-induced hearing loss. The Section of Vestibular Disorders piloted programs with National Aeronautics and Space Administration on the adaptation of the inner ear to the environment of space. The head and neck service investigated adoptive immunotherapy for head and neck cancer. The laryngotracheal reconstruction service developed new techniques of tracheotomy, improving the reconstruction of damaged tracheas and offering new options for patients with severe obstructive sleep apnea. In audiology, outcome studies evaluated the effects of hearing aids and hearing aid use, and, in speech and language pathology, the impact of acid reflux on the voice and the potential for induction of malignancy were under investigation.

In 2000, the Departments of Otolaryngology at Cleveland Clinic Florida in both Weston and Naples came under the directorship of the department in Cleveland. Using the very successful Cleveland regional facilities as the model, three new physicians were recruited, bringing the total staff in Florida to four. The new section flourished under the on-site section head, David Greene, M.D. Shared satellite rounds, joint courses, and frequent on-site visits by Strome strengthened both the section and the department. At present, the otolaryngology group is very successful, and it serves as a possible model for other programs.

An emerging research program is transforming this clinical department into a formidable academic center. Clinical studies have improved the understanding of autoimmune inner ear disease. The new Immunology Genetics Laboratory is carrying out clinical trials for treatment of advanced squamous cell carcinoma of the head and neck.

NEUROLOGICAL SURGERY

From the moment the Department of Neurological Surgery was founded by Charles E. Locke, Jr., M.D., in 1924, it was considered outstanding. The second chairman, W. James Gardner, M.D., enjoyed a long and brilliant career characterized by the combination of innovation with superlative skill. His contributions to the art and philosophy of neurologic surgery earned him a special place in his field. His achievements were not limited to neurosurgery and included development of the pneumatic suit to maintain blood pressure or control bleeding, the pneumatic splint for fractures, and the alternating air-pressure mattress for preventing bedsores. His associate for 30 years was Alexander T. Bunts, M.D., son of one of the four founders, who specialized in the surgery of protruded intervertebral disks and spinal cord tumors.

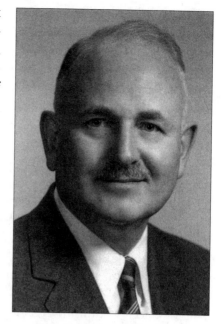

Alexander T. Bunts, M.D., son of Founder Bunts, Neurosurgeon, Co-Editor of the first edition of To Act As A Unit

Gardner was succeeded by Wallace B. Hamby, M.D., who had trained under him and then developed a national reputation in the diagnosis and treatment of brain aneurysms.

After Hamby came Donald F. Dohn, M.D., who maintained the department's reputation for leadership with his proficiency in stereotactic surgery for symptoms of Parkinson's disease, surgery to control excessive sweating, and pituitary destruction with implanted radioactive yttrium (Y^{90}). Dohn left the Clinic in 1981 to enter private practice in Mississippi, but he was coaxed out of retirement in 1988 to start the Department of Neurosurgery at Cleveland Clinic Florida.

Joseph F. Hahn, M.D., who was subsequently appointed chairman of the Division of Surgery in 1987, filled the vacancy Dohn left in Cleveland in 1981. John Little, M.D., held the post of department chairman from 1987 until he left in 1990, whereupon Hahn resumed the department chair in addition to his duties as chairman of the Division of Surgery. During Hahn's tenure, the department grew to include not only clinical neurosurgeons, but also a neurointensivist and a director of neurological research. Hahn developed basic research programs in neuro-oncology, epilepsy surgery, vascular disease, and congenital defects. Taken together with programs in the Department of Neurology, the complete epilepsy program is now ranked among the best in the country. Over the past 17 years, the department established a computer-assisted neurosurgery program, partially funded by a $10 million grant from the Department of Defense, part of a government effort to convert defense technology for civilian applications. The Clinic's program uses targeting software to pinpoint and eradicate lesions in the brain. To better exploit this and other new technologies for treating brain tumors, the department established a Neuro-Oncology Center. Two of the technologies housed in this center are the gamma knife and the Cyberknife®.

The Department of Neurological Surgery also developed the use of subdural and epidural electrodes in epilepsy surgery and the stereotactic wand for brain and spinal surgery. Both procedures are now used throughout the country.

In 1998, Dr. Marc Mayberg was appointed as chairman, succeeding Hahn. Mayberg substantially expanded the department, increasing the staff from eight to seventeen. Subspecialty and multi-specialty programs were developed in cerebrovascular and endovascular neurosurgery, functional neurosurgery, spine, epilepsy, pediatrics, and brain tumor. He developed a community neuro-surgery practice on the west side of Cleveland, serving Lakewood, Fairview, and Lutheran Hospitals. He established the Brain Tumor Institute, under the chairmanship of Dr. Gene Barnett, as an independent department in the Cancer Center.

Mayberg also grew the department's basic research programs. Due to the efforts of both basic scientists and clinician-scientists, the department obtained over $4 million annually in extramural funding to support research projects in cerebrovascular disease, neurodegenerative disorders, spine, hydrocephalus, and neuro-oncology research.

New techniques and medical devices developed and refined in the department since the mid-1990s include frameless stereotactic navigation, deep brain stimulation for movement and behavioral disorders, specialized techniques for endovascular therapy of cerebrovascular disorders, spinal fixation devices, and experimental protocols for treatment of primary brain tumors. Deep brain stimulation is an exciting new intervention in the emerging field of functional neurosurgery. At The Cleveland Clinic, Dr. Ali Rezai, a young staff member, leads this effort and is developing one of the most advanced programs in deep brain stimulation in this country.

ORTHOPEDIC SURGERY

Orthopedic surgery was introduced as a specialty at the Clinic in 1922 by James A. Dickson, M.D., a surgeon of great originality and international repute. Before it became common practice to insert metal hip joints, Dickson had perfected an elegant operation called geometric osteotomy, in which an unhealed fracture of the hip was rotated to promote healing. During his tenure, which lasted until 1954 when he was succeeded by James I. Kendrick, M.D., he witnessed the decline and fall of osteomyelitis as a major orthopedic problem and the development of artificial joints and operations to correct arthritis.

In 1951, George Phalen, M.D., identified carpal tunnel syndrome, a painful disorder that afflicts workers who use repetitive hand and wrist movement. Phalen also developed a test for diagnosing the syndrome, thus enabling its treatment and contributing greatly to the science of occupational health.

Charles M. Evarts, M.D., replaced Kendrick as department chairman in 1970. He was one of the first proponents of internal fixation, the process of holding vertebrae in place by a metal prosthesis. His pioneering work in scoliosis surgery has developed into what is today a broad-based and highly respected spine surgery program. The Clinic pioneered techniques of endoscopic spine surgery as well as the treatment of neoplasms of the spine. During this time, the Clinic took a notable role in the beginning of total joint replacement. In 1970, Evarts performed the first total hip replacement using a metal-on-plastic design. The Clinic received one of the first FDA licenses to use the new methyl methacrylate bone cement.

Another example of the innovativeness of Clinic orthopedists was Dr. Lester Borden's development of instrumentation allowing total hips and total knees to be successfully and precisely implanted by private practitioners. Dr. Borden, a prodigious teacher of joint replacement techniques, also pioneered the development of porous in-growth total hip replacement. This method uses a metal prosthesis with an irregular surface that allows the bone to grow into it and secure it more firmly.

Sports medicine was introduced to the department by H. Royer Collins, M.D., who succeeded Evarts as chairman. Over the years, sports medicine increased in importance and visibility, reaching its peak under the direction of John A. Bergfeld, M.D., who joined the staff in 1973. Bergfeld not only developed techniques of surgery for the treatment of sports injuries, but also developed an organization of medical coverage that helped prevent sports injuries. His ideas on the integration of orthopedic surgeons, sports medical specialists, and on-site athletic trainers have been a model for the rest of the country. Emphasizing conditioning to prevent injury, the Clinic was one of the first centers to make the sports physiologists an integral member of the sports medicine team. Highly respected by athletes and trainers, Bergfeld has fostered many key relationships between the Clinic and major sports teams, including the Cleveland Browns and the U.S. Olympic Ski Team.

Alan H. Wilde, M.D., a surgeon noted for joint replacements, took over the department in 1976 and served with distinction for 15 years.

Since the mid-1980s, the department has added a Foot and Ankle Center, an Upper Extremity Center, and a traumatology program. Musculoskeletal researchers, first housed in the department's biomechanics and biomaterials programs started by Evarts, later merged into the Department of Biomedical Engineering in the Research Institute, collaborate with the orthopedic surgery staff in studies of musculoskeletal biology, gait analysis, neuromuscular control, biomechanics, biomaterials, and image processing. Technology transfer is one of the department's priorities.

A number of new techniques and technologies have been developed in part or wholly at the Clinic. One example is the non-cemented joint prosthesis, which allows bone to grow into pores in the metal surfaces for better fixation. The sports medicine surgeons have led the way in developing techniques for reconstructing knee ligaments. This allows a common but complex operation to be done mostly through an arthroscope, which translates into a shorter hospital stay and quicker recovery.

In 1991, Dr. Kenneth Marks, an orthopedic oncologist and

department member since 1975, succeeded Wilde as department chairman. Under Marks's leadership, the department rose in national rankings and was the first specialty department to expand into the Clinic's Family Health Centers. Ultimately, the family health center offices effectively tripled the department's size.

Prior to 1975, the standard dictum in orthopedics was to amputate sarcomatous limbs. But Marks had been a resident of George "Barney" Crile, M.D., and was impressed with his results with tissue-sparing breast surgery. Inspired, he introduced the same principles to orthopedic oncology. Today, only five percent of cancerous limbs require amputation.

The department's Section of Musculoskeletal Oncology has developed methods for reconstructing the skeleton and soft tissues after massive limb-sparing cancer surgery. These include a new method for the functional attachment of bone or soft tissue to the metal endoprosthetic devices used to reconstruct hips and knees after tumor resection. Fresh and frozen allografts are used often in reconstruction after tumor resection, trauma, and surgery for arthritis, and a new device allows for congenital defects to be gradually reconstructed with vascularized bone segments. A new system for harvesting human osteoblastic progenitor cells by aspiration has played a critical role in the healing of fractures, the incorporation of bone grafts, and maintenance of the skeleton throughout life.

The cerebral palsy clinic helps maximize the function of children with neuromuscular disorders. A Rheumatology/Orthopaedics Clinic improves the care of patients with rheumatoid arthritis, and a Foot and Ankle Clinic aids patients with a broad spectrum of conditions, including those related to diabetes. A geriatric orthopedic program helps patients stay mobile and independent as long as possible. Care for nonsurgical orthopedic conditions of all kinds is provided by the addition of three family practitioners with special training in musculoskeletal disease.

Orthopedic surgery at the Clinic entered a new era of dynamic research and expanded academics with the appointment of chairman Joseph P. Iannotti, M.D., Ph.D., in 2000. The department, which is regularly cited among the nation's top ten by *U.S. News & World Report*, continues to have a single goal: to improve the care of patients with musculoskeletal disorders. At the beginning of the new century, the Department of Orthopaedic[1] Surgery had a growing clinical staff of fifty full-time physicians and surgeons, representing nine general and subspecialty areas of orthopedics. They managed more than 200,000 outpatient clinic visits and performed more than 9,000 surgical procedures annually at the main campus and at nine family health centers.

Iannotti established a Center for Orthopaedic Research, the cornerstone of a restructured and expanded investigative arm. With two major components—musculoskeletal research and clinical outcomes—the center promotes collaboration between clinicians and basic scientists in areas of common interest. Of special interest were bridge programs designed to bring bench research to the bedside. Teams of investigators included surgeons, molecular biologists, bioengineers, and biostatisticians. Recognizing the growing importance of basic research, the orthopedic residency was lengthened from five to six years. All incoming orthopedic residents spend one year performing basic science research. In addition, the curriculum for all residents, fellows, and graduate students now includes an extensive basic science study, emphasizing the principles of the musculoskeletal system and orthopedic surgery.

UROLOGY AND THE GLICKMAN INSTITUTE

During The Cleveland Clinic's existence, scientific developments have transformed urology from a service concentrating on medical treatments and minor surgery to a major surgical specialty. At first, urologists were primarily occupied with treating gonorrhea and performing suprapubic prostatectomies. Then came transurethral resection of the prostate and of bladder tumors. William J. Engel, M.D., Lower's son-in-law, was a master of the transurethral resectoscope. Charles C. Higgins, M.D., who succeeded Lower as head of the Department of Urology in 1948, became renowned for his "acid ash diet," an effective way of preventing, and sometimes dissolving, kidney stones. He also pioneered an operation to transplant the ureter into the lower bowel of children with exstrophy of the bladder. He operated on more of these patients than anyone else in the world, and also had one of the world's largest series of cystectomies for bladder cancer.

In 1934, a Cleveland pathologist (Harry Goldblatt, M.D., of

Western Reserve University) discovered that partial blockage of a renal artery was one cause of hypertension. Acting on this information, Clinic urologist Eugene F. Poutasse, M.D., developed renal arteriography. He discovered that removing the obstruction, grafting a new vessel, or removing the part of the kidney that the diseased artery supplied could correct renal hypertension in many such patients.

After Higgins and Engel retired, Ralph A. Straffon, M.D., became chairman of the department. Straffon was destined for surgical stardom. An All-Star football player during his days at the University of Michigan, he had both the intellectual firepower and the physical stamina to excel in whatever task he set for himself. His achievements were recognized nationally in 1993 by his election to the presidency of the American College of Surgeons, the most prestigious post to which a surgeon can professionally aspire, and one once held by the senior Crile. Collaborating with Willem J. Kolff, M.D., Ph.D., inventor of the artificial kidney and head of the newly formed Department of Artificial Organs, Straffon initiated a kidney transplant program. Within a few years, the Clinic reported more successful transplantations of kidneys taken from cadaver donors than had ever been done elsewhere. Today, the Clinic's renal transplant program remains one of the largest and most successful in the world (see chapter 15); it is supported by a large dialysis program and regional tissue-typing laboratory.

By 1983, the Department of Urology had begun the process of subspecialization. That year, Straffon relinquished his chairmanship to assume the chair of the Division of Surgery, and James E. Montie, M.D., took over. A highly regarded urologic oncologist dedicated to his patients, Montie served only 18 months before deciding that the demands of the position took too much time away from patient care. He returned to his position as a staff urologist, and Andrew C. Novick, M.D., was appointed as department chairman.

Novick had become a national figure in urology through pioneering contributions in kidney disease and reconstructive renal surgery. He developed the technique of extracorporeal or "bench" kidney surgery for repairing complex kidney disorders outside the body and then transplanting the repaired kidney back into the patient. His work on atherosclerotic renal artery disease was the first to demonstrate that this condition was a major cause of kidney failure in older patients and could be successfully treated with surgical renal arterial reconstruction. He pioneered the technique of partial nephrectomy or nephron-sparing surgery for patients with kidney cancer, and he accumulated the largest experience in the world with this approach. Interestingly, much of Novick's work represented an extension of the concept of "conservative kidney surgery" first espoused by Lower.

Under Novick's leadership, the department evolved into one of the largest and most subspecialized programs of its kind in the country, with tertiary care expertise in every urologic subspecialty: female urology, urodynamics, endourology, stone disease, impotence, prostatic surgery, urologic oncology, renal vascular disease, renal transplantation, adrenal disease, male infertility, reconstructive surgery, pediatric urology, and laparoscopic and minimally invasive surgery. Seven basic research laboratories, staffed by full-time urologic scientists, were developed to perform translational investigations in these areas. The urology residency training program was expanded to include an additional year of laboratory research. Several urology staff members gained recognition for their work and were elected to leadership positions in national and international organizations. Novick served as President of the American Board of Urology in 2000 and Chairman of the National Urology Residency Review Committee in 2001-2002.

In August 2000, the institution recognized the excellence of the department's activities by announcing to the trustees that it would henceforth be known as the Cleveland Clinic Urological Institute. In December of that year it was again renamed, this time as the Glickman Urological Institute.

OBSTETRICS AND GYNECOLOGY

James S. Krieger, M.D., introduced gynecology as a specialty at The Cleveland Clinic in 1950. He arrived about the time that the Papanicolaou (Pap) smear became popular. Krieger was interested in the conservative treatment of in situ carcinoma of the cervix by conization. While gynecologists across the country were debating whether the condition should be treated by radical or conservative hysterectomy with or without radiation, Krieger collected data showing that simple conization could be as effective as the more complex procedures if the physician followed the patients with annual Pap tests. At first bitterly criticized, the concept gradually gained broad support.

After Krieger's retirement in 1974, Lester A. Ballard Jr., M.D., assumed the chairmanship. He increased the staff to seven physicians, who covered the areas of general gynecology, gynecologic oncology, child and adolescent gynecology, and microsurgery. He also started a program in assisted reproductive technologies. This program includes both cryopreservation of embryos for later reimplantation as well as routine in-vitro fertilization. In addition, the newest micromanipulation technique of sperm injection into the cytoplasm of the egg has enabled many previously barren couples to achieve pregnancy.

As a natural extension of this program, the Clinic reestablished the obstetrical service under the leadership of Dr. Elliot H. Philipson in 1995 after a 29-year hiatus. The new obstetrics unit was located on the sixth floor of the original hospital building, just around the corner from the old obstetrics ward. The old delivery suite, which had served as an operating pavilion for cardiovascular surgery, then orthopedics, and finally ambulatory surgery, had come full circle with its reconversion to the original use.

Lack of options to treat a large number of patients with defects in the pelvic floor resulted in the establishment of a Center for Pelvic Support. This center unites the efforts of Clinic gynecologists, colorectal surgeons, urologists, and physical therapists to give better care for these difficult problems.

Although the Department of Gynecology always had a strong clinical focus, it began to develop major commitments to research and education in the 1990s with the arrival of a new chairman, Jerome L. Belinson, M.D. The department formed an organized research effort with numerous funded projects in reproductive endocrinology, gynecologic oncology, and general gynecology.

During Belinson's chairmanship, the department expanded rapidly to include all subspecialty clinical services of obstetrics and gynecology. These included maternal-fetal medicine, general obstetrics, midwifery services, reproductive genetics, pediatric and adolescent gynecology, reproductive endocrinology and infertility, general gynecology, gynecologic oncology, and pelvic reconstructive surgery. Minimally invasive surgery procedures expanded rapidly to encompass all the different gynecologic surgical areas. The research effort was expanded to include a basic science laboratory in collaboration with the Urological Institute. This Center for Advanced Research in Human Reproduction, Infertility, and Sexual Function is the laboratory infrastructure for the Obstetrics and Gynecology research program.

After ten years as chairman, Belinson stepped down to focus his practice and research in gynecologic oncology, having a specific interest in cancer prevention in developing countries. Dr. Tommaso Falcone became chairman in 2001 after serving as head of the Section of Reproductive Endocrinology. Falcone and his team at The Cleveland Clinic were the first to conduct a patient trial using robotic laparoscopic surgery. The report is now part of the permanent research collection at the Smithsonian Institution. The department is continuing its objective in outstanding clinical care. The name of the department was changed to "Obstetrics and Gynecology" in 2001 to reflect the growing importance of obstetrical services within the department. A new Women's Health Center opened in 2001 with strong participation from this department. A new Maternal-Fetal Unit also opened in 2002 in collaboration with the Neonatal Intensive Care Unit.

PLASTIC SURGERY

With formal training programs established just before World War II, plastic surgery is one of the youngest surgical specialties. Soldiers wounded in World War I, who had recovered with serious deformities, challenged surgeons in the 1920s and 1930s to develop expertise in repair and reconstruction. These surgeons had a variety of surgical backgrounds, and so the emerging specialty was a hybrid.

Robin Anderson, M.D., was a general surgeon trained in St. Louis by some of the great American pioneers of plastic surgery. Anderson's technical prowess was not limited to the operating room. Like many noted physicians, he had a profound interest in music. He expressed this by building fine harpsichords in his spare time, many of which are still in existence. When Hoerr felt the need to develop plastic surgery at the Clinic, he extended an invitation to Anderson, whom he had known for several years. Anderson joined the Department of General Surgery in 1951. By 1960, a second plastic surgeon had been added, and the department was separated from general surgery with Anderson as chairman.

When Anderson retired in 1979, Melvyn I. Dinner, M.D., succeeded him. A move into more spacious facilities was followed by rapid growth. Dinner recognized the importance of developing subspecialties within plastic surgery and encouraged the development of expertise in craniofacial, pediatric, hand, and microvascular techniques.

When Dinner left the Clinic in 1983 to enter private practice, Shattuck W. Hartwell, Jr., M.D., a long-time member of the department and director of the Office of Professional Staff Affairs, was asked to serve as acting chairman while a search committee looked for a new permanent chairman. Earl Z. Browne, M.D., was appointed in 1985. James E. Zins, M.D., who had been on the staff for the previous nine years, succeeded him. Zins is the department's current chairman. In the ensuing ten years, Zins doubled the size of the plastic surgery staff, adding specialists in aesthetic surgery, and hand surgery, as well as in pediatric, craniofacial, breast, and plastic surgery research.

DENTISTRY

In 1982, a Section of Dentistry and Maxillofacial Prosthetics was established within the Department of Plastic Surgery to provide support for the treatment and rehabilitation of patients with head and neck cancer as well as deformities of the jaw, face, and skull. Salvatore J. Esposito, D.M.D., was recruited to head the section, which included prosthodontists, an oral and maxillofacial surgeon, and a general dentist. Dentistry had existed as a department, led by Dr. Charles Resch, from 1934 until his retirement in 1966. Between 1966 and 1982, consultants provided dental care at the Clinic.

By 1991, the section had regained departmental status, with Esposito as chairman. Under his direction, the department has grown from four to eleven staff members. To support their multidisciplinary approach to patient care, Sections of Maxillofacial Prosthetics, Oral and Maxillofacial Surgery, Oral Medicine, Cosmetic and Implant Dentistry, Dental Oncology, Orthodontics, and Sports Dentistry were established. It became one of the larger hospital programs in the United States.

The department's residency and fellowship positions are highly sought after. It was the first in Ohio to offer a dental oncology fellowship, which, funded by the American Cancer Society, is one of only five in the country. The department's general practice residency, initially funded by the NIH, is now considered one of the finest in the United States. Among the new techniques residents learn are dental implantation, craniofacial implantation, and the carbon dioxide laser for removing intra-oral soft tissue lesions and gingival hyperplasia.

Research activities in the Department have addressed dental implants, periodontal factors in heart disease, effects of mouth guards for athletes, speech prostheses for the patient with neuromuscular compromise, and quality of life for the head and neck cancer patient.

VASCULAR SURGERY

The Department of Vascular Surgery began in 1957, and it was one of the earliest of its kind in the country. In 1952, Crile, Jr., had visited St. Mary's Hospital in London, where he saw the world's first homograft (allograft) artery bank. Impressed with the success of replacing a blocked artery with a patent one from a cadaver, he decided this procedure should be brought to the Clinic. Upon his return, he persuaded Dinsmore to select a surgeon to learn this technique. Since the vessels in the lower extremity would be the main ones grafted, they chose Alfred W. Humphries, M.D., a junior member of the Department of Orthopaedic Surgery. They felt he had the skill, stamina, knowledge of the anatomy, and (perhaps most importantly) would be able to amputate the leg if the graft failed. Fortunately, Humphries proved to be an innovative technician with a keen intellect, and he made bold progress in a new field that was virtually uncharted in the 1950s.

Crile, Jr., was not alone in his interest in establishing this service at The Cleveland Clinic. Victor G. deWolfe, M.D., former chairman of the Department of Vascular Medicine, writes:

> "Early in 1952, I made a visit to Dr. Robert S. Dinsmore, the Chief of the Department of Surgery, and explained to him that, just as heart and kidney surgery were rapidly advancing, so was

the new specialty of vascular surgery, and we should get into the act. Shortly after this, Dr. Barney Crile returned from England with news about Dr. Charles Rob's artery bank and his early work in replacing vessels with freeze-dried arteries. He urged Dr. Dinsmore to take action . . . .

"Due to Barney's enthusiasm, Dr. Dinsmore wasted no more time in solving this dilemma. He came to a very logical solution. On the staff at that time was a young orthopedic surgeon, Alfred Humphries . . . . Initially he would do vascular work in the extremities. Ausey Robnett was a young general surgeon, newly appointed to the staff, who had an interest in abdominal surgery and proved himself to be skillful in that area, and he would work in the belly. These two young surgeons would operate together and each would teach the other about his area of expertise . . . .

"Humphries did his first operation in 1952, when he successfully treated a popliteal aneurysm and replaced it with a section of the patient's saphenous vein. By 1957, 280 patients had been operated on with a 90% success rate in the larger arteries and 80% in the arteries below the groin . . . .

"The department, created from spare parts, has continued the well-established tradition of careful selection, meticulous technology, and outstanding results."

Within a year, Humphries was working full time at vascular surgery, and his knowledge about all types of arterial reconstructions and their complications had become widely recognized. He was the first surgeon in the area with an artery bank. He then promoted the use of plastic grafts, and through the years had great success treating all types of aneurysms. With the assistance of anesthesiologist John Homi, M.D., he devised a technique to increase blood flow to the brain by having patients inhale carbon dioxide, thus enabling operations on their carotid arteries, which previously had often led to brain damage from anoxia.

In 1961, he added a second member to his staff, Edwin G. Beven, M.D., whose surgical skill as a resident was legendary. Beven succeeded Humphries as chairman in 1973. His first staff appointee, Norman R. Hertzer, M.D., was another Clinic graduate who would eventually succeed him as chairman in 1989. Hertzer is a former

President of the Society for Vascular Surgery and also former Associate Editor for the *Journal of Vascular Surgery*.

In 1998, Dr. Kenneth Ouriel was recruited from the University of Rochester to succeed Hertzer as chairman of the department. Ouriel had a long interest in the minimally invasive treatment of vascular disease. His work has examined the use of thrombolytic therapy to treat intra-arterial clots, as well as the minimally invasive treatment of aortic aneurysms with endovascular grafts. Ouriel was the lead author on a landmark multicenter trial comparing thrombolytic therapy to surgery for treatment of acute lower extremity occlusion.

The vascular surgical staff now numbers fourteen surgeons. The department is the largest of its kind and maintains the largest vascular surgical fellowship in the United States. The staff performs the greatest number of aortic endograft procedures of any center in the world and performs almost 4,000 total vascular surgical procedures annually with morbidity and mortality rates that rival those of any other center in the country. The department is active in basic and clinical research, maintaining laboratories within the Lerner Research Institute as well as a clinical research staff that includes nurses, technologists, and a biostatistician. The department has recently added a second operative angiography suite to further its focus of minimally invasive treatment for vascular disease processes.

THORACIC AND CARDIOVASCULAR SURGERY

The growth of cardiac surgery has been one of the most dramatic developments in the history of the Clinic. In 1948, Donald B. Effler, M.D., was appointed head of the Department of Thoracic Surgery. At that time, lung cancers were still rare, and thoracic surgeons were mainly occupied with draining empyemas and lung abscesses and performing thoracoplasties for tuberculosis. With the findings that penicillin was effective in controlling pneumonia and streptomycin reduced the need for thoracoplasties, surgery for these diseases all but vanished. However, the rising incidence of lung cancer, first treated by total pneumonectomy in 1932, soon filled the gap. Then came the pioneering work of surgeons in Boston and California on congenital heart disease and mitral stenosis, and the specialty of cardiac surgery was born. The California surgeon was John Jones, M.D., brother of the Clinic's Chief of Surgery Thomas Jones.

The Clinic's thoracic surgeons were poised to participate in heart surgery. They found that some cardiac defects could be corrected or improved by relatively simple operations, but others required a machine to maintain circulation during surgery. Such machines existed, but they were large and cumbersome. Clinic staff member Willem J. Kolff, M.D., Ph.D., constructed a membrane oxygenator that permitted open heart surgery to be performed on children, who do not have a large volume of blood. Once heart-lung machines were improved, the number of relatively safe operations increased, but other problems remained. Kolff had done animal experiments in which he temporarily stopped the heart's action by injecting a solution of potassium into the coronary arteries. This technique was adapted for clinical use, and open heart surgery became a reality. Congenital and rheumatic valve defects were soon successfully corrected, and prosthetic valves were inserted into the heart.

As soon as Clinic cardiologist F. Mason Sones, Jr., M.D., used his new angiography technique to demonstrate that an internal mammary artery implanted in the heart muscle could form connections with coronary arteries, there was great demand for this operation. Occasionally, a narrowed portion of a coronary artery was excised and a vein inserted, or the narrowed area was slit lengthwise and a tapered gusset inserted to widen the narrowed portion. Both procedures resulted in increased blood flow through the coronary arteries.

In May 1967, Clinic staff surgeon René G. Favaloro, M.D., born and educated in Argentina, began using sections of saphenous veins to bypass coronary artery obstructions. Although isolated attempts at coronary bypass surgery had been attempted previously, Favaloro saw this strategy as a planned, consistent approach to the treatment of large numbers of patients with coronary artery disease, and his colleagues in cardiology and cardiothoracic surgery agreed. The effectiveness of bypass surgery in relieving angina was soon obvious, and coronary bypass grafting rapidly became one of the most common operations performed in the United States. Bypass surgery, an anatomic treatment for coronary artery disease, set the stage for many types of invasive treatments of cardiovascular disease and remains a major contribution to progress in the treatment of cardiovascular disease. The operative mortality associated with these bypass operations was low, and, since 1971, the Clinic's overall

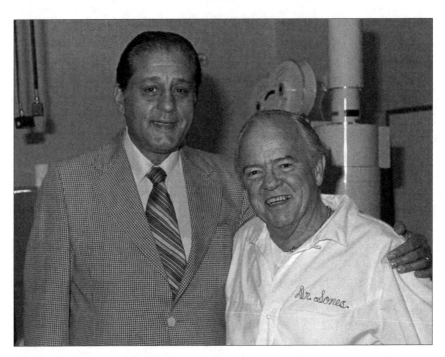

Drs. René G. Favaloro and F. Mason Sones, Jr. (photographed in 1982)

operative mortality rate for non-emergency coronary artery bypass surgery without valvular disease or other serious complications has been less than one percent.

Favaloro returned to his homeland in 1971, where he remained an internationally acclaimed surgical leader until his death in July 2000. Effler retired to a more relaxed practice in 1975 and was succeeded by Floyd D. Loop, M.D. Loop's contributions included development of arterial grafting, improvement of the techniques involved in reoperation, extensive follow-up studies on bypass patients, and approaches to control the cost of hospitalization for cardiac surgery. His confirmation of the superiority of the internal thoracic artery as a bypass graft to the left anterior descending coronary artery was a major advance, and the department has continued to lead the field of cardiovascular surgery in the use of arterial grafting to treat coronary artery obstructions. Clinic surgeons have continued to play important roles in the progress of the field of coronary bypass surgery, including the development of techniques for coronary reoperations and surgery performed without cardiopulmonary bypass. Drs. Joseph Sabik, Gösta Pettersson, and Bruce Lytle have become recognized authorities in these areas.

In addition to bypass surgery, Clinic surgeons have led the world in valve repair and replacement. Delos M. Cosgrove III, M.D., developed techniques to repair the mitral valve in the mid-1980s. He subsequently introduced a mitral valve retractor and annuloplasty ring that afford a more effective repair. With the assistance of intraoperative Doppler echocardiography, the mortality rate of operations for mitral valve repair has been extremely low, and the long-term success has been excellent. The large number of patients with valvular heart disease treated at The Cleveland Clinic has yielded a large experience with a variety of valve procedures, and Clinic surgeons have become expert in the use of homografts (human valve transplants), minimally invasive valve surgery, and aortic valve repair.

Cleveland Clinic surgeons have also become known for the repair

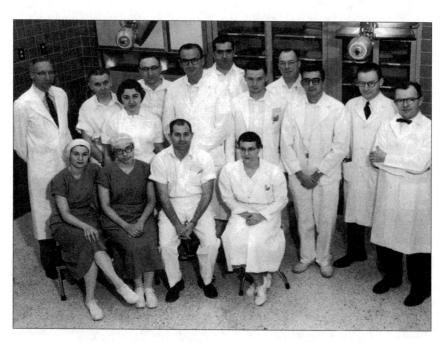

Leaders in the treatment of coronary artery disease. Standing: Willem J. Kolff, M.D., Ph.D., Artificial Organs (far left); Donald B. Effler, M.D., Thoracic and Cardiovascular Surgery (5th from left); Laurence K. Groves, MD., Thoracic and Cardiovascular Surgery (6th from left); Donald E. Hale, M.D., Anesthesiology (4th from right); F. Mason Sones, Jr., M.D., Cardiology (far right) (photographed in 1956)

of thoracic great-vessel aneurysms and aortic dissections. In collaboration with the cardiac perfusionists, Bruce W. Lytle, M.D., introduced and refined a technique that extends the safe interval of total circulatory arrest necessary to perform these complex surgeries without neurological complications. To aid in the continued expansion of techniques for aortic surgery, the department in 2001 recruited Dr. Lars Svensson, a major contributor in the development of this field.

The coalescence of multiple surgical techniques and approaches for the treatment of valvular, coronary, and aortic disease has allowed the Clinic surgeons to treat patients with complicated situations involving combined cardiac diseases, including reoperations. No single breakthrough is responsible for the success in this field, but it results from a combination of improved techniques in anesthesia, perfusion, blood conservation and transfusion, myocardial protection, cerebral protection, and, most of all, the large experience of the surgeons and anesthesiologists involved.

Although surgery for congenital heart disease was performed early in the department's history, the treatment of acquired heart disease demanded the most attention. Progress in the study and correction of cardiac defects accelerated following the appointment of Carl C. Gill, M.D., a congenital heart surgeon, to the staff in 1978. Gill later became Chief Executive Officer of Cleveland Clinic Florida and Chairman of the Department of Cardiothoracic Surgery there. Under the direction of the current head of The Cleveland Clinic's congenital heart program, internationally renowned and legendary Australian surgeon Roger B. Mee, M.B., Ch.B., this program has become one of the largest and most successful in the country.

In the late 1960s, Clinic cardiac surgeons performed two successful heart transplants. But it was not until 1984 that consistent transplantation activity was launched. Initially directed by Robert W. Stewart, M.D., by the mid-1990s the transplantation team was performing more than sixty heart transplants a year, making it one of the top four programs in the country (see chapter 15).

In 1997, The Cleveland Clinic established the Kaufmann Heart Failure Center, with surgeon Patrick M. McCarthy, M.D., and cardiologist James Young, M.D., as co-directors. The heart failure concept brings together multiple medical and surgical treatments for heart failure, including transplantation, in one area. Additional options offered include left ventricular remodeling, mitral valve repair, revascularization for patients with ischemic cardiomyopathies, and the use of mechanical-assist devices. Also participating in this heart failure team are surgeons Nicholas Smedira, Michael Banbury, and José Navia.

In December 1991, the Clinic joined a multicenter group using the HeartMate implantable left ventricular assist device (LVAD) as a bridge to transplantation. Patients who were candidates for a heart transplant, but who were not expected to survive the wait for a donor, received the LVAD. Despite the fact that all were in cardiogenic shock and many were moribund, 75% recovered and subsequently underwent transplantation. The Clinic's program quickly became the most active in the United States and obtained some of the best clinical results.

In 1993, The Cleveland Clinic was one of three centers selected by the National Institutes of Health to continue research towards an electrically powered total artificial heart. This device will be used on patients who are not candidates for an LVAD, and will initially be used as a bridge to transplantation. Both the HeartMate® and total artificial heart are designed to serve as an alternative to heart transplantation as well as therapy for patients with end-stage heart disease.

In 1986, the Board of Governors established a formal Section of Thoracic Surgery under the leadership of Thomas W. Rice, M.D. This section has recorded significant achievements, including the first lung transplant in Ohio and, since then, approximately 176 single and 101 double transplants. The lung transplant program is currently under the direction of Malcolm DeCamp, M.D. In addition, pioneering work in video-assisted, thoracoscopic lobectomies and the use of ultrasound to further the clinical staging of esophageal cancers has improved results, and with the input of Drs. Rice, DeCamp, and Sudish Murthy, the volume of the Section of Thoracic Surgery has grown to almost 1,300 cases per year.

The department's extensive surgical activity has provided a fertile resource for its computerized cardiovascular information data bank (Cardiovascular Information Registry [CVIR]). Established in 1971, it is the oldest and one of the country's largest. The data, entered on every patient, have helped the surgeons to track the results of the procedures they perform. In 1986, the CVIR was instrumental in confirming the long-term benefits of the internal thoracic artery bypass graft, thus influencing the choice of grafts for future patients.

In 1989, Loop became chairman of the Board of Governors and Chief Executive Officer. Paul C. Taylor, M.D., then served as acting chairman of the Department of Thoracic and Cardiovascular Surgery until Delos M. Cosgrove III, M.D., was selected as chairman the following year. Under Cosgrove's direction, The Cleveland Clinic has become the largest open-heart surgery center in the United States, also performing the largest number of valve operations. In addition to caring for several thousand patients a year and conducting extensive research, members of the Department of Thoracic and Cardiovascular Surgery have tackled the challenges of a more efficient and cost-effective surgical practice. Despite the facts that 48 percent of the patients are over age 65, that 30 percent undergo reoperations, and that the majority of cases are complex, the department has reduced overall length of stay by admitting stable patients to the hospital on the day of surgery and discharging many earlier than is traditional. A total quality management program ensures consistency in the quality of care. For this reason, The Cleveland Clinic is proud to have been the first hospital in the country to voluntarily release outcomes data and mortality statistics to the public. The first of the Cleveland Clinic's award-winning *How to Choose a Doctor and Hospital* series dealt with coronary artery surgery. In these brochures, various Clinic services are evaluated according to six quality indicators (credentials, experience, range of services, research and education, patient satisfaction, and outcomes) showing Clinic data vs. national benchmarks.

CONCLUSION

An overview of the Division of Surgery shows that Clinic surgeons have been both innovative themselves and quick to exploit the best ideas of others. Moreover, some have shown how medical or office treatment could replace an operation previously considered necessary. This ability to think of surgery as only one way of treating the patient is encouraged by the fact that there is no incentive for Clinic surgeons to perform a large number of operations; their salaries depend more on their peers' estimation of the quality of their work than on the dollars received as a result of it. It has been helpful, too, to have the cooperation of skilled colleagues who spend their time in research as well as readily available, high-quality support from medical services. The tradition of innovation started so many years ago by Bunts, Lower, Crile, and Phillips has flourished in an environment well suited to the study of clinical problems and to the discovery of their solutions in the operating room, clinic, and laboratory.

---

[1] The department affects the British spelling, with an "a" in its official name, but American usage eschews the "a"; hence the inconsistency of spelling of orthop(a)edics in this section and elsewhere.

14. DIVISION OF ANESTHESIOLOGY AND CRITICAL CARE MEDICINE

BY FAWZY G. ESTAFANOUS AND JOHN TETZLAFF

*We are more sensible of
one little touch of a surgeon's
lancet than of twenty wounds
with a sword in the heat of fight.*
—Montaigne, 1588

THE BEGINNINGS OF ANESTHESIA HAD A DISTINGUISHED PLACE AT THE Cleveland Clinic. Around 1910, one of the four founders, Dr. George Crile, coined the term "anoci-association," later shortened to "anociation," which denoted the removal of pain and defined the role of anesthesia in safety and survival of patients undergoing surgery. Crile created the expression anoci-association to explain why the prevention of the perception of pain was an essential element to the practice of surgery, placing the importance on the preoperative preparation of the patient.

From 1921 to 1946, the administration of anesthesia at The Cleveland Clinic was handled by three or four nurses, who dropped ether onto gauze laid over the patient's airway or used chloroform to "put them under." This was done at the direction and under the supervision of the staff surgeon. Physicians did not begin to specialize in anesthesiology until just before World War II.

THE HALE YEARS, 1946-1967

Following the war, the Clinic established a Department of Anesthesiology in the Division of Surgery. Donald E. Hale, M.D., was appointed chairman in January 1946. Fully trained in surgery at the Mayo Clinic, Hale obtained board certification in both surgery and anesthesiology and later published an important textbook on anesthesia (Hale, Donald E., ed. *Anesthesia, by Forty American Authors*, Philadelphia: Davis, 1954). In this work, Hale wrote: "The anesthesiologist must have a thorough knowledge of the various surgical needs which he must meet. He must be a diagnostician and therapist; his diagnosis must often be instantaneous and must be followed by immediate and accurate therapy. To give anesthesia is not difficult; but to give safe anesthesia is." Among his numerous innovations while at The Cleveland Clinic were the first ventilator used in the state of Ohio and the first EKG machine that could be used in the operating room to support the developing area of open-heart surgery.

THE WASMUTH YEARS, 1967-1969

To complement his efforts to establish physician anesthesia at the Foundation, Hale initiated a residency program in anesthesiology in 1946. One of his early trainees (1949) was Carl E. Wasmuth, M.D., who replaced him as chairman in 1967, but served only two years before being elected chairman of the Board of Governors. Wasmuth also served as president of the American Society of Anesthesiologists (1968-9).

THE POTTER-VILJOEN YEARS, 1970-1977

J. Kenneth Potter, M.D, filled Wasmuth's vacancy in the Department of Anesthesiology. Under Potter's chairmanship, anesthesiology achieved divisional status at The Cleveland Clinic. John F. Viljoen, M.D., a specialist in the care of patients undergoing surgery for heart disease, succeeded Potter. Viljoen was one of the founders of the Association of Cardiac Anesthesiologists, an elite group of 50 physicians. When Viljoen stepped down in 1976, Potter was called out of retirement to lead the division until a replacement could be found.

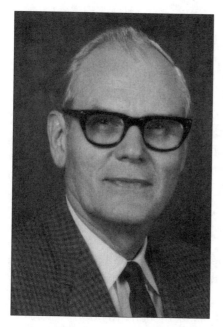

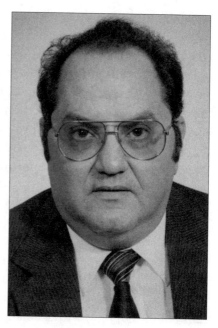

J. Kenneth Potter, M.D., Chairman,
Division of Anesthesiology,
1970-1973

Fawzy G. Estafanous, M.D., Chairman,
Division of Anesthesiology and
Critical Care Medicine, 1987-

THE BOUTROS YEARS, 1977-1986

The Board of Governors appointed a search committee that recommended Azmy R. Boutros, M.D., a professor of anesthesiology at the University of Iowa, who accepted the position and assumed the chair in May 1977. Boutros subsequently reorganized the division and added staff to accommodate increasing clinical and educational responsibilities. He had a special interest in critical care and functioned as its director. In addition, he reestablished the anesthesiology residency program.

THE ESTAFANOUS YEARS, 1986-

Fawzy G. Estafanous, M.D., who came to The Cleveland Clinic in 1970 and became chairman of the Department of Cardiothoracic Anesthesiology in 1977, was appointed chairman of the Division of Anesthesiology upon Dr. Boutros' retirement in 1986. To reflect the scope of its services, Estafanous changed the name of the division to the Division of Anesthesiology and Critical Care Medicine. In 2003, the division oversaw 70 operating rooms and more than 70 critical care beds. The division contains four departments (General Anesthesiology, Cardiothoracic Anesthesiology, Pain Management, and Regional Practice) and three centers (clinical engineering and information systems, anesthesiology research, and anesthesiology education) reporting to the division chairman. The division has become one of the largest anesthesiology groups in the world.

CARDIOTHORACIC ANESTHESIOLOGY

In response to the Clinic's growing recognition as a heart center, the Section of Cardiothoracic Anesthesiology, founded by Viljoen, became a department in 1976, the first subspecialty department of its kind in the country, with Estafanous as its first chairman. As a cardiac anesthesiologist with an active interest in clinical and basic research, Estafanous played an important role in the evolution of cardiac anesthesia as a specialty. Not only did he build his department into one of the most respected in the world, but also he made significant contributions in the areas of post-myocardial-revascularization hypertension, hemodynamic and clinical effects of opioids and muscle relaxants, blood conservation, and limitations of hemodilution. In 1979, the department started one of the first fellowships in cardiothoracic anesthesiology, and this fellowship has become the largest of its kind in the United States. In 1986, the department offices moved to the new hospital wing, adjacent to eleven modern cardiac operating rooms and three cardiovascular intensive care units.

Upon Estafanous's appointment to the chair of the Division of Anesthesiology, Norman J. Starr, M.D., a staff member since 1979, became chairman of the Department of Cardiothoracic Anesthesiology. Under Starr, the department has grown to include 20 full-time, board-certified cardiac anesthesiologists, nine certified registered nurse anesthetists, 43 respiratory therapists, and a five-member clinical engineering department.

In addition, the Clinic's recognition as a major center for heart and lung transplantation has enabled the cardiac anesthesiologists to gain extensive experience in the use of advanced ventricular support devices, the forerunners of an artificial heart. At the Clinic, surgeons regularly implant cardiac assist devices and perform lung reduction surgery, arrhythmia surgery, and valvuloplasty. The section for congenital heart anesthesia, headed by Dr. Emad Mossad, participates in more than 500 open heart procedures on infants and children each year. It also provides anesthesia for an equal or greater number of patients undergoing diagnostic and therapeutic procedures in the pediatric catheterization laboratories. In 2002, the approximate number of patients anesthetized by the members of the Department of Cardiothoracic Anesthesiology exceeded 6,190. By 2003, under the direction of Jean Pierre Yared, M.D., the 55-bed cardiovascular intensive care unit accommodated 14,000 patient-days per year, providing the department's twelve-year-old registry with a rich resource for outcomes research.

GENERAL ANESTHESIOLOGY

Although committed to subspecialization in anesthesia, one of Estafanous' first acts as chairman of the Division of Anesthesiology was to reestablish a Department of General Anesthesiology. Arthur Barnes, M.D., was selected chairman. Barnes formalized the department structure, establishing clinical subspecialty sections, appointing section heads, and creating new protocols to distribute resources. He also arranged for additional space to accommodate pre-surgical evaluation and the School of Nurse Anesthesia. In 1993, Barnes stepped down as chairman of general anesthesiology to dedicate all his time and efforts as director of the residency program.

Armin Schubert, M.D., a neuroanesthesiologist with a strong background in clinical research, succeeded Barnes as department chairman in 1993. Schubert expanded the acute postoperative pain service to make epidural analgesia routinely available. By 2003, the Department of General Anesthesiology was a dynamic group of more than 50 physicians with a remarkable breadth and depth of talent, and 36 nurse anesthetists supported it.

The department met the rapidly growing need for sophisticated post-surgical intensive care through its Section of Critical Care, with four staff members certified in critical care medicine as well as anesthesiology and full responsibility for the 18-bed surgical intensive care unit (SICU). Shahpour Esfandiari, M.D., current director of the unit, was one of the original members, serving continuously for 28 years. In 1989, the department developed an ambulatory anesthesia service headed by R. John Anderson, M.D. This unit cared for 45 percent of all non-cardiac surgical patients at The Cleveland Clinic.

In 1995, Walter Maurer, M.D., became director of pre-anesthesia testing. He transformed this system into the pre-anesthesia consultation and evaluation (PACE) clinic. He established uniform algorithms for disease assessment and guidelines for laboratory testing. Maurer also served the institution as director of the Office of Quality Management. Universal use of HealthQuest, the computer-based health-screening tool developed by the division's clinical engineering group, was initiated by Dr. Sara Spagnuolo and accepted by the Division of Surgery.

The chair of the Department of General Internal Medicine (the late Joseph Cash, M.D.) agreed to participate in pre-surgical testing in 1995 and created the internal medicine pre-anesthesia consultation and therapy (IMPACT) clinic, which now evaluates approximately 9,000 patients per year.

The Departments of Orthopaedic Surgery and Plastic and Reconstructive Surgery have added procedure rooms in the Crile Building to accommodate more patients. In 1995, the Division of Anesthesiology acquired new space on the third floor of the Emergency Medicine and Access Center Building. In 1999, the Cole Eye Institute added a section of ophthalmic anesthesia under the leadership of Mark Feldman, M.D.

In the 1990s, pediatric surgery grew rapidly. The Clinic built two pediatric operating rooms in 1994 for congenital heart surgery and five for general pediatric surgery in 1997. Dr. Julie Niezgoda, the section head for pediatric anesthesiology, and Mossad, the section head for congenital heart anesthesiology, established the pediatric anesthesiology fellowship in conjunction with Akron Children's Hospital.

In 1960, the south wing of the sixth floor of what is now known as the M building housed the obstetrics unit. Interestingly, as noted in chapter 9, the space committee selected the same location (with some additional space on the same floor) as the site for the new obstetrics unit, which opened in April 1995. The late Dr. Gerald A. Burger started the obstetric anesthesia service. Steady growth in volume of service had led to a number of expansion projects, including the establishment of a level-3 neonatal nursery in 2002. In 1999, Jonathan Waters, M.D., became the head of the section of anesthesia for obstetrics.

PAIN MANAGEMENT

In the 1970s, The Cleveland Clinic established a formal program for the management of postoperative pain. In 1988, the program was expanded to include chronic pain. Michael D. Stanton-Hicks, M.B., B.S., was appointed director of the Pain Management Center. The center's activities rapidly outgrew the capacity of its original space in the original hospital building and moved to the second floor of the former Woodruff Hospital. In 1998, the center moved again into a 25,000-square-foot space at the William O. Walker Center. Because of its increasing importance and rapid growth, the center became the Department of Pain Management in 2001, with Nagy Mekhail, M.D., Ph.D., as its first chairman. The department worked closely with the Reflex Sympathetic Dystrophy Syndrome Association, and The Cleveland Clinic's Spine Center, Cancer Center, Department of Physical Medicine and Rehabilitation, and Department of Gynecology. The most current pain management techniques were available, including spinal cord stimulation, the implantation of infusion systems, and the introduction of highly specific diagnostic tests using enhanced fluoroscopic imaging. Pain management expanded beyond the Clinic's main campus, providing diagnostic and therapeutic services at Lutheran Hospital, Lakewood Hospital, Marymount Hospital, Lorain Community Hospital, and others.

Postoperative pain management was a key service. The staff oversaw the placement of epidural catheters prior to anesthesia, allowing patients to continue analgesia postoperatively as long as necessary. The fellowship in pain management, established in 1993, has grown to be the largest pain management fellowship in the United States.

CLINICAL ENGINEERING AND INFORMATION TECHNOLOGY CENTER

In 1977, the Department of Cardiothoracic Anesthesiology formed the nation's first clinical engineering group. Headed by John Petre,

Ph.D., the group was charged with providing instrumentation management for cardiac anesthesia as well as the cardiac surgical intensive care units. This role rapidly expanded to the selection of equipment, round-the-clock maintenance, invention of new medical equipment, and planning for construction of new clinical spaces in the division. In the late 1990s, the clinical engineering group assumed the responsibility for the division's information systems. Estafanous encouraged the clinical engineering group to develop a computerized anesthesia record, the automated record-keeping system (ARKS). They formed a partnership with General Electric to commercialize the product.

EDUCATION CENTER

Hale started the first residency program, which continued under Wasmuth's leadership, and it combined with the residency program at Huron Road Hospital with the cooperation of William Dornette, M.D. When Boutros arrived in 1977, the division applied for an independent residency program that received approval the following year. The first class of two residents included Zeyd Ebrahim, M.D., who subsequently joined the staff and became vice-chairman of the Department of General Anesthesiology.

Estafanous delegated the responsibility for the residency program to Barnes. Under his direction, the program achieved a high level of excellence, having repeatedly received five-year unconditional approvals by the national Residency Review Committee in 1990, 1995, and 2000. Graduates of the program are highly sought after and continue to attain prominent positions. In addition to residency training, the Division of Anesthesiology initiated fellowships in cardiac anesthesiology (1979), anesthesiology critical care medicine (1989), anesthesiology pain management (1993), pediatric anesthesiology (1999), and obstetric anesthesiology (2002).

The opening of the E Building in 1995 provided sufficient space to establish the Center for Anesthesiology Education, including library space, a multimedia classroom seating 150, and dedicated on-call rooms. The division acquired a full-scale anesthesiology human patient simulator, created fully electronic residency information systems as well as an education website, and developed several software programs for resident selection, tracking of cases, and evaluation. In 2000, the center applied for an increase in the residency and received permission to train 30 more residents for a total capacity of 90 residents. Upon Barnes's retirement in 2001, Estafanous appointed Dr. John Tetzlaff as director of the residency program.

In 1969, Wasmuth and Marietta (Del) Portzer started The Cleveland Clinic School of Nurse Anesthesia. Portzer was the first director of the school, which graduated its 216th student in July 1995. It was a hospital-based, 24-month certificate program until 1989, when it affiliated with the Frances Payne Bolton School of Nursing to offer an M.S. degree. Paul Blakeley, C.R.N.A., M.S.N., is the current director of the school. More than half of the graduates join the division.

RESEARCH CENTER

In 1994, the division established its first endowed chair, the Carl Wasmuth Endowed Chair in Anesthesiology and Critical Care Medicine for basic science research. In 1996, the Michael J. Cudahy Chair for Clinical Engineering was endowed for research in biomedical engineering. The division's research projects have attracted significant funding from the pharmaceutical and medical technology industries as well as the National Institutes of Health and American Heart Association.

In 1995, the division established the Carl Wasmuth Center for Anesthesiology Research and recruited Paul Murray, Ph.D., to coordinate and administer all research activity. The center occupies 3,500 square feet and includes six laboratories and six offices. Its goal is to maintain active investigation within the basic sciences of anesthesiology and to coordinate clinical research within the division.

Murray's own research focused on the mechanisms of pulmonary vascular regulation and the effects of anesthetic agents on pulmonary vasoregulation. A program for basic science research in pain management resulted in the recruitment of Manju Bhat, Ph.D., Salim Hayek, M.D., and Leonardo Kapural, M.D., Ph.D.

15. CENTERS, INSTITUTES, AND EMERGING DIVISIONS

By Daniel J. Mazanec, Richard A. Rudick, J. Michael Henderson, Maurie Markman, and Hilel Lewis

> *Men of genius do not excel in any*
> *profession because they labour in it, but*
> *they labour in it because they excel.*
> —*William Hazlitt, 1823*

THE COMBINATION OF EXPONENTIAL GROWTH OF THE INSTITUTION THROUGH addition of increasingly talented individuals, the emergence of new technology, and refinement of the team approach to complex clinical problems has begun to strain the traditional departmental and divisional structure of The Cleveland Clinic. To accommodate the special needs generated by these factors, the Board of Governors has designated several centers and institutes (some with their own endowments secured through philanthropy) and has created some new divisions as well. A few of these, such as the Lerner Research Institute, are long-established entities within the Clinic's structure, renamed to recognize specific benefactors. Others, like the Post Acute Medicine Division, are totally new structural entities, formed to better coordinate previously fragmented, or even unavailable, services. Some are so new that their histories are very short, and others are as yet in a somewhat fluid state and still works in progress. A few others are described in enough detail in other sections of this book that they do not require further description here.

While the Board of Governors has applied the designations

"Institute" or "Center" (or occasionally both) to some of these entities, there exist as yet no formal definitions of these terms. Some institutes are divisions, others are departments, and still others are neither. Most are multidisciplinary in some way: either multiple departments (sometimes crossing divisional lines), or strong, wholly contained research components may be incorporated into them.

This chapter describes a group of these entities that do not fit into the more traditional structural formats. Perhaps in future editions of this book, some or all of them may appear elsewhere, or, indeed, the entire basic structure of The Cleveland Clinic could be different. Time will tell what the best structure is, but it is certain that the Clinic will continue to experiment and fine-tune its structure as long as potential improvement in function appears possible.

THE CLEVELAND CLINIC SPINE INSTITUTE

The Center for the Spine was established in November 1984 as a cooperative effort of the Departments of Orthopaedic Surgery and Neurosurgery under the joint leadership of Frank Boumphrey, M.D., and Russell Hardy, M.D. Specialists from the Departments of Neurology and Rheumatic and Immunologic Disease who shared an interest in studying and treating patients with spinal conditions readily joined them in this effort. This "center without walls" relied on a central triage system to refer patients to the appropriate physician. The entire group met regularly to discuss and develop new approaches to the diagnosis and management of patients with back pain.

In 1990, a task force appointed by the Board of Governors recommended that the Center for the Spine be reorganized as a medical department "with walls." They concluded that placing a medical director, physicians, and physical therapists at a single location, devoting their practices to disorders of the spine, would further the Center's development as a model program for the treatment of spinal disorders through conservative patient management and rehabilitation. Its core concept was initial evaluation by a medical specialist rather than a surgeon.

In July 1991, rheumatologist Daniel J. Mazanec, M.D., became director of the Center for the Spine. Shortly thereafter, he developed a close collaboration with the recently reconstituted Department of Physical Medicine and Rehabilitation (housed at that time in the Division of Medicine, later in the Division of Post Acute Medicine). In 1994, this collaboration resulted in the WERC (Work Evaluation and Rehabilitation Clinic), an innovative, multidisciplinary program for injured and disabled back patients aimed at restoring function and returning patients to work. The WERC has become one of the most successful programs of its kind in the country, with more than 90% of the patients who complete the program returning to work.

The Center for the Spine attracted a growing number of workers' compensation patients seeking alternative approaches or second opinions on work-related injuries. Center physicians collaborated extensively with the Department of Physical Medicine and Rehabilitation and the Pain Management Center to meet these patients' needs.

The interdisciplinary nature of the Center for the Spine enabled it to serve as a focal point for clinical activities, research, and education. The participating members of the Departments of Orthopaedic Surgery, Neurosurgery, Radiology, Pain Management, Psychiatry, and Rehabilitation Medicine focused on the development of clinically superior, cost-effective diagnostic and management methods for spinal disorders, emphasizing the appropriate use of technology.

In August 2002, a section of occupational health and employee health was created in the Spine Center headed by Dr. Richard Lewis. This clinical area served the health needs of both Cleveland Clinic employees and injured workers requiring ongoing follow-up care and rehabilitation.

In March 2003, the Center for the Spine joined the Spine Surgery sections in Neurosurgery and Orthopedic Surgery in a newly created Cleveland Clinic Spine Institute (CCSI), headed by neurosurgeon Edward C. Benzel, M.D. This new entity combined

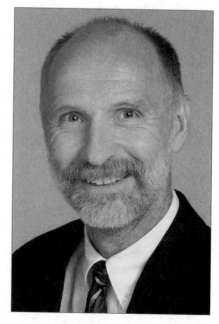

Edward C. Benzel, M.D., Director, Cleveland Clinic Spine Institute, 2002-

the medical and surgical spine programs at The Cleveland Clinic into one organizational structure for the purpose of streamlining patient care, promoting treatment pathways, and ultimately facilitating the most efficient model of spine healthcare delivery. Its goal was to facilitate clinical and academic collaboration among medical and surgical staff as well as strengthen research and educational activities in existing departments. It enabled further development of The Cleveland Clinic as a leader in the field of spine disorders.

MELLEN CENTER FOR MULTIPLE SCLEROSIS

A comprehensive center for the treatment of multiple sclerosis was the brainchild of Neurology chairman John Conomy, M.D., who had a special interest in the disease. The generosity of the Mellen Foundation and Mr. John Drinko made the dream a reality.

The Mellen Center for Multiple Sclerosis opened on February 11, 1985, occupying two rooms in the Department of Neurology. In addition to Conomy, the staff included three neurologists, each of whom dedicated one day a week to multiple sclerosis patients. Within three months, the Center also had a full-time nurse, occupational therapist, physical therapist, psychologist, and social worker, making it one of the most comprehensive clinical teams ever assembled to handle the various neurological and psychosocial aspects of the disease. Conditions were so crowded that staff members often saw patients together. Each team member evaluated every patient, resulting in comprehensive treatment recommendations. This mode of operation continued for about two years, until the increasing demand for services made it impractical. By mid-1986, the Mellen Center had moved into its own facility in the former Woodruff Hospital. A search committee recruited Richard A. Rudick, M.D., as the full-time director of the Mellen Center, and the program began a rapid growth phase.

Space and resources allowed the development of novel clinical programs, including special aerobic exercise, functional electrical stimulation, and adapted cooking. Staff members formed psychology groups for stress management and development of coping strategies, as well as specialized programs for children and adults. They also developed educational programs to teach patients and their families about multiple sclerosis, often in conjunction with the local Multiple Sclerosis Society. The Center began to train students in nursing, occupational therapy, and social work to help non-Mellen patients cope with the disease. Outpatient services expanded to include neuropsychological assessments and counseling about the functional effect of multiple sclerosis-related cognitive impairment. A project to design and fabricate custom seating was implemented along with programs designed to help patients maximize their independence. In 1990, the Center started a day treatment program to provide social and therapeutic activities for patients with severe physical or cognitive impairment, and to afford a respite for their caregivers.

In 1999, the Mellen Center opened a Multiple Sclerosis Learning Center in the lobby of the U building to augment the educational focus of the Mellen Center. Several generous donors made this unique facility possible, and it became a collaborative effort among the local chapter of the National Multiple Sclerosis Society, the Multiple Sclerosis Women's Committee, and the Mellen Center itself. A full-time health educator staffed the Learning Center, providing resources in various formats, including a website and both drop-in educational sessions and scheduled programs.

In 1998, the Mellen Center began to explore the possibility of communicating with established patients about their care and concerns via the Internet. The result was establishment of the Mellen Center Care On-Line. Mellen Center Care On-Line allowed patients to communicate securely with their healthcare providers without having to wait by the telephone. It made use of preformatted, fill-in-the-blank questions to assist patients in providing the information necessary to address their needs. The system routed questions to

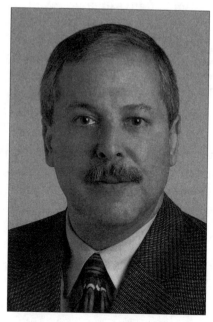

Richard A. Rudick, M.D., Director,
Mellen Center for Multiple Sclerosis,
1987-

the appropriate member of the care team and tracked response time.

The Mellen Center helped found the Consortium of Multiple Sclerosis Centers. Conomy was named its first executive director, and subsequently two other Mellen staff members, Jill S. Fischer, Ph.D. (1992 to 1993), and Marie Namey, R.N., M.S.N. (2000 to 2001), served as presidents of the organization.

In 2002, the Mellen Center expanded its imaging capability by adding an MRI facility adjacent to the existing outpatient clinic.

Research programs began in 1988 at the Mellen Center and soon included studies of medications, memory impairment, cognitive function, physical function, and emotional status. The Center received grants to develop new devices to assist in managing symptoms and adapting computer equipment. Center scientists played a key role in developing interferon therapy, the first treatment proven to slow multiple sclerosis disease progression. The Center recruited Dr. Jeffrey Cohen to direct and develop experimental therapeutics.

In the realm of basic research, Dr. Richard Ransohoff, one of the founding neurologists at the Mellen Center and a world authority on brain inflammation, established a multidisciplinary group of investigators. Ransohoff and Rudick recruited a well-known myelin researcher, Bruce Trapp, Ph.D., to chair the newly formed Neuroscience Department in 1994. By 1998, the combined efforts of researchers in the Departments of Neuroscience, Immunology, Radiology, and Biomedical Engineering teamed with Mellen Center researchers to win a $5-million program project grant from the National Institutes of Health to study the pathogenesis of multiple sclerosis.

In summary, the Mellen Center has developed a reputation as a leading multiple sclerosis center. The team approach has enabled the Center to fulfill its mission to provide compassionate, innovative care to patients and families affected by multiple sclerosis, to conduct important clinical and basic research, and to educate other clinicians, scientists, and the public about the disease.

TRANSPLANT CENTER

The concept of organ transplantation had long interested Clinic surgeons looking for ways to extend natural organ function without the use of artificial materials. The first successfully transplanted organs were the kidneys. Ralph A. Straffon, M.D., started the Clinic's renal transplant program while he was chairman of the Department of Urology, and this program was the precursor of the Transplant Center. Since the 1980s, major technical improvements, advances in immunosuppression, and better patient selection criteria enabled establishment of successful transplant programs for bone, bone marrow, cornea, heart, larynx, liver, lung, and pancreas.

The Cleveland Clinic views transplantation as an essential component of a broad strategy to

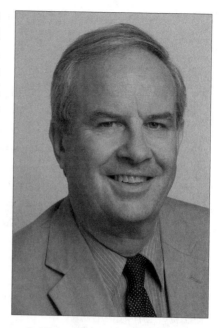

J. Michael Henderson, M.B., Ch.B.,
Director, Transplant Center, 1992-

offer all patients with advanced diseases the most appropriate therapy. To coordinate all activities in this rapidly developing specialty, the Clinic opened a Transplant Center in 1985, under the direction of Andrew C. Novick, M.D. Since 1992, it has been directed by J. Michael Henderson, M.B., Ch.B., a liver transplant surgeon who also chaired the Department of General Surgery.

Kidney Transplantation

The kidney transplant program, initiated in January 1963, was an outgrowth of Dr. Willem Kolff's pioneering efforts to develop and refine hemodialysis. At that time, renal transplantation was considered experimental and had relatively low patient and graft survival rates. From 1963 to 1967, The Cleveland Clinic, under Straffon's direction, performed about 10 percent of all cadaver kidney transplants. Advances in tissue matching techniques, the use of living donors, and a reduction in the surgical morbidity gave the program an edge, which resulted in more successful transplants than any other institution.

Andrew C. Novick, M.D., became director of renal transplantation in July 1977. The following year, he initiated the first approved postgraduate fellowship-training program in transplantation. As the first program to receive approval by the Education Committee of the American Society of Transplant Surgeons, it has trained 28 urologists in renal transplantation. Many went on to direct their own programs. In 1985, he was appointed chairman of the newly established Cleveland Clinic Organ Transplant Center, a position he held until Henderson assumed the role in 1992.

During the 1980s, the Clinic made important contributions to the field of renal transplantation, including use of pediatric cadaver kidneys for transplantation, development of microvascular surgical techniques to enable the transplantation of kidneys with abnormal vascular supply, and use of antilymphocyte globulin for immunosuppression.

By 2003, Clinic surgeons were performing approximately 200 kidney transplants a year at The Cleveland Clinic's main campus in Cleveland and its affiliated transplant programs in Youngstown, Akron, and Charleston, West Virginia. These programs, staffed by full-time Clinic kidney transplant surgeons, were developed to serve patients better and to improve acquisition of cadaver kidneys. The Cleveland Clinic's patient- and graft-survival rates following kidney transplantation were above the national average: the one-year patient survival rate was 95 percent, and the one-year graft survival rate was 93 percent following live-donor transplant. The graft survival rate was 86 percent following cadaver transplantation.

Kidney/Pancreas Transplantation

In the mid-1980s, physicians realized that a combined kidney and pancreas transplant could be used to improve management of diabetic renal disease in some patients. The Clinic performed its first kidney/pancreas transplant in 1985, and had done 14 by 1989, when the procedure was put on temporary hold due to the high rate of complications. After reassessing the immunologic and surgical aspects of the procedure, the kidney/pancreas program was resumed in 1993 under the direction of James Mayes, M.D. In 2000, Venkatesh Krishnamurthi, M.D., assumed the directorship and also initiated a pancreas-only transplant program. Today, improved patient selection and better understanding of immunosuppressive agents make these procedures a viable option for selected patients with diabetes mellitus.

Bone Marrow Transplantation

The Cleveland Clinic's first bone marrow transplant took place in 1977, but the program did not begin to grow in earnest until the arrival of Roger Herzig, M.D., in 1982. Brian Bolwell, M.D., became director of the program after Herzig left the Clinic in 1988. During the 1990s, under Bolwell's dynamic leadership, bone marrow transplantation experienced remarkable growth. The Clinic was a founding member of the National Marrow Donor Program, which coordinates the search for unrelated donors for patients in need of allogeneic marrow transplants but lacking sibling donors. The Clinic became one of America's most active bone marrow transplantation centers performing transplants from unrelated donors.

In the 1990s, the use of stimulated peripheral blood progenitor cells, or stem cells, revolutionized autologous bone marrow transplantation. Researchers at the Clinic pioneered the application of novel growth factors to stimulate hematopoietic stem cells, thus bringing international recognition to the organization as a research leader in this field. The most common indication for autologous transplantation is non-Hodgkin's lymphoma.

Allogeneic bone marrow has the potential to yield an anti-tumor effect known as the graft-versus-tumor effect. This concept has led to non-myeloablative allogeneic hematopoietic cell transplantation, in which donor cells are utilized to confer an anti-tumor effect. Clinical application of the graft-versus-tumor effect became a major focus of the program.

Heart Transplantation and the Kaufman Center for Heart Failure

Cardiac transplantation is the most effective treatment for patients with truly end-stage heart failure. The cardiac transplant program, as we know it today, began in 1984 and has sustained tremendous growth since that time. Indeed, in 1999, Clinic surgeons performed 113 cardiac transplants, the most at any single center in the United States in one year. More important than volume, however, are the outcomes. The survival rate exceeded the national average and was higher than expected, given the Clinic's liberal donor and recipient criteria.

Patrick M. McCarthy, M.D., joined the Department of Cardiovascular Surgery in 1990. He became a pioneer in the field of heart-failure surgery. He developed the Left Ventricular Assist Device (LVAD) program at the Clinic, the largest such program in the United States. Utilized primarily as bridge-to-transplant, the LVAD improved survival and quality of life for the most critically ill patients awaiting a donor heart. The Clinic participated in the early clinical trials for both the Novacor® and HeartMate®, now FDA-approved. In 2001, The Cleveland Clinic became the second center in the United States to begin a clinical trial with the Jarvik 2000® assist device.

The cardiac transplant program underwent significant personnel changes after its inception in 1984. James B. Young, M.D., joined the Department of Cardiology to head the Section of Heart Failure and Transplant Medicine. McCarthy became Director of the program in 1998. Three additional surgeons, Nicholas G. Smedira, M.D., Michael K. Banbury, M.D., and José L. Navia, M.D., eight cardiologists, and thirteen nurse coordinators worked with him.

For all its success, cardiac transplantation remained but a small part of the multitude of medical and surgical options available to treat heart failure. Recognizing the enormity of the heart failure epidemic, George M. and Linda H. Kaufman established the Kaufman Center for Heart Failure in 1998. The Center provided for collaboration across departments, bringing together cardiologists, cardiothoracic surgeons, research scientists, and allied health professionals to advance the treatment of congestive heart failure.

Lung and Heart/Lung Transplantation

Cleveland Clinic surgeons performed Ohio's first single lung transplant in February 1990 and the state's first double lung transplant 16 months later.

In February 2000, the Clinic's Lung Transplant Program entered its second decade, riding an impressive wave of growth. With the recruitment of thoracic surgeon Malcolm DeCamp, M.D., in 1998, the program doubled its annual volume. By 2003, performing more than 40 transplants each year, the Clinic continued to have the most active lung transplantation program in Ohio and ranked in volume among the top five in the country. To sustain such volume, the surgical cadre grew to include four experienced transplanters. DeCamp joined Nicholas Smedira, who was also active in the cardiac transplant program and served as Director of the Heart/Lung Transplant Program. B. Gösta Pettersson, M.D., who initiated and directed Denmark's flagship heart and lung transplant center, was recruited to the Clinic in 1999. His pioneering work with bronchial artery revascularization at the time of lung transplantation enriched the spirit of innovation within the Clinic's program. General thoracic surgeon Sudish C. Murthy, M.D., Ph.D., also joined the team in 1999.

By 2003, the program had evaluated more than 1,100 patients with advanced lung disease. Almost 300 individuals received replacement lungs. Patients with a variety of end-stage respiratory diseases are potential lung transplant recipients and can expect survival rates approaching 80 percent after one year and 50 percent after five years. An ongoing shortage of donors has stimulated the evolution of a comprehensive advanced lung disease program. Directed by Atul C. Mehta, M.D., this collaboration identified alternatives to transplantation for patients with chronic respiratory failure. Drs. Jeffrey Chapman and Omar Minai assisted Mehta in the evaluation of selected patients with emphysema for lung volume reduction surgery, selected patients with pulmonary hypertension for pulmonary thromboendarterectomy, continuous prostacyclin or endothelin-antagonist therapy, and interstitial lung disease patients for antifibrotic or immune modulative drug therapy.

The success of The Cleveland Clinic's lung transplant program as well as the advanced lung disease center was the result of a multidisciplinary effort by experts from the Departments of Pulmonary and Critical Care Medicine, Thoracic and Cardiovascular Surgery, Cardiothoracic Anesthesiology, Infectious Disease, Pathology, Endocrinology, Nursing, and Social Services as well as the allogen laboratories. Surgical mortality for lung transplantation steadily decreased from nearly 30% in the early 1990s to less than 5% by

2000. In 2001, all 40 patients transplanted left the hospital alive. Such results are a testament to the success of an integrated transplant center concept.

On February 14, 1992, McCarthy performed the first heart-lung transplant in Ohio. Candidates for this rare type of transplant have either complex congenital heart disease with severe pulmonary hypertension, or combined end-stage heart and lung disease. Due to the lack of donors, only 30-50 of these operations have been performed in the entire country every year.

Liver Transplantation

Robert E. Hermann, M.D., and Edwin G. Beven, M.D., performed the first liver transplant at The Cleveland Clinic in the late 1960s. It was an auxiliary transplant, and the patient's own liver remained in place. The patient, a child, died 24 hours after the operation. This was one of only 100 liver transplants that had been attempted worldwide by 1975.

Cleveland Clinic physicians performed the Clinic's first orthotopic (in the normal position) liver transplant in November 1984. The operation followed several months of planning and training of the liver transplant team. Hermann, along with David Vogt, M.D., and William Carey, M.D., visited the University of Pittsburgh to observe Thomas Starzl's liver transplantation program before the Clinic's program began. Additionally, the surgeons carried out several transplant procedures in the laboratory setting to become familiar with both the donor and recipient procedures. From 1985 to 1992, Vogt and Thomas Broughan were the Clinic's liver transplant surgeons. In 1992, Broughan left The Cleveland Clinic, and Dr. J. Michael Henderson, an experienced liver transplant surgeon from Emory University, came aboard as chairman of the Department of General Surgery and Head of the Transplant Center. In 1993, the liver transplant surgical staff was further augmented by the arrival of James T. Mayes III, M.D.

Between November 1984 and December 2001, the Clinic's team did 586 liver transplants on 542 patients, including four patients who had combined liver/kidney transplants, one patient who had a liver/pancreas transplant, and thirteen adult patients who received a right lobe from a living donor. In 2002, the overall one-, five-, and ten-year survival rates were 84.7%, 72.6%, and 55.2%, respectively. The limiting factor in liver transplantation was always insufficient availability of cadaver organs. To address this, in October 1999, after several months of preparation and planning, the Clinic's liver transplant team began using liver tissue from adult living donors. By 2003, 14 living-donor liver transplants had been performed at The Cleveland Clinic without serious complications for the donors. The survival results for the recipients were also very good.

Corneal Transplantation

The corneal transplant program, co-directed by David M. Meisler, M.D., and Roger H.S. Langston, M.D., in the Cole Eye Institute, was initiated in 1970. By 2003, surgeons in the Cole Eye Institute performed more than 100 corneal transplants annually.

Meisler has sat on the national advisory committee of the Eye Bank Association of America and has been a long-standing member of the medical advisory committee for the Cleveland Eye Bank. He has authored many articles and chapters on corneal transplantation. He has participated in national collaborative studies and is currently the principal investigator for The Cleveland Clinic in the National Eye Institute-sponsored Cornea Donor Study. Current research efforts, in part supported by the Eye Bank Association of America, include investigating the effect that nitric oxide has on corneas in corneal storage media.

Laryngeal Transplantation

Marshall Strome, M.D., joined The Cleveland Clinic in 1993, having been recruited from the Brigham and Women's Hospital in Boston to head the Department of Otolaryngology and Communicative Disorders. Strome's primary research focus from the mid-1980s had been on laryngeal transplantation. The Clinic's laryngeal transplantation laboratory opened soon after his arrival. Five more years of research data supported consideration of a human procedure, which was controversial because the organ was considered "non-vital." After an exhaustive review by the Institutional Review Board, Strome received a green light to proceed. The screening process for the "perfect" recipient took one year. Donor screening was similarly rigorous.

Strome performed the transplantation on January 4, 1998, and, as of 2003, it remained viable. This represented the first-ever total laryngeal transplantation. The thyroid gland and parathyroid glands were transplanted as well, also firsts. Interestingly, 80% of the patient's thyroid function today is from the donor organ. Calcium metabolism is normal. The patient uttered his first words in many years, "Hello Mom"—very hoarsely—three days after the procedure. Today his voice is normal with pitch control, inflection, and normal volume. His occupation is motivational speaking!

Bone Transplantation

The Department of Orthopaedic Surgery has restored limbs using large-segment bone allografts, allograft prosthetic composite reconstructions, and osteoarticular allografts since the 1980s. In 1983, the department established a full-service Musculoskeletal Tissue Bank, under the direction of Michael Joyce, M.D., since 1993. Services included donor screening, serological testing, procurement, processing, and hospital-based patient surgical implantation, coordinated through a national Musculoskeletal Tissue Organization, working with The Cleveland Clinic to ensure quality and safety by meeting federal guidelines and standards of the American Association of Tissue Banks. The Musculoskeletal Tissue Bank stored tissues such as demineralized bone, freeze-dried small segments of bone, and frozen large bone segments, including whole bones, hemipelvises, and fresh osteochondral grafts. These allografts were commonly used in prosthetic hip revisions, reconstruction of long bones affected by previous tumor resection, and restoration of cruciate knee ligaments.

Allogen Laboratories

The Cleveland Clinic's kidney transplant program was in its infancy when the Department of Immunopathology opened a tissue-typing laboratory to support it. William E. Braun, M.D., arrived in 1968 to head the laboratory, with a joint appointment in the Department of Hypertension and Nephrology. Under Braun the laboratory achieved international prominence in HLA typing for solid organ and bone marrow transplants as well as disease associations and paternity testing. In recognition of these achievements, the American Society of Histocompatibility and Immunogenetics elected Braun as its first president in 1974.

Under the direction of Daniel J. Cook, Ph.D., the allogen laboratory used advanced technology, such as flow cytometry, to perform more than 60,000 tests annually. These techniques were used to identify the presence of antibodies recognizing a potential organ donor's histocompatibility antigens, possibly indicating a heightened risk of organ rejection. In addition, they enabled monitoring of the effectiveness of post-transplant treatment in preventing rejection. The laboratory's use of high-resolution HLA typing to identify HLA gene products at the molecular level was critical in obtaining a contract to type the DNA of potential bone marrow donors through the National Marrow Donor Program.

TAUSSIG CANCER CENTER

Throughout its history, Cleveland Clinic physicians have contributed significantly to advances in the care of cancer patients. George Crile, Jr., M.D., was one of the earliest and most influential advocates of limited surgery for breast cancer, having begun to doubt the need for radical mastectomy in the early 1950s. Rupert P. Turnbull, Jr., M.D., discovered that isolating diseased tissue during surgery for colon cancer would prevent the further spread of cancer cells. By the 1980s, his "no-touch" technique was widely accepted as reducing the risk of death from metastatic disease following colorectal surgery.

Since the term "cancer" refers to a group of more than 100 diseases characterized by the abnormal growth and spread of cells, many departments incorporated the treatment of patients with cancer into their programs at The Cleveland Clinic. Pathologist William A. Hawk, M.D., first attempted to organize a centralized cancer program in the 1970s. Hawk's vision focused on aspects of malignant

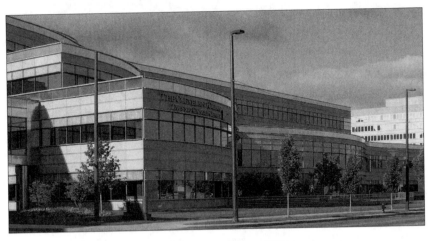

Taussig Cancer Center, 1999

disease that were not yet well represented within the institution, such as basic research, epidemiological studies, cancer rehabilitation, and continuing care. He conceived the program in collaboration with Case Western Reserve University, which had an established program in basic cancer research and could contribute to the community-wide efforts necessary for epidemiological studies and rehabilitation. Unfortunately, this resulted in an initial activity that had little relationship to the cancer treatment services under way in the clinical departments.

In the early 1980s, the Board of Governors perceived the need for a Cancer Center that could coordinate all cancer treatment and research at The Cleveland Clinic. The Departments of Hematology and Medical Oncology and Radiation Therapy had already established distinct programs. Surgical oncology fell under no specific departmental umbrella. The Board of Governors recruited general surgeon John H. Raaf, M.D., in 1985 to be the center's first full-time director.

As the cancer program expanded, surgical departments began to create formal oncology sections. This increased the number of cancer patients. To serve them best, the Department of Hematology and Medical Oncology, then chaired by James K. Weick, M.D., began to recruit staff members with special organ expertise. The first was David J. Adelstein, M.D., an expert in digestive tract malignancies, who joined the group in 1989. After Weick transferred to Cleveland Clinic Florida, Maurie Markman, M.D., a medical oncologist with a major interest in gynecologic malignancies, was recruited as chairman of the Department of Hematology and Medical Oncology and director of the Cancer Center in 1992.

In the mid-1980s, the opening of the A Building, later rechristened as the Crile Building, had a significant impact on the Cancer Center. Several departments vacated space in the original and main Clinic buildings when they moved to their new quarters. Fortunately, this space was adjacent to Radiation Therapy. Weick immediately recognized the value of such space, where related clinical specialties could practice in proximity, and he decided to relocate Hematology and Medical Oncology to the third floor of the original Clinic building. A portion of this floor was reserved for interdepartmental use, where related services, such as neurological assessments and postoperative follow-up of cancer patients, could take place.

Even in the absence of physical proximity, some oncologists had organized interdepartmental clinics before 1985 by making departmental space available for cancer patients scheduled to be seen by physicians from other departments. One example is urologic oncology, where a team that included a urologic oncologist from the Department of Urology and a medical oncologist from the Department of Hematology and Medical Oncology saw patients weekly. The area was renovated and dedicated as the Cleveland Clinic Cancer Center in June 1987. The subsequent catalytic impact of the physical identity for the Cancer Center resulted eventually in the creation of several additional discrete centers, including the Breast Center on the ground floor of the Crile Building, and the Center for Prostatic Diseases in the Department of Urology.

By 1994, the Cleveland Clinic Cancer Center had the largest cancer treatment program in Ohio and surrounding states. In only 10 years, the number of patients treated at the Clinic for cancer had grown from one in six to one in four inpatients, and from one in twelve to one in nine outpatients. This volume permitted subspecialists to develop substantial expertise in dealing with some relatively rare forms of cancer.

Besides coordinating existing cancer programs, the Cancer Center collaborated with other departments to develop new programs. One successful example was the establishment of screening and detection programs for patients without symptoms within departments that previously focused on the diagnosis and treatment of symptomatic patients. By 1994, the Clinic was offering site-specific screenings for cancers of the breast, cervix, colon and rectum, mouth, prostate, and skin.

Treatment advances since 1971 have increased the number of patients surviving five or more years by one-third. Many of these patients at The Cleveland Clinic participated in a peer-support group, which was founded in 1988 by Cancer Center nurse counselor Barbara Gustafson. They also celebrated National Cancer Survivors Day yearly with major festivities on campus.

Unfortunately, the lack of basic understanding about how to control cancer means that progression of the disease is still a reality for many patients. For this reason, the Cancer Center is committed to helping patients with a poor prognosis control their symptoms. The Palliative Care program began in 1987 when T. Declan Walsh, M.D., was recruited jointly by the Cancer Center and Department of Hematology and Medical Oncology. Initially established as a consulting service for hospitalized patients, the program grew to include a dedicated outpatient clinic, home care services, and certified hospice. In 1994, a generous gift from the H. R. H. Family Foundation made it possible to add a 23-bed inpatient unit, which has been recognized by the World Health Organization.

Comprehensive cancer care required a team approach that combined the contributions of physicians with those of allied health professionals, especially nurses and social workers. In 1985, the Division of Nursing established a Cancer Nursing Section with six clinical nurse specialists assigned to interdepartmental cancer teams. By 2003, cancer nursing care throughout The Cleveland Clinic had been carefully coordinated. Social workers, who were available only to hospitalized cancer patients and their families before 1985, were provided in the Cancer Center clinics for outpatient counseling, follow-up in the community, and leadership of peer support groups.

Since the analysis and interpretation of results were recognized to be critical in controlling cancer, the Department of Biostatistics and Epidemiology, then in the Research Institute, established a new Section of Biostatistics in the Cancer Center in 1985 to help with this process and track cancer patients enrolled in clinical trials. Beginning in 1986, the section directed the work of the Cleveland Clinic Tumor Registry, which collected baseline and follow-up information on all cancer patients seen at the Clinic. In 1994, it was expanded to include a registry for studies involving families with a strong history of cancer. In 2003, the Section of Cancer Biostatistics, under the leadership of Paul Elson, D.Sc., supported collaboration of clinical researchers with biostatisticians, systems analysts, and data management study coordinators.

In 1993, the Cancer Center assisted in recruiting Roger Macklis, M.D., to chair the Department of Radiation Therapy. A funded investigator in radiation biology and radiation physics as they related to targeted delivery of cancer therapy, Macklis was interested in many of the Cancer Center's programs. For this reason, the new department was transferred from the Division of Radiology to the Cancer Center and renamed the Department of Radiation Oncology. Within the first two years, the new department received a gift that allowed it to begin planning a Center of Oncologic Robotics and Computer-Assisted Medicine, where a prototype linear accelerator mounted on a robotic arm (Cyberknife®) was housed. This design was intended to reduce the need for rigid immobilization of patients undergoing lengthy and recurring treatments for brain cancer.

New basic research insights have been applied to the care of cancer patients at the Clinic for over a quarter of a century and have been an integral part of the Cancer Center's success. Cancer research reached a new level of institutional prominence when Bernadine Healy, M.D., was named chair of the Division of Research (soon thereafter renamed the Research Institute) in 1985. She immediately established a Department of Cancer Biology in the division and recruited Bryan R. G. Williams, Ph.D., to head it. Its importance was further underscored when George R. Stark, Ph.D., a researcher with interests in gene amplification and interferon, succeeded Healy as chairman. He received the Research Institute's first National Cancer Institute basic sciences program project award for an interdepartmental investigation into signal transduction (for more about the Research Institute, see Chapter 20). By 2003, dozens of Clinic researchers were working closely with Cancer Center clinicians to find better ways of preventing and treating all forms of this group of diseases.

In September 2000, the new 162,000 square-foot Taussig Cancer Center opened, with modern facilities for both treatment and research. The design included accommodations for patient comfort, including individual rooms for patients receiving chemotherapy.

The highlight of the building was an entire floor devoted to multidisciplinary outpatient clinics where the various specialists caring for cancer patients could work as a team to optimize management. The building, designed by Cesar Pelli, also included ten laboratories where researchers focused on translating basic discoveries from the bench to the clinic could work in close proximity with oncologists and their patients.

In the new century, the Clinic continued to build upon its leadership role in the care of cancer patients through a wide array of experts and specialized services. The Cleveland Clinic's Taussig Cancer Center provided a single, integrated approach to the control of cancer for patients throughout the Foundation.

COLE EYE INSTITUTE AND DIVISION OF OPHTHALMOLOGY

Ophthalmology was introduced at The Cleveland Clinic in 1924 under A. D. Ruedemann, M.D., a capable surgeon with a dynamic personality. He acquired an enormous following and saw an extraordinarily large number of patients on a daily basis. An independent thinker who often locked horns with the chief of surgery, Ruedemann left the Clinic in 1947 and was succeeded by Roscoe J. Kennedy, M.D., a respected physician who served with distinction.

When Kennedy retired in 1969, Froncie A. Gutman, M.D., a vitreoretinal specialist, was appointed department chairman. The only other staff member at that time was a general ophthalmologist named James Nousek, M.D., whom Kennedy had hired in 1957.

Under Gutman's leadership, the Department of Ophthalmology began to expand and modernize, adding subspecialty-trained physicians, implementing new technology, strengthening the educational programs, and expanding clinical research activity. By 1988, the department included specialists in corneal and external disease, neuro-ophthalmology, uveitis, pediatric ophthalmology, glaucoma, ophthalmic plastic and reconstructive surgery, and general ophthalmology, in addition to a vitreoretinal staff of four. They developed busy and challenging clinical practices that provided the resources and environment for resident and fellowship training as well as clinical investigation. Many of the staff members were recognized as

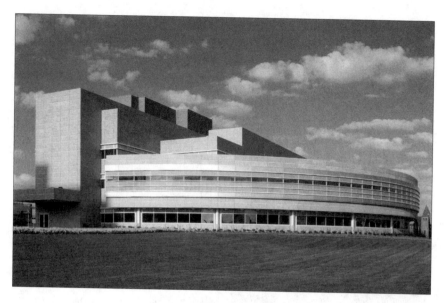

Cole Eye Institute, 1999

leaders through their appointment or election to office in professional ophthalmic organizations. Gutman himself was elected chairman of the American Board of Ophthalmology and served as president of the American Academy of Ophthalmology.

Ophthalmic technicians, laboratory services, and optometry were introduced to support the clinical programs. In 1970, the Department of Ophthalmology opened the first ophthalmic laboratory in Cleveland with a full-time staff of photographers who performed fluorescein angiography studies. New laboratories for ophthalmic electrophysiology and ultrasonography soon made additional diagnostic services available. The department established an ophthalmic technician training program to supply a pool of trained individuals who could assist in patient evaluations and ancillary testing. The addition of optometrists and an optical dispensary rounded out the department's primary care service.

In 1993, Hilel Lewis, M.D., a highly regarded vitreoretinal specialist and researcher from California, succeeded Gutman as chairman. With his appointment, the Ophthalmology Department left the Division of Surgery and formally became a new division and an institute in October 1994. Lewis envisioned the creation of a world-class center for vision science that would be preeminent in patient care,

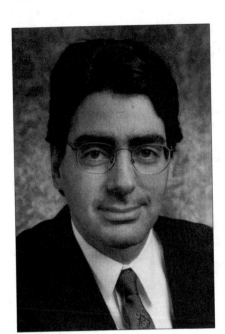

Hilel Lewis, M.D., Chairman,
Cole Eye Institute (Division of
Ophthalmology), 1992- (© Janine
Bentivegna, used with permission)

research, and education. His goals were to create the leading eye research and patient care institute in the world, and to train the future leaders in ophthalmology.

Lewis immediately began recruiting both experienced and established as well as young and ambitious ophthalmologists and highly credentialed basic researchers to staff 10 clinical departments and the newly formed basic and clinical research programs. He encouraged all of them to participate in clinical trials, to conduct original research, and to involve themselves in basic research.

To solidify a national and international academic reputation, Lewis planned a series of disease-specific summits, continuing medical education courses, and other education activities. He placed new emphasis on the residency-training program and added fellowships in vitreoretinal diseases and surgery, pediatric ophthalmology, uveitis, neuro-ophthalmology, refractive surgery, and glaucoma. By 1998, the program was recruiting from the top 10% of the applicant pool.

It was clear that top-notch facilities would be needed to accommodate the ophthalmology initiative. The Clinic made the decision to build a freestanding, comprehensive facility that would house all Eye Institute activities. Lewis envisioned an innovative facility that would foster provision of the best outcomes and service for patients, close and effective interactions between clinicians and scientists, and meeting the Institute's goals. After two years of program planning, the Clinic hired Cesar Pelli and Associates to design the building according to the plan.

Beginning in 1994, Lewis led fundraising efforts for the $60-million Eye Institute. After a successful campaign, construction began in May 1997, and the building opened in 1999. A naming gift that year from the Cole National Corporation gave the campaign a major boost. By 2003, the clinical and research faculty numbered 70. The Cole Eye Institute provided care to more than 130,000 patients in 2001, more than any other eye institute in the country. Its physicians were providing care to heads of state, royalty, and industry leaders, as well as everyday people. Scientists were working in all Cole Eye Institute laboratories, and an additional 3,000 square feet of lab space in the 1974 Research Building (FF) had to be renovated for research in corneal wound healing and gene therapy. Multi-million dollar grants from the National Institutes of Health, foundations, and industry provided support for this work.

Lewis understood that, to be effective, the Cole Eye Institute would need to integrate into the community. He established ophthalmology practices at the Clinic's Family Health Centers to provide regionally convenient access to eye care. An Eye Care Network, established in 1995, enables the Eye Institute to provide services under managed care contracts.

By 2003, initial staffing was complete. Cole Eye Institute physicians provide clinical services in the departments of Comprehensive Ophthalmology, Vitreoretinal Services, Corneal and External Disease, Refractive Surgery, Neuro-Ophthalmology, Uveitis, Pediatric Ophthalmology and Adult Strabismus, Oculoplasty and Orbital Surgery, Glaucoma, and Ocular Oncology, supported by departments of Optometry, Low Vision and Rehabilitation, and Ophthalmic Anesthesia. The Institute has clearly made excellent progress toward its ambitious goal of world leadership in eye care and related research.

DIVISION OF POST-ACUTE CARE

In September 2002, the Board of Governors brought together several clinical operations under the rubric of post-acute care, directed by Declan Walsh, M.D. These included rehabilitation medicine (physical medicine and rehabilitation), palliative care, home care services (including hospice care and infusion therapy), subacute care, discharge planning, and long-term acute care (Grace Hospital). A main driver for the creation of this division was the recognition that, although consumers of post-acute care services accounted for about 25% of hospital discharges, they incurred 40% of hospital days with the attendant high costs. Another reason for combining these services was the similarity of Medicare reimbursement issues that affected them all, as the federal government continued to develop prospective payment systems to cover all services. Appropriate operation under these payment systems requires special administrative expertise, which Walsh had accumulated in setting up palliative care and hospice care under the Cancer Center, as discussed in the Taussig Cancer Center section of this chapter.

Rehabilitation Medicine merits special mention, having existed for many years as a department in the Division of Medicine. Recognizing the necessity of rehabilitation for continuity of care, the Clinic established a free-standing Institute of Rehabilitation Medicine in 1990. Vinod Sahgal, M.D., a respected neurologist and rehabilitation specialist, was recruited from Northwestern University Medical School to head the new program. The institute later became a department in the Division of Medicine and finally in the Division of Post-Acute Care in 2002. It is physically located at Euclid Hospital, a member of the Cleveland Clinic Health System. It now has 150 employees and collaborates with nearly every department in the Clinic. A measure of the department's excellence is the recent philanthropic funding and establishment of the Glickman Chair in Rehabilitation Medicine, currently held by Sahgal.

DIVISION OF CLINICAL RESEARCH

As previously noted (Chapter 10), the Board of Governors created the position of Chief Academic Officer in March 2001 and appointed Eric Topol, M.D., to this job. At the same time the Board established the Office of Clinical Research and made Rudick the head of it. In December 2002, the Board of Governors made this office a division and placed two departments (Biostatistics and Bioethics) into it.

In addition to the two departments, the new division contained three centers: (a) Integrative Medicine, headed by Joan Fox, Ph.D.; (b) the General Clinical Research Center (GCRC); and (c) Clinical Trials. The GCRC, as of this writing (2003) had $17 million of outside funding.

The Division of Clinical Research, the Division of Education (see Chapter 19), the Lerner Research Institute (see Chapter 20), and the Lerner College of Medicine (see Chapters 10 and 19) report to the Chief Academic Officer. Together, these constitute the "academic enterprise" of The Cleveland Clinic.

DIVISION OF REGIONAL MEDICAL PRACTICE

We have described this new division, created in 1995 and headed by Dr. David Bronson, in Chapter 10.

CONCLUSION

Each of the above entities brought together professionals from a variety of disciplines, often in a common setting but in some cases more dispersed, to address all aspects of an identified clinical problem. Group practice lends itself well to the creation and smooth operation of team approaches to medicine, and The Cleveland Clinic has been particularly successful in implementing this matrixed approach to health care delivery, research, and education.

16. DIVISION OF PATHOLOGY AND LABORATORY MEDICINE

By William R. Hart, M.D.

The fruit of healing grows on the tree of understanding.
Without diagnosis, there is no rational treatment.
—*Carl Gerhardt, Wurzburg, 1873*

DURING ITS LONG AND ILLUSTRIOUS HISTORY, THE CLEVELAND CLINIC'S Division of Pathology and Laboratory Medicine has undergone remarkable growth and development. Since 1992, the division has been consolidated into two departments: Anatomic Pathology and Clinical Pathology. The apparent simplicity of this structure belies the complexity of the division's specialty and subspecialty laboratories, which have routinely produced staggering amounts of laboratory data for diagnosis and treatment.

The Department of Anatomic Pathology provides diagnostic services based primarily on the gross and microscopic features of tissue and cellular samples obtained by biopsy, smear, surgery, or autopsy. The Department of Clinical Pathology is composed of six sections: Clinical Biochemistry, Clinical Microbiology, Hematopathology, Molecular and Immunopathology, Thrombosis and Hemostasis, and Transfusion Medicine. Also housed in the Division Office are Laboratory Information Systems, responsible for all computerization activities in the division, the Division Business Office, the Pathology Residency program, and The Cleveland Clinic Reference Laboratory.

Under the leadership of William R. Hart, M.D., who became

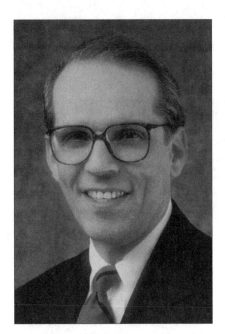

William R. Hart, M.D., Chairman,
Division of Pathology, 1992-

chairman in 1992, the division supports a highly specialized professional staff of about three dozen pathologists and clinical laboratory scientists, and a technical and clerical staff of about 540 employees. They perform nearly all laboratory testing for The Cleveland Clinic hospitals and clinics, as well as for the off-campus Family Health Centers and ambulatory surgery centers. By 2003, more than 5.5 million tests were reported annually, including more than 76,000 surgical pathology and 81,000 cytopathology cases. These volumes surely could not have been foreseen in 1921. At one time, the clinical laboratories were scattered in different buildings around the Clinic's campus, but in 1980, essentially all diagnostic anatomic and clinical pathology laboratories and offices were brought together in the 185,000 square-foot Laboratory Medicine Building.

Each of the five physicians who have occupied the position of division chairman has also held leadership roles in national and international organizations devoted to pathology and laboratory medicine. The first chair, Dr. J. Beach Hazard (1958-70), was President of the U.S. and Canadian Academy of Pathology (USCAP). Dr. Lawrence J. McCormack (1970-81) was President of the College of American Pathologists (CAP). Dr. George C. Hoffman (1981-86) was President of the American Society of Clinical Pathologists (ASCP). Dr. Thomas L. Gavan (1986-91) was President of the National Committee for Clinical Laboratory Standards (NCCLS) and a member of the Board of Directors of the CAP. Dr. William R. Hart (1992-present [2004]) was President of the International Society of Gynecological Pathologists, a member of the Board of Directors of ASCP, and a member of the Governing Councils of both the USCAP and the Association of Directors of Anatomic and Surgical Pathology (ADASP).

ANATOMIC PATHOLOGY

In the early days, Allen Graham, M.D., who joined the organization in 1928 as head of tissue pathology, provided the sole pathological support for Cleveland Clinic surgeons. Everyone respected him for his abilities as a diagnostician, teacher, and expert in diseases of the thyroid. Trained first as a surgeon, he was a valued consultant in the operating room. An acute observer, he was able to identify several abnormal conditions whose corresponding diseases were not described until many years later. He preferred to work alone, even doing his own photomicrography and developing his own prints and films. However, this often delayed pathology reports by months. Faced with a growing workload and unable to delegate, Graham became overwhelmed by his burden and left The Cleveland Clinic in 1943.

During the next few years, pathology services were supplied by Harry Goldblatt, M.D., an outstanding pathologist at the Western Reserve University School of Medicine. Routine activities within the department were carried out by Betty Haskell, one of the original technologists. Although Clinic surgeons felt the quality of pathology reports was excellent, they missed having the support of a pathologist in the operating room. Fortunately, several staff surgeons had become acquainted with a pathologist named John Beach Hazard, M.D., either through shared service during World War II or through Boston City Hospital. In 1946, Hazard joined the staff as head of the Department of Tissue Pathology. As part of the Division of Surgery, the department was located in a small area adjacent to the operating room where surgeons could freely seek consulta-

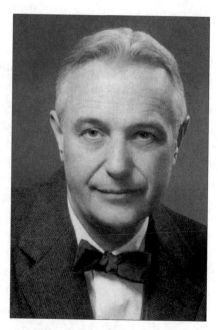

John Beach Hazard, M.D., Chairman, Division of Laboratory Medicine and Chief of Pathology, 1946-1970

tions. In the beginning, Hazard was the only physician in a department of technicians.

Hazard set about organizing his department with the enthusiasm and good will that characterized his leadership of 24 years. He made pathology come alive. Growth of the Clinic's hospital and surgical facilities eventually created a demand for additional pathologists. In 1951, Lawrence J. McCormack, M.D., joined Hazard. It was a good match, since Hazard specialized in diseases of the thyroid, and McCormack's interests encompassed diseases of the lung, kidney, bone, and brain, as well as the developing field of cytology. William A. Hawk, M.D., became the third member of the team in 1955, specializing in gastrointestinal and thyroid diseases. Surgical pathology activities continued to expand at a rapid pace. To ensure an orderly development in this rapidly growing specialty, the Division of Surgery relinquished the Department of Tissue Pathology. The Board of Governors created a new Division of Pathology in 1958 with Hazard as chairman. For the first time, the Division contained both anatomic pathology and the clinical laboratories.

McCormack took over as head of Tissue Pathology (later the Department of Anatomic Pathology) in 1968. Upon Hazard's retirement in 1970, he became chairman of the division, which he renamed the Division of Laboratory Medicine. In contrast to the mild-mannered Hazard, McCormack was an imposing figure with a booming voice. Residents shuddered at the prospect of incurring his wrath. In truth, he was a gentle soul at heart, and those who worked closely with him held him in affectionate esteem. Hawk became the anatomic pathology department chair. In the early part of that decade, Howard S. Levin, M.D., and Bruce A. Sebek, M.D., joined the staff. Their interests in the fields of genitourinary, endocrine, breast, and head and neck pathology expanded the department's growing expertise. These stalwart pathologists carried the bulk of the caseload themselves for years. The division added sections of dermatopathology and neuropathology to meet the needs of the growing departments of neurology, neurological surgery, and dermatology.

In 1981, William R. Hart, M.D., became the department chairman. McCormack had recruited him to the Clinic from the University of Michigan, where he was professor of pathology specializing in surgical pathology and gynecologic pathology, after stints at the Armed Forces Institute of Pathology and the University of Southern California-Los Angeles County Medical Center. Under his direction, growth of the department accelerated. New staff members (Norman B. Ratliff, M.D., Ralph T. Tuthill, M.D., Steven N. Becker, M.D., Thomas W. Bauer, M.D., Ph.D., Robert E. Petras, M.D., Melinda L. Estes, M.D., Charles V. Biscotti, M.D., Mark H. Stoler, M.D., and John R. Goldblum, M.D.) with subspecialty expertise were recruited from around the country to develop cytology, cardiovascular pathology, dermatopathology, gastrointestinal pathology, gynecologic pathology, hematopathology, hepatic pathology, nephropathology, neuropathology, orthopedic pathology, and soft-tissue pathology. James T. McMahon, Ph.D., expanded the use of diagnostic electron microscopy. Under the leadership of Raymond R. Tubbs, D.O., the department rapidly incorporated new technologies into the diagnostic armament, including immunohistochemistry, flow cytometry (pioneered a few years earlier in the Department of Immunopathology), DNA cell-cycle analysis, and morphometry. The addition of tissue-based molecular techniques and liquid-based thin-layer cytology helped keep the department at the forefront of technological advancement in anatomic pathology.

During the 1980s, the anatomic pathology department emerged as one of the strongest such departments in the country, specializing in diagnostic pathology and clinical research. Scientific publications from the staff coupled with high-visibility lectures at major educational conferences and leadership positions held in national and international pathology organizations established the department as a leader in academic pathology. The department also became one of the first fully computerized anatomic pathology facilities of its kind in the country.

In 1993, after Hart was appointed chairman of the renamed Division of Pathology and Laboratory Medicine, Robert E. Petras, M.D., was promoted to chairman of Anatomic Pathology. He had joined the staff after completing his residency training at the Clinic and had developed expertise in gastrointestinal pathology. Petras continued to build on the department's strengths, as the volume of surgical and cytology specimens exploded. He expanded the training of histotechnologists as physician extenders to enhance efficiency. Petras recruited additional staff pathologists (Jonathan L. Myles, M.D., Richard A. Prayson, M.D., Diana Fischler, M.D., Carol F. Farver, M.D., Terry L. Gramlich, M.D., Andrea E. Dawson, M.D., and Jennifer A. Brainard, M.D.) to bolster the subspecialty expertise of the staff. Petras also introduced "telepathology" to provide real-time consultation to off-site pathologists.

In early 2001, Petras resigned as chairman and Hart replaced him as acting chairman until John R. Goldblum, M.D., was appointed chairman in 2002. Goldblum, a prolific contributor to the surgical pathology literature, had established himself as an authority on soft-tissue tumors and gastrointestinal pathology

CLINICAL PATHOLOGY

The original clinical laboratories were designed by David Marine, M.D., who never occupied them. They opened in 1921 under the medical supervision of Henry J. John, M.D., a diabetologist with an interest in chemical analysis. After John left the Clinic in 1933, Russell L. Haden, M.D., head of the Division of Medicine, supervised the clinical laboratories for 10 years. He also organized and led a laboratory for the study of hematologic diseases in the Research Building while carrying a heavy clinical load as well. The various other clinical laboratories were also under Haden's direction, but technicians actually ran them.

Although Clinical Pathology was said to have been "inaugurated" in 1930,[1] it was not until 1944 that the Division of Medicine created a new Department of Clinical Pathology, and appointed Lemuel W. Diggs, M.D., to head it without formally designating him as chairman. The organization incorporated his ideas into the design of the modern laboratories in a new clinic building. After Diggs left in 1947, John W. King, M.D., Ph.D., became head of the department in 1950. King was a one-man faculty at first, but soon the department began to grow, with the additions of Drs. Adrian Hainline (1952), Willard Faulkner (1956), and Devina Tweed (1957). In order to ensure a steady supply of well-trained technologists, King also founded the School of Medical Technology (later to be designated the John Weaver King School of Medical Technology), which graduated hundreds of students.

In 1958, the Board of Governors transferred the Department of Clinical Pathology from the Division of Medicine and combined it with the Department of Tissue Pathology to form the new Division of Pathology with Hazard as chairman and King as vice chairman. Each of the clinical laboratory specialties was established as a separate department in 1970. This arrangement continued until Hart restructured the division in 1992. The Department of Clinical Pathology was then resurrected by combining the departments of biochemistry, blood banking, immunopathology, laboratory hematology, and microbiology into a single department where they became sections. John A. Washington, M.D., became the department chairman, a position he held until 1997, when health problems caused him to relinquish it. Raymond R. Tubbs, D.O., was then promoted to chair the department.

Section of Transfusion Medicine

The Clinic's Blood Bank, originally established by Diggs, came under King's direction in 1950. The Blood Bank prospered under his leadership, meeting the enormous need for blood required by the Clinic's expanding surgery program. Between 1975 and 1981, the Blood Bank resided administratively within the Department of Laboratory Hematology and Blood Banking. Following King's retirement, the Department of Blood Banking separated from Hematology in 1981, and Gerald A. Hoeltge, M.D., became its chairman. The demand for blood products escalated as the overall volume of cardiac surgical procedures rose and organ transplants became commonplace. The Clinic's Blood Bank has become the largest user of blood products supplied by the American Red Cross in the United States. With the divisional reorganization in 1992, Hoeltge became the head of the Section of Transfusion Medicine, which additionally included the growing intraoperative autotransfusion service and the cytogenetics laboratory.

Section of Clinical Biochemistry

King, who had originally established the Section of Biochemistry, later added an endocrine laboratory and named Adrian Hainline, M.D., as head. Charles E. Willis, M.D, a practicing general surgeon who had developed an interest in clinical chemistry and had a talent for working with automated machinery, replaced him in 1961. After Willis' retirement, Robert S. Galen, M.D., joined the Clinic in 1982 to head Biochemistry. Galen recruited several experienced staff Ph.D.s and developed a number of specialized functional sections: Quality Control, Lipids, Nutrition and Metabolic Diseases, Automated/Acute Care Chemistry, Applied Clinical Pharmacology, and Enzymology. He introduced automated instrumentation capable of handling high volumes of routine as well as specialized chemical analyses, and these became the laboratory standard. Galen left in 1988, and Frederick Van Lente, Ph.D., a clinical biochemist the former had appointed to head the automated and acute care laboratories, replaced him. Van Lente later became vice chairman of the Department of Clinical Pathology under Tubbs in 1997. He further advanced laboratory automation, culminating in the installation of a robotic modular automation laboratory system in late 2000. Point-of-care testing, a burgeoning activity throughout the Clinic, also came under Van Lente's supervision.

Section of Hematopathology

George C. Hoffman, M.D., became head of the hematology section in 1959 after a two-year fellowship in clinical pathology at the Clinic. For many years, the hematology laboratory (called Special Hematology) was Hoffman's domain alone. Five colleagues eventually joined him, each specializing in different hematologic diseases. The andrology laboratory initially found its home there. Hoffman was named division chairman in 1981 and recruited Ralph G. Green, M.D., from the Scripps Clinic, who succeeded him as head of laboratory hematology in 1983. Green's research focused on Vitamin B_{12} metabolism. Andrew J. Fishleder, M.D., who later became the chairman of the Division of Education, introduced molecular techniques for the diagnosis of hematologic and lymphoid diseases.

Green served until 1993, when he returned to California and was replaced by Michael L. Miller, D.O., a former fellow in laboratory hematology and member of the staff. He incorporated the reporting of lymphomas and related conditions, previously done in Anatomic Pathology, into the section and renamed it the Section of

Hematopathology. Eric Hsi, M.D., recently recruited from the Loyola University faculty and medical director of the flow cytometry laboratory, was promoted to section head in 1999 when Miller left. Research into various lymphoid diseases expanded under his leadership. Dr. Karl S. Thiel arrived from Ohio State University and also took over as director of the Stem Cell Laboratory for bone marrow transplantation. After more than a decade of research and development of sophisticated coagulation assays, the division created a new Section of Hemostasis and Thrombosis in 2001. Kandice Kottke-Marchant became its first section head.

Section of Clinical Microbiology

King, who also had a doctorate in microbiology, established the bacteriology and serology laboratory when he became head of clinical pathology. He led this informal section, along with the blood bank, until 1961 when Donald A. Senhauser, M.D., took over the microbiology laboratory. Senhauser introduced new immunologic techniques. When Senhauser left the Clinic three years later, Thomas L. Gavan, M.D., joined the staff as a clinical pathologist in microbiology and later became chairman of the Department of Microbiology in 1970. Gavan loved calculators and computers, which were just then coming into use around the laboratory, and he soon established himself as the laboratory's resident consultant for any issues that arose with these new-fangled devices. He took pride in his ability to calculate chi-square from a two-by-two contingency table on a hand-held calculator faster than anybody else. The department incorporated the bacteriology and serology laboratory. As the scope of microbiology expanded, Gavan recruited additional staff to head anaerobic microbiology, parasitology, mycobacteriology, mycology, and clinical virology. Under his direction, the staff actively pursued interests in computerization, automation, and antibiotic susceptibility testing, and the laboratory established a national reputation.

Following Gavan's appointment as division chairman in 1986, John A. Washington, M.D., was recruited from the Mayo Clinic to head Microbiology. Washington, an acknowledged authority in microbiology before joining the Clinic, expanded the laboratory's activities and continued his highly-regarded microbiology fellowship program. The virology laboratory, directed initially by Max R. Proffitt, Ph.D., and later by Belinda Yen-Lieberman, Ph.D., became a leader in the development and use of molecular techniques for the identification of viruses, most notably the human immunodeficiency virus (HIV). Geraldine S. Hall, Ph.D., focused her activities in mycobacteriology and mycology, while Isobel Rutherford, M.D., took responsibility for parasitology and serology. Washington continued as microbiology section head after being appointed chairman of Clinical Pathology in 1992, until his retirement in 1998. Gary W. Procop, M.D., trained in microbiology at the Mayo Clinic, replaced him as section head. Procop's broad-based training in anatomic pathology as well as clinical pathology led to increased collaborative clinical and research activities with his colleagues in molecular pathology, cytology, and surgical pathology. He became a strong advocate for the transformation of the specialty into molecular microbiology.

Section of Molecular and Immunopathology

In 1964, McCormack established a Department of Immunopathology with Sharad D. Deodhar, M.D., Ph.D., as head. Deodhar, originally from India, had received his training at Western Reserve University and was a protégé of Harry Goldblatt. Deodhar, himself a fine tennis player, was the son of one of India's most famous cricket players. The senior Deodhar had been immortalized on an Indian postage stamp, which his son was fond of displaying when the opportunity arose. He led the laboratory from its inception until his retirement in 1993. Under his guidance, the Clinic became a national leader in the field of immunopathology. With the assistance of John D. Clough, M.D., William E. Braun, M.D., Manjula K. Gupta, Ph.D., Barbara Barna, Ph.D., and Rafael Valenzuela, M.D., the laboratory developed expertise in the functional aspects of the immune system, cellular immunity, endocrine immunology, autoimmunity, and cancer immunology. Deodhar instituted the histocompatibility laboratory under Braun's direction for the organ transplantation program. He also started the flow cytometry program under the leadership of Valenzuela. Raymond R. Tubbs, D.O., a member of the anatomic pathology staff and a former fellow in immunopathology, succeeded Deodhar. Tubbs recognized the looming importance of molecular techniques in the laboratory and accepted Hart's challenge to spearhead the development of molecular pathology for the entire division. The section was renamed the Section of Molecular and Immunopathology, and Ilka Warshawsky, M.D., Ph.D., was recruited to expand the menu of molecular assays. In 1998, Tubbs succeeded Washington as chairman of the Department of Clinical Pathology and continued his role as section head.

THE CLEVELAND CLINIC REFERENCE LABORATORY

When The Cleveland Clinic built the Laboratory Medicine Building in 1980, McCormack began a regional laboratory to provide high-quality, cost-effective laboratory services to the community. In 1989, Gavan formed the Reference Laboratory by partnering the Regional Laboratory with an expanding reference laboratory developed at the University of Utah. The intent of the joint venture was to provide esoteric clinical laboratory testing to hospitals and institutions

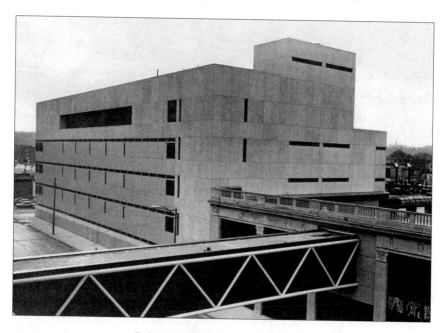

Laboratory Medicine Building, 1980

within a six-state area. Gavan appointed Washington as medical director. The growth of the partnership business, however, was slow and did not meet expectations.

In 1994, Hart developed a new business plan calling for dissolution of the partnership and the creation of an independent Cleveland Clinic Reference Laboratory. The Board of Governors enthusiastically adopted the plan. Hart became the Medical Director. He quickly developed an infrastructure, including sales and marketing, couriers, account representatives, a client services center, and a business office with computerized billing capabilities. The Cleveland Clinic Reference Laboratory (CCRL) eventually became the major provider of esoteric clinical laboratory testing for the hospitals of northeast Ohio and also has clients outside the region, as well as in nearby states. In addition, the CCRL provided surgical pathology and cytology services to physician offices and second-opinion consultations in anatomic pathology to hundreds of clinicians and pathologists throughout the country. Couriers drive about 300,000 miles annually to pick up and deliver specimens for testing.

LABORATORY INFORMATION SYSTEMS

Over the years, the laboratory became a major generator of data for the medical record. As the Clinic expanded, the volume of laboratory data eventually threatened to overcome routine systems for ordering laboratory tests and distributing results to the treating physicians. Under McCormack's leadership as division chairman, the arduous task of planning for the systematic computerization of the clinical pathology laboratories began. The microbiology laboratory was the first to be computerized, followed by anatomic pathology, the blood bank, the histocompatibility laboratory, and the acute care laboratory.

In 1984, McCormack recruited David Chou, M.D., a clinical pathologist and informatics specialist, to implement an innovative, one-of-a-kind general laboratory computer system developed by Kone, a Finnish company. Chou was named Director of Laboratory Information Systems (LIS) upon McCormack's retirement the following year. Chou successfully managed and maintained the system despite its being orphaned by the company that had developed it. He also implemented a computer system for the Reference Laboratory. In

1995, Chou replaced the general laboratory system with a more comprehensive and sophisticated computer system that incorporated the previously independent microbiology and blood bank systems and interfaced with the newly installed hospital information system, thereby allowing direct order-entry of clinical laboratory tests.

The anatomic pathology system, which remained as a standalone system, was also interfaced with the hospital information system. Since then, all clinical pathology and anatomic pathology reports have been electronically available to the entire medical staff, regardless of their location in the hospital, clinic, or off-site family health centers. Walter H. Henricks, M.D., replaced Chou as LIS director in 1997. He expanded the LIS, implemented electronic interfaces with numerous Reference Laboratory client hospitals, and upgraded both the clinical pathology and the anatomic pathology computer systems to client-server, graphical-user-interface platforms.

CONCLUSION

The Division of Pathology and Laboratory Medicine developed from small disparate laboratories in the medical and surgical divisions into an integral component of the Clinic and one of the largest clinical laboratories in the country. Analytic methods have evolved from simple chemical reactions to complex molecular studies. Diagnoses previously based solely on light microscopy have been enhanced by sophisticated adjunctive techniques. The division has responded to the challenges of a rapidly changing medical environment by increasing subspecialization of its staff, adopting modern automation systems, maximizing computerization, and continually implementing innovative strategies to stay at the forefront of diagnostic medicine. Clinical research and development by the staff have kept the division in the vanguard of pathology and laboratory medicine. The division has always been dedicated to providing accurate diagnoses and timely test results for physicians and their patients within and beyond The Cleveland Clinic.

---

[1] Rowland, Amy. The Cleveland Clinic Foundation. 1938, p 58.

17. DIVISION OF RADIOLOGY

By George H. Belhobek

Beware lest you lose the substance by grasping at the shadow.
—*Aesop, Sixth Century B.C.(?)*

WHEN THE CLEVELAND CLINIC FIRST OPENED, RADIOLOGY WAS A RELATIVELY young medical specialty. At least one of the founders of The Cleveland Clinic had reason to believe that good diagnostic radiology was essential to the practice of medicine. In 1902, when Crile was still operating at St. Alexis Hospital (known in its later years as St. Michael Hospital), one of the trustees of the hospital woke up at midnight, choking, and felt certain that he had swallowed his lower denture. For an hour and a half he clawed at his throat, mistaking the hyoid bone for the missing teeth. He succeeded in so traumatizing the throat that he could no longer swallow, even his saliva. A roentgenogram was made (this was only seven years after Roentgen's discovery of the x-ray), and the film showed some calcifications in the aortic arch which were interpreted as being the missing teeth. The patient was by this time in serious condition as a result of his own and his physicians' attempt to locate and remove the teeth. Finally Crile was called and was prevailed upon to operate.

Shortly after the operation the teeth were found in an obscure corner of the patient's room. The next day the patient died, and the story hit the headlines throughout the country: "Death Due to Operation. Patient Who Didn't Swallow His Teeth Is Dead." Crile in his autobiography summarized the diagnostic problem as follows:

"The positive statement of an intelligent man, a benefactor of the hospital, one whom we had known for a long period, that

279

he had not only swallowed his teeth but that he had touched them a number of times with his fingers and at one time had almost succeeded in removing them; the firm belief of his doctor, a physician of wide experience, that the teeth were still in the throat; the statements of the family that the teeth were not in the room, and their reiterant belief that the teeth had been swallowed; the rapid increase and gravity of the symptoms of the patient during the first day, seemingly out of proportion to the exploratory traumatism; and lastly the positive x-ray diagnosis, overruled our negative findings at the exploration. In consultation the various doctors who had been interested agreed that an operation was indicated."

The founders selected Bernard H. Nichols, M.D., to be the first head of the Department of Radiology, which was positioned in the Division of Medicine. This choice was a singularly fortunate one, for Nichols was one of the country's pioneers in diagnostic radiology. He practiced medicine first in Youngstown, Ohio. He then moved to White Hospital (now Robinson Memorial Hospital) in Ravenna, Ohio. There he met Bunts, Crile, and Lower, who were also on the staff and often operated there. Nichols became interested in radiology when a Ravenna manufacturing company began making x-ray machines of the primitive hand-cranked variety and one of these machines was put at his disposal.

Nichols entered the Army Medical Corps during World War I and, after completing a course in bone pathology, served as a radiologist. With this background, he joined the staff as a specialist in radiology in 1921. Over the next 15 years, he wrote 50 papers on diagnostic radiology, 23 of which concerned the diagnosis of diseases of the genitourinary tract. Energy, honesty, and an amused affection for people combined to make him a popular member of the staff. He had a goatee that gave him such a distinguished air that he was commonly referred to as the "Duke of Ravenna," the town in which he lived.

In 1922, the Department of Radiology was strengthened by the appointment of U. V. Portmann, M.D., as director of radiation therapy and by the purchase of the Cleveland area's first 250,000-volt radiation therapy machine. Tall, massively built, handsome, and somewhat intimidating, Portmann generated confidence. He soon became a national figure in radiotherapy, writing as extensively as Nichols did, chiefly on the measurement of radiation dosage and its use in treating cancers of the thyroid and breast. He also wrote a widely read textbook on radiotherapy.

A third pioneer in radiology, Otto Glasser, Ph.D., was a biophysicist and a member of the Research Division. He was described by a colleague as "a giant radiation physicist." Glasser first formulated the concept of a condenser dosimeter for measuring the amount of radiation delivered by a diagnostic or therapeutic radiation device. This instrument was used for calibrating x-ray equipment, a safety measure for the patient and medical personnel. Previously, radiothera-

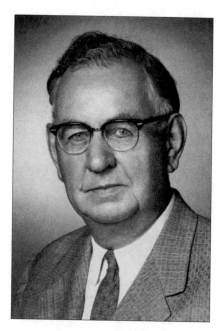

Otto Glasser, Ph.D., Head, Department of Biophysics, 1923-1964

pists estimated the dosage on the basis of reaction of the skin, the amount of radiation required to redden the skin being considered to be an "erythema dose." Glasser's concept was implemented by the Clinic's brilliant engineer, Mr. Valentine Seitz, who constructed a practical unit that Portmann used clinically. Thus, the talents of a radiotherapist, a biophysicist, and an engineer were combined to produce one of the fundamental advances in radiology. A prototype of the dosimeter is in the collection of scientific discoveries in the Smithsonian Institution.

Glasser was responsible for control of the radon (radium) seeds used in the treatment of certain types of cancers. He was also a prolific writer of scientific papers and editor of a massive three-volume work entitled *Medical Physics*. In addition, he wrote a definitive biography of Wilhelm Conrad Roentgen, the man who discovered the x-ray in 1895. Later in his career, Glasser's interest turned to radioactive isotopes, and again he made important contributions. He was urbane but not pretentious, and he was kindly and considerate to all, relating to those of modest station in life as easily and sincerely as to those of exalted status. His human qualities matched his scientific achievements.

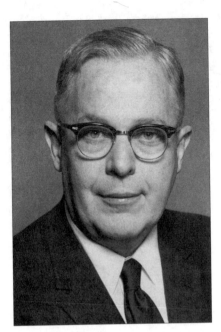

C. Robert Hughes, M.D., Chairman, Division of Radiology, 1960-1969

C. Robert Hughes, M.D., became head of the Department of Radiology in 1946. Hughes had trained in surgery before his interests changed to radiology, and this clinical background, combined with his technical knowledge, gave him insights valued by both internists and surgeons, who consulted him frequently about problem patients.

Hughes was a born planner and inventor whose talents were not confined to medicine. At the time of his appointment, the Clinic was on the threshold of an explosion in growth, and Hughes, working with Charles L. Hartsock, M.D., of the Department of Internal Medicine, designed a new and innovative x-ray department. Hughes wanted original ideas to supplement proven concepts, so the two planners came up with a unique department design that served efficiently for many years with little modification—a great accomplishment in an ever-changing field. The Department of Radiology was originally confined to the Clinic Building. Only "portable" equipment was used in the hospital, at the bedside, or during operations. An additional radiology facility was opened in the hospital in 1947. Surgical operations were becoming more complex, and often it was desirable to obtain intraoperative radiological examinations, and so x-ray facilities were included in many of the operating rooms when a new surgical pavilion was built in 1955.

In 1960, the Board of Governors established a Division of Radiology, removing Radiology from the Division of Medicine. Hughes was appointed to head this new division. In 1966, the Board further subdivided the Division of Radiology into a Department of Hospital Radiology, including radiology performed in the operating pavilion, a Department of Clinic Radiology, and a Department of Therapeutic Radiology and Isotopes.

At this time, the Board of Governors appointed Thomas F. Meaney, M.D., a former radiology fellow under Hughes, to chair the Division of Radiology and manage the hospital department, with Hughes taking responsibility for the clinic department, and Antonio R. Antunez, M.D., chairing therapeutic radiology and nuclear medicine. Hughes continued as clinic department chairman until 1970 when he was replaced by Anthony F. Lalli, M.D. George H. Belhobek, M.D., assumed the responsibility of chairman of the Department of Clinic Radiology in 1983. Meaney turned the hospital department chair over to Ralph J. Alfidi, M.D., in 1970 and continued on as division chairman until 1987. Gregory P. Borkowski, M.D., was appointed chairman of the Department of Hospital Radiology in 1985. With the retirement of Belhobek as clinic chairman in 2002, the hospital and clinic departments were combined into a single Department of Diagnostic Radiology. Borkowski assumed responsibility for this unit.

Meaney, an innovative young man with great vision, became division chairman coincident with tremendous advances in x-ray technology and practice. He had already achieved recognition for his work with the newly developed procedure of angiography, a technique with which he had become familiar during a sabbatical leave in Sweden in 1963. Over the next several years, Meaney was instrumental in developing angiographic and interventional procedures for use not only at The Cleveland Clinic but across the nation. His collaborative work with Harriet Dustan, M.D., in the Department of Hypertension and Nephrology and Lawrence McCormack, M.D., in the Department of Tissue Pathology in the mid-1960s yielded multiple publications outlining the role of renal vascular disease in hypertension.

Over the next 35 years, radiologists expanded their arsenal of interventional procedures to include biliary drainage, abscess drainage, tumor embolization and clot lysis, venous access procedures, and percutaneous lung, kidney, and bone biopsies. Thus, radiologists emerged with an active role in patient treatment as well as diagnosis.

DIAGNOSTIC RADIOLOGY

In 1972, Meaney visited England to evaluate a new device that was capable of directly imaging pathology of the brain in a cross-sectional display. The technique, computerized axial tomography (CAT), was just being introduced to the world at that time. Seeing its great promise, Meaney purchased the fourth such device in the world for the Clinic. This original machine, which was limited to scanning the brain, quickly had a profound effect on the practice of neurology and neurosurgery. Ten months later, a computed axial tomography (CAT) scanner (now referred to as a CT scanner) designed for body imaging was installed at the Clinic, greatly increasing the scope of this technology. Numerous generations of CT scanners have been developed since that time, with the latest technology providing images of very thin tissue thickness obtained with sub-second imaging times. Current machines also provide sophisticated multi-planar reconstruction capabilities.

Digital subtraction angiography was the next innovative technology to hold a primary research focus in the Division of Radiology during Meaney's tenure. This computerized technology allowed individual arteries to be visualized with a generalized injection of intravenous water-soluble contrast material, thereby decreasing the need for the more invasive catheter arteriography in some cases.

Meaney brought a third technological breakthrough to The Cleveland Clinic in the early 1980s. Nuclear magnetic resonance imaging, later called magnetic resonance imaging (MRI), was first used to examine internal organs in 1973. Although the development of this technique was slow, by the early 1980s, recognition was growing that this non-invasive means of visualizing internal organs without exposure to the ionizing radiation characteristic of x-ray-based techniques would have great promise in examining the tissues of the body, especially the brain and spinal and musculoskeletal structures. Meaney once again recognized the potential value of an emerging technology and purchased a unit for the Clinic in 1983. The Cleveland Clinic's Department of Diagnostic Radiology led the way in developing this major imaging technology.

A corollary of the dramatic growth of radiology activities in the 1970s and 1980s was the need to enlarge the physical facilities of the diagnostic radiology departments. In 1974, the Hospital Radiology Department moved from the eighth floor of the original hospital to a vastly expanded facility in the basement of the new hospital building. Further expansion of radiology facilities came with the development of an outpatient radiology facility in the Crile Building, which opened

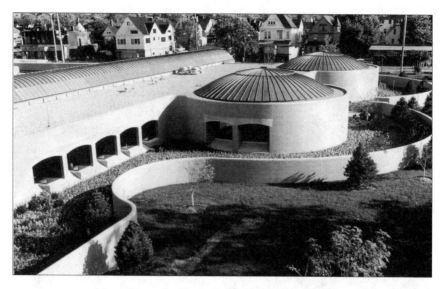

Meyer Center for Magnetic Resonance Imaging, 1983

in 1985. A philanthropic gift from Mr. E. Tom Meyer (president of The Cleveland Clinic Foundation from 1969 to 1972) enabled the construction of the Meyer Center for Magnetic Resonance Imaging in 1983, a building constructed without the use of iron-containing materials (such as steel nails), designed to house the Clinic's magnetic resonance scanners. The department installed plain radiographic, CT scanning, and ultrasound capabilities in the expanded emergency department facility that opened in 1994.

Following Meaney's retirement in 1987, the Board of Governors convened a search committee to identify a new division chairman. After an intensive review of nationally known candidates, the Board selected Michael T. Modic, M.D., a former resident in diagnostic radiology at the Clinic, to fill this important position. Modic, a neuroradiologist, was well known for his MRI research, especially for its application to diseases of the spine. He had a reputation for clear, decisive thinking. He enthusiastically accepted the challenges of maintaining The Cleveland Clinic's leading position in diagnostic imaging and of supporting a research-friendly environment while providing excellent clinical care and educational opportunities. With a growing staff of subspecialty-oriented diagnostic radiologists, Modic forged ahead into the 1990s.

New challenges soon arose, however. While the traditional goals

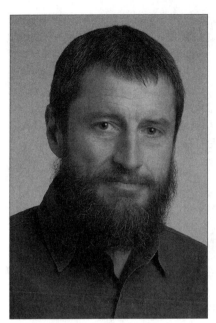

Michael T. Modic, M.D., Chairman,
Division of Radiology, 1989-

of excellent patient care, productive research, and effective education were still considered high priorities, stricter control of operational costs also became increasingly important. The addition of eight off-campus family health center radiology facilities, along with management and professional staffing responsibilities for five Cleveland Clinic Health System community hospital radiology departments, further increased demands on the Division of Radiology. In 2002, the division added a Department of Regional Radiology to coordinate and direct the activities of these off-campus facilities. Gregory Baran, M.D., assumed leadership for this new department. Modic also agreed to oversee the operations of the two Cleveland Clinic Florida hospital radiology departments.

Modic recognized that traditional radiology practice had to be reevaluated and that new practice methods, including electronic transfer of digital-based images, voice recognition transcription, and filmless radiography (digital or computed radiography), needed to be considered. He initiated soft-copy interpretation of CT, MR, and ultrasound images on workstations and developed plans for progressive installation of digital or computed radiography units in various departments. The conversion to digital-based imaging processes would not only improve the operational efficiency of each department, but also eliminate significant film purchase costs.

Electronic image transfer capabilities would also lead to new radiology ventures, such as contractual arrangements to interpret examinations performed at independent imaging centers across the country. The growth and success of these operations necessitated the development of an additional department in the radiology division (eRadiology). Dr. Michael Recht assumed leadership of this business unit. The demands of modern practice would also require more plain hard work. The division was ready to accept these challenges and move ahead.

RADIATION ONCOLOGY

After Portmann's retirement, several radiologists led the radiation therapy activities within the Department of Radiology until Antunez was appointed chairman of the Department of Therapeutic Radiology and Nuclear Medicine in 1963. Like Meaney, Antunez was a builder. As in the case of diagnostic radiology, radiation physicists and engineers were developing new equipment, and Antunez acquired the latest equipment, sometimes raising funds to pay for new devices by personally attracting large gifts from philanthropists and grateful patients.

Antunez' department acquired a modern cobalt therapy unit and high-voltage linear accelerators. He obtained computers for treatment planning and a simulating device to permit calculation of the maximal dose delivery to the desired location. He also arranged for the Lewis Research Laboratories of the National Aeronautics and Space Administration to make their Cleveland cyclotron available for neutron beam treatment of Clinic patients. In 1991, a major expansion of radiation therapy space became necessary to keep up with increasing practice demands.

Two chairmen (Frank Thomas, M.D., and Melvin Tefft, M.D.) each led the department for brief periods after Antunez' departure.

In 1993, shortly after the arrival of the present department chairman, Roger Macklis, M.D., radiation therapy was moved administratively from the Division of Radiology into the Cleveland Clinic Cancer Center. Radiation oncologists and medical oncologists had long been combining their talents to provide effective treatment protocols for the Clinic's cancer patients. The positioning of these two groups within the Cancer Center further strengthened this working relationship. With the recruitment of Macklis from the Harvard Joint Center for Radiation Therapy, the renamed Department of Radiation Oncology began another expansion phase. By 1995, it had become the largest and most technically sophisticated clinical radiation therapy department in Ohio, treating over 2,500 patients a year at the main campus and satellite sites. New personnel, new equipment, and a new clinical and research pavilion constructed at the corner of Euclid Avenue and East 90th Street added to the department's momentum.

NUCLEAR MEDICINE (MOLECULAR AND FUNCTIONAL IMAGING)

The use of radioactive iodine in treating thyroid disease had interested Glasser, who headed the Department of Bio-Physics in the early days, prior to the formal establishment of the Division of Radiology. With his knowledge of physics and the technical skills of Mr. Barney Tautkins, a hand-constructed rectilinear scanner for imaging the thyroid gland following the uptake of radioactive iodine was developed. The device worked well, and thus isotope imaging studies at The Cleveland Clinic began. A physician was needed to interpret these scans, and since the Radiation Therapy Department was near the scanner, this responsibility naturally fell to the department's staff.

Eventually the gamma camera replaced the slower rectilinear scanning devices, and a multitude of radioisotopes useful for organ imaging were developed. The scope of nuclear medicine was rapidly increasing so that in 1978 a separate Department of Nuclear Medicine was created within the Division of Radiology. Sebastian A. Cook, M.D., became its first chairman.

Raymundo Go, M.D., succeeded Cook as chairman in 1983, a position he held until 2000. During his tenure, Dr. Go added the sophisticated computerized technology necessary for the practice of modern nuclear medicine. Under the direction of W. James MacIntyre, Ph.D., an internationally respected authority on nuclear instrumentation, the department embarked on investigations of cardiac radionuclide imaging and positron emission tomography (PET) imaging techniques.

Following Go's retirement, Dr. Jean Luc Urbain was recruited to chair the department. He brought to The Cleveland Clinic, among other things, a fine reputation for innovative research. He soon instituted additional nuclear medicine capabilities, such as second-generation single-photon emission computed tomography (SPECT) scanning and gene-expression imaging techniques. The department changed its name to Molecular and Functional Imaging to reflect the new dimensions of the specialty. Subsequent to Urbain's resignation in June 2003, the search for a new chairman began.

CONCLUSION

Nichols, Portmann, and Glasser would be amazed that from their small beginnings the Division of Radiology has grown to include 74 staff physicians, six physicists, two computer scientists, 19 informatics personnel, and 359 employees who support their work. They have achieved many significant accomplishments over the years, and many accolades have been bestowed on individual staff members. Under Modic's leadership, the Division of Radiology is shaping itself to meet the challenges of the future. We expect that the next 80 years will be as productive and promising as the previous 80 have been.

18. DIVISION OF NURSING

BY SANDRA S. SHUMWAY

I enjoy convalescence. It is the part
that makes the illness worth while.
—*George Bernard Shaw, 1921*

THROUGHOUT THE HISTORY OF THE CLEVELAND CLINIC, THE IMPORTANCE OF nursing in providing "better care of the sick" has always been recognized. It is universally acknowledged that the dedication, professionalism, and compassion of Cleveland Clinic nurses have played a key role in making it one of the world's leading health care institutions. Nursing, like all health care professions, has changed drastically over the years as a result of advances in medical technique and technology as well as changes in the way health care is financed. Florence Nightingale could never have foreseen many of the duties and programs undertaken today by Cleveland Clinic nursing personnel.

IN THE BEGINNING

The Cleveland Clinic opened in 1921 with four clinic nurses on staff. Secretaries at the Clinic took care of many of the clerical functions usually handled by a doctor's office nurse in private practice. The 184-bed hospital, which opened in 1924, had a nursing staff of 75, which included seven head nurses, 42 general-duty nurses, and four operating room nurses. Graduate (i.e., registered) nurses, assisted by orderlies and ward maids, provided all direct patient care. For many years, private-duty nurses, who contracted directly with patients, supplemented the hospital nursing staff. At first, nurses were mostly white women. This began to change slowly in the 1950s, gaining momentum thereafter, as racial and ethnic minorities (especially African Americans) and men appeared in larger numbers in registered nurse, nursing unit assistant, and patient care assistant positions.

The position of the ward maid eventually evolved into that of the nursing unit assistant (NUA). The Clinic added floor hostesses, the precursors of unit secretaries, in 1947. The hospital hired the first practical nurses in 1954, and five years later there were as many practical nurses as general duty registered nurses on the hospital staff. The ambulatory nursing staff also added practical nurses in the 1950s. The hospital added patient care assistants (a new title) in 1977. These were nursing assistants who received additional training to assist the nurse with patient care at the bedside.

With a nurse-superintendent supervising all departments in the hospital, nursing was represented at the highest level of hospital administration. However, when long-time superintendent Abbie Porter, R.N., retired in 1949 and was replaced by hospital administrator James Harding (not a nurse), the heads of the nursing and operating room departments became the Clinic's highest-ranking nurses. In 1970, the Clinic decentralized the Department of Nursing into seven areas headed by directors, leaving the hospital without a unified nursing department.

THE DANIELSEN ERA, 1981-1986

This situation lasted until 1981, when the Board of Governors reunified nursing activities under the leadership of Sharon L. Danielsen, M.S.N., R.N. The new Department of Nursing encompassed operating-room nursing as well as nursing education and nurse recruitment. Within the next few years, Danielsen organized the department according to a clinically oriented scheme.

By 1985, the department consisted of three clinical divisions—surgical nursing, medical nursing, and operating room and treatment areas—and a support division called nursing resources. The number of nursing personnel had risen to 150 in the outpatient departments and 1,725 in the hospital. They attended to more than 400 patients daily in the operating rooms and treatment areas alone. Increasing numbers of nurses were breaking with traditional roles and practicing as clinical nurse specialists or departmental assistants in outpatient medical departments. Certified registered nurse anesthetists (CRNAs) worked outside the Department of Nursing. From the first, they had administered all anesthetics at the Foundation until a physician-headed Department of Anesthesiology came into being in 1946. Nurse anesthesia was never phased out as it was in many hospitals after World War II, and the Clinic established a school for nurse anesthetists in 1969.

Danielsen met regularly with the four division heads, the director of program planning, and the fiscal coordinator as the nursing administrative group to make decisions about nursing policy and practice. Surgical nursing was headed by Linda J. Lewicki, M.S.N., R.N.; Medical Nursing by Francine Wojton, M.S.N., R.N.; operating room and treatment areas by Isabelle Boland, M.S.N., R.N.; nursing resources by Shirley Moore, M.S., R.N.; and program planning by Sandra S. Shumway, M.S.N., R.N.

The next year was a busy one for nursing as the hospital's new wing opened in January 1986. Several older inpatient units in the original hospital building underwent a phased transfer to the new building. The first unit in the new building to open was G80. The new wing, part of the Century Project (see chapter 8), added needed beds to the hospital especially in the cardiac area. The census at this time ranged from 750 to 800.

Danielsen left the Foundation in July 1986. Isabelle Boland, head of the operating room and treatment areas, served as acting head of nursing during a nationwide search for a new director.

THE COULTER ERA, 1987-1997

Sharon J. Coulter, M.S.N., M.B.A., R.N., was chosen for the position and assumed her duties in May 1987. The Board of Governors immediately approved her request for divisional status for nursing. The new Division of Nursing encompassed all inpatient facilities, surgical services, and the emergency department. It did not, however, include clinic nursing or departmental assistants.

Coulter reorganized the administrative structure of nursing to reduce its management hierarchy to three levels: head nurse, clinical director, and division chairperson. She retained nursing operations managers (similar to nursing supervisors) and assistant head nurses to handle administrative and managerial responsibilities on the off-shifts. She also streamlined the department of nursing resources and the operating room nursing structure. She focused quality management efforts at the unit level. Her team annually identified and tracked quality indicators to keep practice standards high. She also initiated patient satisfaction efforts.

By 1988, Coulter chaired the nursing management group (successor to the nursing administrative group and predecessor of the nursing executive council), which included the clinical directors for medical nursing, neurosurgery/orthopedics/otolaryngology nursing, critical care nursing, surgical nursing, operating room nursing, cardiac nursing, and the support department directors for physical and environmental resources, nursing research, and nursing education, the fiscal coordinator, and the assistant to the chairman. Clinical directors for oncology and critical care nursing were added in 1989 and 1991.

By 1988, the nursing management group had the following membership: Coulter as chair; clinical directors Mary Ann Brown, M.S.N., R.N. (medical nursing), Cathy M. Ceccio, M.S.N., R.N. (neuro/ortho/ENT nursing), Angela Janik, M.S.N., R.N. (critical care), Linda Lewicki, M.S.N., R.N. (surgical nursing), Marian K. Shaughnessy, M.S.N., R.N. (operating room nursing), and Gayle Whitman, M.S.N., R.N. (cardiac nursing); support department directors Kathleen Lawson, B.S., R.N. (physical and environmental resources), Deborah M. Nadzam, Ph.D., R.N. (nursing research), and Elizabeth Vasquez, M.S.N., R.N. (nursing education); and two staff, Amy Caslow Maynard (fiscal coordinator) and Sandra S. Shumway, now assistant to the chairman. Meri Beckham (Armour), M.S.N., R.N., was named clinical director of oncology in 1989. Marlene Donnelly, M.B.A., R.N., was named director, center for nursing, in 1990. Madeline Soupios, R.N.C., served as acting director of critical care nursing for most of 1991 until a permanent director,

Deborah Peeler (Charnley), M.N., R.N., was hired.

Coulter subsequently modified the basic table of organization. By 1993, the Division of Nursing had six departments: medical/surgical nursing, cardiothoracic nursing, critical care nursing, surgical services, the center for nursing (which included nurse recruitment and retention, nursing education, quality management, staffing and scheduling, nursing operations managers, and information systems), and nursing research. At that time, medical/surgical nursing was headed by Armour, cardiothoracic nursing by Whitman, critical care nursing by Charnley, surgical services by Betty Bush, M.B.A., R.N., the center for nursing by Donnelly, and nursing research by Christine Wynd, Ph.D., R.N. To top it off, in 1993 the Division of Nursing broadened its scope, adding the pharmacy and the patient support services operations department. At the same time, the division changed its name from the Division of Nursing to the Division of Patient Care Operations.

In May 1994, the Clinic opened a new Emergency Department (see chapter 9). It included a clinical decision unit designed for observation of selected patients to determine the need for hospitalization. Also in 1994, a new palliative care service opened in the hospital, and plans were afoot to open an obstetrical service. This occurred in May 1995, after a 28-year hiatus. Staffing efforts were successful during this period because of a large local and regional supply of nurses. In 1994 the vacancy rate was just 4.2% at The Cleveland Clinic, while nationally it was 5%.

By 1996, the Division of Nursing had three vice-chairs for nursing (two for clinical units and one for surgical services), 25 unit directors, 69 unit clinical coordinators (formerly head nurses), and ten managers in surgical services.

In 1997, Coulter left the Clinic. Sandra Shumway was appointed interim chair from September 1997 through March 1998. At this same time, the Division of Nursing's reporting structure moved from the Division of Operations, directed by Frank Lordeman, to the Office of Medical Operations, directed by Dr. Robert Kay, soon to become Chief of Staff. The structure of the division reverted to the old Division of Nursing, and the pharmacy, itself becoming upgraded, administratively separated from nursing. Kay immediately initiated a search for a new division chair.

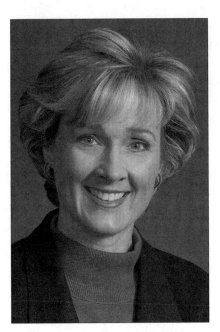

Shawn M. Ulreich, M.S.N., R.N.,
Chairwoman, Division of Nursing,
1998-2003

THE ULREICH ERA, 1998-2003

Shawn M. Ulreich, M.S.N., R.N., became Chief Nursing Officer and chair of the Division of Nursing effective April 1, 1998. Ulreich had fourteen years of nursing practice and management experience at The Cleveland Clinic. She announced a new and flatter organizational structure later that year. It consisted of four clinical directors and two non-clinical directors: one for systems/resources/operations and one for education and research. The clinical directors then were Debbie Albert for surgery and post-acute care, Dawn Bailey, M.A.O.M., R.N., for medicine and children's services, Peggy Kuhar, M.S.N., R.N., for cardiac and emergency services, and Lois Bock, B.S.N., R.N., for surgical services. Non-clinical directors were Lorraine Mion, Ph.D., R.N., for education/research and Donnelly for systems/resources/operations. Also included were nurse managers and assistant nurse managers for each unit. One operations analyst, to assist with financial and other support functions, was added for each department. Further changes in leadership personnel continued until the final additions in November 2001.

In 1998, Cheryl Adams, R.N., B.A., C.P.H.Q., was appointed director of case management. In 1999, her reporting relationship changed from Kay to Ulreich, and Adams joined the nurse executive council. In December 1999 Mion left the Clinic, and Lewicki served as interim director of education/research. In May 2000, Michelle Dumpe, Ph.D., M.S.N., R.N., joined the staff as director of nursing education, research, and advanced practice. In August 2000, Albert assumed a chief nursing role at the Cleveland Clinic Health System's Euclid Hospital and was replaced in January 2001 by Andi

Wasdovich, R.N., B.S.N., B.A., who brought much experience from leadership positions in ambulatory clinics at The Cleveland Clinic and University Hospitals of Cleveland. On September 11, 2000, Bock moved to the Division of Human Resources to assume responsibility for nurse recruitment and retention, and Bush was appointed to head the surgical services. On November 5, 2001, a fifth clinical director, Sharon Kimball, R.N., M.S., M.B.A., was appointed to lead nursing practice in the newly formed Cleveland Clinic Children's Hospital and birthing services.

Along with the new organizational structure, Ulreich formed the nurse executive council (NEC), which included all directors, the finance manager, the assistant to the chairman, and a nurse manager representative. The NEC met twice monthly to set nursing policy and to manage nursing operations. By 2002 a task force of its members had completed revision of contemporary policies and procedures for administration of the division. The NEC's standards committee, composed of clinical nurse specialists, also developed contemporary nursing practice policies and procedures. The division focused on enhancing its quality monitoring of patient care outcome indicators including patient satisfaction, patient education, continuing education for the staff, and nursing research to improve practice.

New services added in subsequent years included a heart failure unit in January 2000 and a neonatal intensive care unit in July 2001. Opening a new cardiothoracic fast-track unit and a cardiac stepdown unit also enabled the division more efficiently to meet the needs of special patient populations.

The expansion of care-delivery sites, along with increased patient volume and acuity, contributed to the need for additional personnel in nursing and other professions. At The Cleveland Clinic, pressure for more patient beds continued, as patient volumes often strained capacity. Signs of a nursing shortage became apparent in 1999, with a vacancy rate of 17% at The Cleveland Clinic (national range: 4-12%). We discuss the nursing shortage and the Clinic's response to it in greater detail later in this chapter under "The Nursing Shortage."

In 2000, Ulreich formed the Cleveland Clinic Health System Nurse Executive Council (CCHS-NEC) with its membership consisting of all system hospitals' chief nursing officers. The purpose of the group was to manage system-wide planning for nursing practice.

Clinic Nursing

Throughout the years, Clinic Nursing remained separate from hospital nursing. The clinic nurses traditionally reported directly to the medical departments for which they worked and had no nursing management *per se*. After World War II a Director of Nursing was appointed, but it was not until the long tenure of Corinne Hofstetter, R.N., that the department firmly established its own identity and stability. After Hofstetter's retirement in 1986, E. Mary Johnson, B.S.N., R.N., assumed the directorship.

In 1990, a significant gap between clinic and hospital nursing closed when Johnson, who had long supported the idea of closer ties among Cleveland Clinic nurses, accepted an invitation to join the nursing management group as a voting member. This improved communication for policy-making between the Division of Nursing and Clinic Nursing. Ambulatory (clinic) nursing, however, remained administratively separate from the Division of Nursing. With decentralization in 1991, the nurses reported directly to the medical department chairmen. In August 1999, Johnson retired as director of ambulatory nursing. Jan Fuchs, M.S.N., R.N., served as the interim leader and was appointed director in 2000.

By 2003, a medical director, administrator, and ambulatory-nursing manager managed the ambulatory clinics. Patient care delivery and its quality were their responsibility. Ambulatory nursing managers had a matrix reporting relationship, which included the medical departments and ambulatory clinic nursing. Ambulatory clinic nursing was integrated with the Division of Nursing through the director's membership on the NEC.

Health care financing and technology had a substantial effect on ambulatory nursing, as many procedures moved to the outpatient setting. Diagnostic and interventional procedures carried out under sedation became common, including cardiac catheterization, cardioversion, pacemaker change, ablation, bronchoscopy, pump insertion for pain management, and many gastrointestinal procedures.

Also by 2003, outpatient nursing incorporated ambulatory nursing practice at 67 outpatient desks, at 14 family health centers located throughout northern Ohio, and at 25 regional surgical practices in off-campus facilities. There were 108 advanced practice nurses (APNs) working in outpatient clinics on the main campus.

Another 30 APNs staffed six of the 14 family health centers, located in Independence, Wooster, Lorain, Strongsville, Westlake, and Beachwood.

Changes in Delivery of Nursing Care

As in all other areas of medicine, The Cleveland Clinic's nursing staff had to evolve in response to the scientific and technological advances. In the 1920s, no antibiotics were available to treat post-operative patients or those with infections. Today, nurses administer antibiotics daily by mouth as well as parenterally. Better infection control removed one obstacle to the performance of increasingly complex surgical procedures. Operating room nurses, who had themselves manufactured some of the supplies and equipment used in the operating room well past the mid-century, now became responsible for the purchase, care, and readiness of an extensive array of surgical instruments and supplies. But high costs of care in the hospital raised the pressure for cost containment and fostered a new emphasis on outpatient care.

In the hospital, the delivery of nursing care was originally organized according to function: nurses received specific assignments, such as pouring and passing medications for all patients on their units. During the 1960s and 1970s, nursing leadership implemented team nursing, with registered nurses heading small teams that included licensed practical nurses and nursing unit assistants, who were responsible for the complete care of a group of patients. In the late 1970s, the Nursing Department began to encourage "primary nursing," whereby a nurse was assigned to each patient. The idea was that primary nursing would enable each patient to identify his or her nurse, give nurses increased responsibility for patient care, and provide better continuity of care. Later, many of the less technical nursing functions became the domain of specially trained non-registered nurses, while nurses continued to perform more demanding patient-care services and administrative functions.

In the 1980s, each unit had a head nurse and, in most cases, two assistant head nurses. In 1992, the title of head nurse was changed to nurse manager, clarifying the responsibility for managing 50 or more employees as well as the unit's patients and budget. The following year, the title of ambulatory nursing coordinator was also changed to nurse manager, to reflect the same level of responsibility within the clinic.

The patient care technician (PCT) position was developed in the early 1990s. First proposed by the cardiothoracic nursing department in the late 1980s, the intensive care units had adopted it by 1992. The intensive care units used PCTs to perform some technical tasks along with the traditional duties of the nursing unit assistant, freeing registered nurses to concentrate on patient assessment, care planning, and patient education.

By the late 1980s, the effect of managed care on nursing had become obvious. Nurses understood the importance of documentation in tracking the patient's progress and response to nursing interventions. But lack of nurse documentation developed financial implications as, in some cases, third-party payers would refuse reimbursement if portions of the record had not been completed properly. For better compliance, the division replaced old forms with new ones and adopted new charting methods. By 1992 the PIE charting system, which focused on a "nursing progress record," was in use. This provided a format for recording the nursing assessment, planning, intervention, and evaluation (PIE) for the individual patient. An associated "problem list" recorded the results of the assessment in terms of nursing diagnoses, and followed the problems to record their resolution—or lack thereof—during the patient's hospital stay.

In 1988, the Division of Nursing began to focus on a case management system for care delivery. Nurse case managers would be assigned to track patients throughout the course of their care, ensuring that they were recovering according to schedule. In 1994 the information systems staff implemented "order entry phase I" throughout the hospital and clinical areas. Work on coordinated care tracks (CCTs), or care maps, began in the same year. In 1995 the information systems department implemented "order entry phase II" and "results reporting," requiring extensive design and educational training efforts.

Facing the impact of managed care, the Division of Nursing was under pressure to control costs while managing a significant increase in numbers of patients. Capacity management became an issue, and increasing the efficiency of patient discharge and admission was a goal.

Nursing Education and Research

In the 1920s, the largest Cleveland hospitals had their own "nurses' training" schools. At the best schools, nurses received education in both the classroom and clinical settings. At the better hospitals, graduates might serve as head nurses. But in hospitals with training schools, the staff nurses were often students. Early on, Cleveland Clinic leadership decided not to follow this pattern, but to staff both the clinic and hospital with graduate nurses. The founders felt that an experienced nursing staff would provide the best patient care.

Formal educational opportunities for nurses at the Clinic existed from the beginning, but these were limited to a few postgraduate positions on staff. However, a severe nursing shortage caused by World War II led to the hiring of a few undergraduate nurses. In 1954, the hospital entered into its first formal affiliation with a nursing school, which allowed students to receive clinical experience at The Cleveland Clinic's hospital. In subsequent years, a number of local diploma, associate degree, bachelor's degree, and graduate programs as well as licensed practical nursing schools arranged to send their students to the Clinic for clinical observation and practice.

At first, overseeing these affiliation programs fell to the assistant director of nursing, who was also responsible for orientation and continuing education as well as for nurse recruitment, staffing, and scheduling. In the late 1960s, this position was divided into three parts: recruitment, continuing education, and patient care. The Departments of Nurse Education and Nurse Recruitment grew from the first two, and the Division of Nursing absorbed them in the mid-1980s. In response to the severe nursing shortage that began in the late 1990s, the division created a Nurse Recruitment and Retention Department, which was moved to the Division of Human Resources in September 2000, with a dual reporting relationship to nursing.

By the 1988-89 academic year, the Division of Nursing had affiliated with seven college- and university-based nursing programs, including Case Western Reserve University's Frances Payne Bolton School of Nursing, and the schools of nursing at Cleveland State University, Cuyahoga Community College, Kent State University, Lakeland Community College, the University of Akron, and Ursuline College. Thirty-three Cleveland Clinic nursing staff members were pursuing A.D.N., B.S.N., or M.S.N. degrees with the help of tuition grants administered through the division. By 2002, that number had increased to sixty-two.

The division strengthened its ties with the Frances Payne Bolton School of Nursing at Case Western Reserve University when the latter reinstated its B.S.N. program in 1990. The Clinic, along with University Hospitals of Cleveland and Cleveland Metropolitan General Hospital (now called MetroHealth Medical Center), agreed to collaborate in the program by providing tuition support and clinical experience to the students, who would commit to serve at the sponsoring hospitals after graduation. Because of high costs, all hospitals eventually discontinued financial support for this program. The last graduates completed their studies in the late 1990s.

In addition to educating students, the Division of Nursing provided ongoing education for its own nursing staff in a number of ways. Nurse educators oriented all new nurses, and unit-based preceptors worked with the new staff to facilitate their entry into practice. Clinical instructors provided education for staff when practice changes were required, for example, with the introduction of new equipment and procedures. Finally, 34 advanced practice nurses worked with hospital nursing staff to enhance patient care practices in the Clinic's many specialty areas.

The Division of Nursing also offered education to nurses outside the Clinic. Nurses from around the world visited the Clinic regularly to observe nursing practice and organization. Cleveland Clinic nurses traveled widely, offering their expertise in clinical specialties, procedures, and management to clinics, hospitals, and professional groups at home and abroad. An international nurse scholar program offered clinical fellowships to nurses from other countries.

A formal program for nursing research was established under the jurisdiction of nursing resources in the mid-1980s. First, a process for approving nursing research proposals was established, then a nursing research committee was formed. The committee reviewed research proposals with an eye towards projects that would enhance the quality of nursing and institute new approaches to patient care. The program was housed in the Nursing Education and Research Department. Initially, the director of nursing was a member of The Cleveland Clinic's Institutional Review Board. More recently, the senior nurse researcher has filled that role.

The Nursing Shortage

The national nursing shortage of the late 1990s extended well into the early 2000s. Projections for the future indicated an aging nursing work force, a decline in available graduates from schools of nursing, and continued shrinkage of the registered-nurse pool, as well as a decrease in the availability of other professionals. In 2001, in response to the nursing shortage, the Clinic made major financial investments in nursing and in the operations that support nursing. For example, one million dollars was allocated to support a tuition assistance program for nursing students. Students accepted in this program obtained loans of $5,000 or $10,000 per academic year. The Clinic's commitment was to forgive $5,000 of a student loan for each year the graduate worked in the Clinic's hospital. In 2002 this program had 55 enrolled students.

Nursing leadership concluded that various types of flexible scheduling would increase nurse satisfaction and improve recruitment and retention. In response to the challenge, they implemented a "Weekender Option Program" in 1990. It attempted to solve one part of the problem by allowing part-time registered nurses and licensed practical nurses to work two 12-hour shifts during the weekend, as well as additional hours during the week. The option was so popular that by 1991, full-time nurses in most areas were working only one out of every three to six weekends. When the division instituted a shift-incentive program that year to encourage more nurses to work straight evenings or nights, 130 nurses signed up to participate. This helped stabilize staffing and reduced the need for rotating shifts.

Economic constraints resulted in discontinuation of the weekender program, but it was re-introduced in a modified form in 2001, along with other incentives. These incentives included premium pay for nurses, unit secretaries, and other staff working extra shifts, an hourly rate premium for division registered nurses, and a retention bonus for registered nurses with two years of continuous service. These incentives demonstrated the Clinic's commitment to attracting and retaining their experienced and talented staff.

The nursing shortage became a national and international crisis in 2001, and the Clinic invested approximately $5 million in additional incentives to retain nurses. These included a retention bonus, an hourly differential for nurses working in the Clinic's main campus hospital, premium pay, the reinstated weekender program mentioned above, and three 12-hour shifts. Recruitment investments included financing for job fairs, sign-on bonuses, international recruitment, a program to attract retired nurses, a program to attract nurses working in other roles at the Clinic, and a summer work program for nursing students.

The Clinic initiated an educational program designed to serve as a long-term approach to the shortage in 2002. This was an accelerated B.S.N. curriculum resulting from a collaboration between The Cleveland Clinic and the Cleveland State University nursing department. It afforded persons with bachelor's degrees in other fields the opportunity to complete their study of nursing in an accelerated format. Students in this program received their clinical practice experience in the Cleveland Clinic Health System.

The April 2002 registered nurse position vacancy rate was 15.2%, up from 14.7% in January 2002. Significant recruitment and retention efforts continued. Retention efforts included leadership training through a Nursing Leadership Academy to enhance the skills of front-line managers, since research had demonstrated their significant impact on staff nurse decisions to remain in current positions. These and other efforts helped to ensure that the Clinic recruited and retained the nurses needed to deliver the quality care for which The Cleveland Clinic has always been known.

In June 2003, the Clinic received designation as a Magnet hospital from the American Nurses Credentialing Center (ANCC). This prestigious designation (one of 82 nationally and only three in Ohio) recognized the strength of the administrative priority on quality of care, delegation of management authority to clinicians, involvement of nursing staff in continuing education, and creation of a satisfactory working environment. Peggy Kuhar led the project that resulted in this designation.

LOOKING AHEAD

In 2003, Ulreich announced her resignation as the Clinic's Chief Nursing Officer. In September of that year, as this book was going to press, the Clinic announced that Claire Young, R.N., M.B.A., would be her successor. At that time, the Division of Nursing had a staff of close to 3,000, caring for approximately 57,000 patients admitted to the hospital, 35,000 patients requiring surgery, and 435,000 patients receiving ambulatory care. Nurses were working in all 50 inpatient units, in 59 operating rooms, perioperative areas, the emergency department, infection control, and in ambulatory clinics. Annually, nurses received and triaged 260,000 calls through the Nurse-On-Call program.

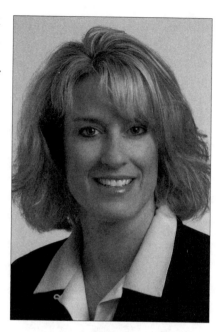

Claire Young, R.N., M.B.A., Chairwoman, Division of Nursing, 2003-

Although many of their duties were changing, Cleveland Clinic nurses remained focused on their nursing mission: to help patients perform activities contributing to health or its recovery (or to a peaceful death), and to help patients become independent as quickly as possible. Clearly nurses have been an essential part of the care delivery team at The Cleveland Clinic from the beginning. Their roles will continue to change and expand as clinical innovations follow successful research endeavors here and elsewhere. Nursing and medicine will continue their collaborative efforts to enhance the practice environment for patient care and to attract and retain nursing staff in spite of the serious shortage. The future for nursing at The Cleveland Clinic has never been brighter.

19. DIVISION OF EDUCATION

By Andrew J. Fishleder

The roots of education are bitter, but the fruit is sweet.
—*Aristotle, Fourth Century B.C.*

THE EARLY YEARS, 1921-1944

AT THE OPENING OF THE CLEVELAND CLINIC IN 1921, DR. FRANK BUNTS said, "We hope that as we have after many years been allowed to gather together able associates and assistants to make this work possible, so in time to come, those men, taking the place of their predecessors, will carry on the work to higher and better ends, aiding their fellow practitioners, caring for the sick, educating and seeking always to attain the highest and noblest aspirations of their profession."

It is not surprising that the founders placed so much emphasis on teaching, since all served on the clinical faculties of one or more Cleveland medical schools. From the time it opened, the Clinic had graduate fellows-in-training, now called residents. The first medical resident was Charles L. Hartsock, M.D., who trained from June 1921 to June 1923, then joined the staff and served with distinction until his death in 1961. The first surgical resident was William O. Johnson, M.D., who spent June 1921 to June 1922 at the Clinic, then returned in 1924 after the hospital opened and served with another surgical resident, Nathaniel S. Shofner, M.D. The Clinic also established fellowships in research soon after the institution opened, and a number of traveling fellowships were awarded for residents to visit other clinics and medical centers in this country and abroad.

In the Clinic's early years, the absence of American specialty boards made training programs more flexible than they are today. Residents could finish a year or two at one hospital and then apply to another to train with someone else. In those days the terms "residents" and "fellows" were used interchangeably. Because the training programs at the Clinic were called "fellowships" then, the term "fellow" was normally used where we would now use the term "resident." The system had no formal rules, rotations, or examinations. Today, the rigid requirements of the various specialty boards make transferring from one institution to another difficult. In the 1920s, most interns and residents in teaching hospitals were underpaid or not paid at all. The Clinic paid relatively high salaries for that era and supplied competent technicians to perform time-consuming laboratory studies. Consequently, there was no shortage of applications for the limited number of fellowships offered. Both residents and staff benefited from an apprentice-like arrangement.

Dr. William Proudfit, retired former chairman of the Department of Cardiology, recalls, "The entire formal educational experience when I was in training was a weekly lecture for fellows—all the fellows, regardless of specialty. This was held in the evening, and the same program was repeated annually (an advantage, for we learned what lectures to miss!). How that contrasts with the present programs! An internist or a surgeon was expected to be competent in all subspecialties (except, perhaps, allergy for internists and neurosurgery and orthopedics for surgeons)."

Although formal postgraduate courses had not been established, more than 12,000 physicians spent various periods of time at the Clinic between 1924 and 1937. To support teaching, lecturing, and the presentation of papers, a medical library, medical illustrators, and medical photographers were available.

In 1935, the Clinic formalized education by establishing the Frank E. Bunts Educational Institute with Cleveland Clinic staff as faculty. The stated purpose of the new institute was "to maintain and conduct an institution for learning, for promoting education, and giving instruction in the art, science, and practice of medicine, surgery, anatomy, hygiene, and allied or kindred sciences and subjects."

During the Clinic's early years, a fellowship committee, which was organized in 1924, administered the fellowship program. Robert S. Dinsmore, M.D., of the Department of General Surgery served as chairman until 1936. Founder Frank Bunts's son, Alexander T. Bunts, M.D., a neurosurgeon, who held the post with distinction for 10 years, succeeded him. After Bunts came William J. Engel, M.D., of the Department of Urology. Engel's service ended with the establishment of the Cleveland Clinic Educational Foundation in 1962.

By 1944, expanding educational activities pointed out the need for a full-time director of medical education. Howard Dittrick, M.D., a well-known Cleveland physician, was chosen for

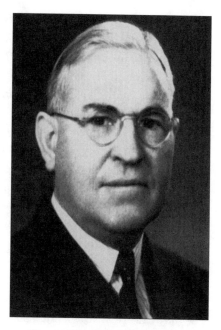

Howard Dittrick, M.D., Director, Frank E. Bunts Educational Institute (now Division of Education), 1944-1947

the role. For the next three years he was in charge of the editorial department, library, postgraduate courses, preparation of exhibits, and art and photography departments. He also became editor of the *Cleveland Clinic Quarterly*, which had been publishing scientific papers by the Clinic staff since 1932.

In 1982 the *Cleveland Clinic Quarterly* published its fiftieth anniversary issue. The following remarks are summarized from an article by James S. Taylor, M.D., editor-in-chief, on the history of the *Quarterly*.

"In the first year of publication, the Quarterly published six original articles and the balance consisted of reprints. Because of the Great Depression, the Quarterly did not appear in 1933 or 1934. On November 28, 1934, the Medical Board met and decided that the Quarterly would no longer publish papers that had appeared in other journals.

"Some outstanding contributions to the world literature have been published in the *Quarterly*. The *Quarterly* is distributed without charge to physicians and medical libraries throughout the world. In 1982, circulation exceeded 16,000. It is sent to approximately 2,600 alumni of The Cleveland Clinic Educational Foundation and to 1,000 medical libraries and medical schools. The remainder are sent to other physicians requesting the journal.

"The *Cleveland Clinic Quarterly*, a refereed, indexed journal, is an integral part of the educational activities of the Cleveland Clinic and is underwritten solely by The Cleveland Clinic Educational Foundation. The journal is indexed in *Index Medicus, Chemical Abstracts, Biological Abstracts, Current Contents*, and *Nutritional Abstracts*. It is also microfilmed by University Microfilms International."

Upon Dittrick's retirement, Edwin P. Jordan, M.D., an editor at the American Medical Association, was appointed to replace him. He held the position from 1947 to 1950, when he was replaced by Stanley O. Hoerr, M.D. Then Fay A. LeFevre, M.D., served as acting director of education from 1952 until 1955, when Col. Charles L. Leedham, M.D., was recruited from the Armed Forces to assume the directorship.

THE LEEDHAM YEARS, 1955-1962

When Leedham took over, with the development of American specialty boards and increased regulation by the American Medical Association's Council on Medical Education, formal training programs had to be established for candidates to meet the requirements of the various specialties. Leedham established a Faculty Board within the Bunts Educational Institute in 1956 to oversee the quality of the educational programs and develop policies governing them. The nine-member group comprised the division chairmen, director of research, chairman of the Board of Governors, director of education, and two members-at-large. They made appointments and promotions within the Clinic teaching staff, determined educational policies and curricula for graduate education, established criteria for their selection, and established standards for granting certificates for academic work performed.

THE ZEITER YEARS, 1962-1973

In 1962, the name of the Bunts Education Institute was changed to The Cleveland Clinic Educational Foundation to help physicians here and abroad more closely recognize its relationship with The Cleveland Clinic. Walter J. Zeiter, M.D., a physiatrist and former Executive Secretary to the Board of Governors, was appointed director and held the position until 1973. There was another reason for changing the name: Crile did not wish to be memorialized in any way that would set him apart from the other founders. Some felt that this policy should extend to Bunts as well. Also, with Dr. Alexander Bunts' retirement, Dr. George Crile, Jr., was the only remaining descendant of the founders on the staff. Dr. William Engel, who was soon to retire, was Lower's son-in-law.

As the years passed, the growth of The Cleveland Clinic led to an expansion of educational activities. However, the Clinic lacked adequate physical facilities to support them. The solution came in the form of a generous gift from the estate of Martha Holden Jennings, which provided funds for the construction of a seven-story Education Building and an endowment to maintain it. The building, which opened in 1964, contained an auditorium, seven seminar rooms, a medical library, editorial and administrative offices, and on-call accommodations for house staff.

THE MICHENER YEARS, 1973-1991

In 1973, the Board of Governors appointed William M. Michener, M.D., director of education following Zeiter's retirement. A former Clinic staff member, Michener returned after spending five years as a professor of pediatrics and assistant dean of graduate education at the University of New Mexico.

Under Michener's leadership, education programs flourished. By 1981, the division clearly needed reorganization, and he formed a task force to accomplish this. Two years later, the task force made many excellent recommendations, which the Board of Governors adopted. These included replacing the Faculty Board and its committees with a peer review group. Called the Education Governing Group, it was charged with reviewing, monitoring, and evaluating all existing and proposed education activities and training programs; establishing educational policies and program priorities; and proposing programs and budgets to the Division of Education.

At the same time, the division formed councils for allied health and nursing education, management and training, and physician education. Michener also appointed a vice chairman to oversee the Physician Education Council. Later, a Continuing Medical Education Council was added.

The Board of Governors also agreed that The Cleveland Clinic Educational Foundation should formally function as a division of the institution. Patient education became a department within the new Division of Education. Most importantly, the Board of Governors affirmed that teaching should become an integral part of the annual professional review process for staff members involved in education, and that consideration should be given to the quality and quantity of their educational performance. With great foresight, the task force recommended that Cleveland Clinic training programs in collaboration with one or more medical schools be considered in the future.

Graduate Medical Education (GME) programs also thrived during Michener's tenure. With advances in medical technology stretching the curriculum of core residencies to capacity, the Clinic expanded subspecialty fellowships in a broad range of medical and surgical areas. Residency training programs grew in size, reflecting the growth of the institution and its professional staff. In order to ensure the maintenance of high-quality education programs, the Clinic responded to recommendations from the Accreditation Council on Graduate Medical Education (ACGME) by establishing an internal review of training programs and documenting the evaluation of resident performance and staff teaching. By 1994, 650 residents were registered at the Clinic, with approximately 250 graduating each July.

Clinic graduates have gone on to practice in a broad range of medical environments throughout the United States and the world. Under the jurisdiction of the Division of Education, the Office of Alumni Affairs maintained contact with more than 7,600 alumni throughout the United States and 72 other countries in an effort to help the institution remain responsive to their evolving needs.[1]

In addition to the strong focus on residency training, the education of medical students began to play a more prominent role starting in 1974. The first year, 125 students enrolled in the senior medical student electives at the Clinic. In 1975, the number jumped to 280. By 1994, 400 third- and fourth-year students from American medical schools were rotating through the Clinic. They provided a broadened academic stimulus to the residents and staff and served as an important source of candidates for residency positions. An average of 26 percent of the Clinic's first-year positions in the National Residency Match were annually filled by these students, who knew firsthand the value of training at The Cleveland Clinic.

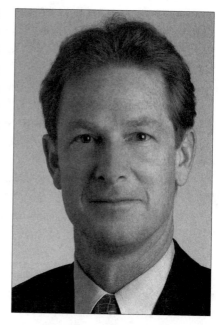

Andrew J. Fishleder, M.D., Chairman, Division of Education, 1991-

In 1986, the Clinic expanded its medical student commitment through a formal affiliation with the Pennsylvania State University Medical School in Hershey. The agreement provided for third-year medical students to spend required clerkships in neurology, internal medicine, and pediatrics at the Clinic. Both students and faculty rated the experience highly, and it helped enhance the academic focus of residency training in these areas.

THE FISHLEDER YEARS, 1991-

In 1991, the Board of Governors appointed Andrew J. Fishleder, M.D., chairman of the Division of Education. A graduate of the Clinic's pathology training program, Fishleder's interest in education was well known through his service on the Physician Education Council and Education Governing Group. In recognition of the tremendous growth that had taken place in education, and with a desire to develop new programs to support the institution's educational mission, Fishleder added directors of patient education, medical student education, and allied health education to those in graduate medical education and continuing medical education. Vice chairpersons appointed to oversee these areas were charged with developing strategic initiatives aimed at enhancing the quality and diversity of their educational activities. At the same time, he focused significant energy on ensuring appropriate recognition for staff educational efforts through the development of an annual educational activities report provided to the Office of Professional Staff Affairs during the Annual Professional Review process.

The enactment of a broad-based academic partnership with Ohio State University in 1991 was a milestone for The Cleveland Clinic. Prompted by interests in medical student education and research, the agreement facilitated cooperation in many areas of mutual benefit. By 2000, more than 200 Clinic staff members had obtained full faculty appointments at the Ohio State University School of Medicine. The partnership, entitled The Cleveland Clinic Health Sciences Center of the Ohio State University, also facilitated the development of several joint research programs, most notably in biomedical engineering. Although the partnership was a major academic affiliation, it was not exclusive, and strong relationships continued with Case Western Reserve University.

The Clinic's strong commitment to medical education also extended to practicing health care professionals. With the opening of the original Education Building and Bunts Auditorium in 1964, the number of continuing medical education courses offered at the Clinic increased substantially. In the 1970s and '80s, growth was stimulated by state requirements that licensure renewal be accompanied by documentation of attendance at continuing medical education courses. Taking that cue, programs sponsored by The Cleveland Clinic grew from 20 per year in the mid-1970s to more than 90 per year in 2001, with over 7,800 physicians, nurses and allied health professionals attending annually from throughout the medical community.

Continuing education outreach was further strengthened under the leadership of William Carey, M.D., who expanded the range of continuing medical education (CME) offerings by the institution. Non-traditional programming including videoconferencing, online activities, and *Cleveland Clinic Journal of Medicine*-related CME provided more than 45,000 CME credits in 2001. The division established a new Center for Continuing Education in 1998, incorporating both the CME and Media Services departments, to support increasingly complex programs. The division also formed Unitech Communications in 1996, a new subsidiary, to capitalize on the education-related intellectual property of the Clinic's faculty. In 2000, the Center started a new website, www.clevelandclinicmed-ed.com. By 2001, 8,500 visitors per month, on average, accessed online CME content at this site. This initiative responded to the increasing demands by physicians for online education program access and complemented the continued strength of the Clinic's live, onsite courses.

When the *Cleveland Clinic Quarterly* began publishing in 1932, there were relatively few medical research journals that provided an opportunity for physicians to share scientific expertise gained at the Clinic with other physicians. In 1987, the division changed the name of the *Cleveland Clinic Quarterly* to the *Cleveland Clinic Journal of Medicine*, and publication increased to six times per year. John Clough, M.D., was appointed editor-in-chief of the *Journal* in 1996. Under his leadership the *Journal* refocused editorial content from original research to education, dealing with the practical challenges of medical care faced by office-based physicians everywhere. The *Journal* "relaunched" itself, with a new look, increased publication frequency, and more aggressive sales of advertising space. This strategic change helped greatly to advance readership among office-based internists and cardiologists, the primary audience of the *Journal*. Deputy editor Brian Mandell, M.D., Ph.D., brought an additional strong educational commitment to the *Journal's* editorial staff.

In 1994, the division created an Office of Faculty and Curriculum Development in an effort to support the continuing enhancement of education program quality. The first director of that office, Mariana Hewson, Ph.D., was appointed in January 1995 and started the Clinic's Seminars in Clinical Teaching program. This office has evolved into a Center for Medical Education Research and Development (CMERAD) with an additional three part-time staff members. In 2001, Alan Hull, M.D., Ph.D., assumed responsibility as Director. CMERAD offered a diverse range of seminars for faculty and trainees including programs on teaching skills, curriculum development, doctor-patient communication, and clinical research topics.

In 1999, the Division of Education occupied new quarters within the Lerner Research Institute complex. These new facilities stood as a monument to the institution's commitment to education and research. Funded through philanthropy, the new Education building included classrooms, an 85-seat amphitheater, a 30,000 square-foot medical library with seating capacity for 311, and administrative space to consolidate the majority of the Division's resources. The MBNA Conference Center, located across the street in the Inter-Continental Hotel, which opened in April 2003, further enhanced the resources available to support the Clinic's academic programs and educational outreach.

With this strengthened foundation of academic commitment in place, the Clinic has embarked on plans for the establishment of a new medical school. On May 13, 2002, The Cleveland Clinic Board of Trustees approved the formation of The Cleveland Clinic College of Medicine of Case Western Reserve University. The mission of this enterprise will be to train physician investigators and scientists who will help to assure the development and application of future biomedical advances. This collaboration, linking two great academic institutions, marked a major milestone for the Clinic. On June 19, 2002, an unprecedented philanthropic gift of $100 million by Mr. and Mrs. Alfred Lerner secured the financial foundation of this initiative. In recognition of the generosity and vision of the Lerner family, the new medical school was renamed The Cleveland Clinic Lerner College of Medicine of Case Western Reserve University. Although the challenges of this exciting endeavor are many, the establishment of The Cleveland Clinic Lerner College of Medicine, slated to enroll its first students in 2004, will help to propel the institution into the new millennium with a renewed commitment to scientific investigation and academic achievement.

---

1 The Alumni Association was transferred back to the Division of Education in 1993 after being revived and reinvigorated under Frank Weaver's leadership during the 1980s.

20. LERNER RESEARCH INSTITUTE

By Paul DiCorleto and George Stark

*Science is the attempt to make the chaotic
diversity of our sense-experience correspond
to a logically uniform system of thought.*
—*Albert Einstein, 1950*

EARLY ACTIVITIES

Both basic and clinical research have been fundamental to the mission of The Cleveland Clinic since the beginning. The Clinic's founders were convinced that they could only provide the best patient care by conducting active programs of medical research in the new Clinic. In 1921, they agreed among themselves that no less than one fourth of the net income from the new organization would be devoted to research and indigent care. Later, this percentage substantially increased, and in 1928, the trustees approved construction of a building for medical research.

All of the Clinic's founders participated in research, but George Crile, Sr., M.D., was its strongest advocate. He believed that laboratory discoveries provided the essential scientific basis for modern clinical practice. From his investigations had come the original thesis linking the activity of the adrenal glands to physiologic stress.

Hugo Fricke, Ph.D., was the first scientist in charge of research in biophysics, a field that interested Crile. The latter's "bipolar theory of living processes" was based on the differences in electrical

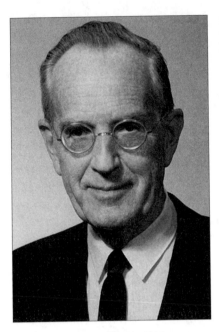

Irvine H. Page, M.D., Chairman,
Research Division, 1945-1966

charges between the brains and livers of animals, as well as between the nuclei and cytoplasms of individual cells. Fricke, and later Maria Telkes, Ph.D., measured the thickness of cell membranes and showed their relationship to electrical charges in living cells. Their studies were widely recognized contributions to this complicated field.

In 1930, a team of biochemists headed by D. Roy McCullagh, Ph.D., replaced the biophysics group. McCullagh persistently tried to isolate a hormone from the testicle believed to inhibit the enlargement of the prostate gland. Although the quest was tantalizing, no solid results ever materialized. McCullagh did, however, become a pioneer in the measurement of thyroid function through iodine levels in the blood. He collaborated with his brother, Clinic endocrinologist E. Perry McCullagh, M.D., in studies of pituitary and sex hormones.

The original Research Building was designed for types of research that no longer exist today. By 1945, it was largely empty except for a few small laboratories. During the late 1930s and early years of World War II, Crile's leadership waned, and although the laboratories remained partially serviceable until the end of the war, they had neither the resources nor the inspiration they enjoyed during the peak of Crile's influence.

THE PAGE ERA, 1945-1966

By the mid 1940s, it had become clear that the Clinic needed a research leader. In 1945, to the everlasting credit of the trustees, they persuaded Irvine H. Page, M.D., to become chairman of the Clinic's new Research Division. They had become acquainted with

Page through his treatment of Charles Bradley, a prominent Clevelander, for high blood pressure. Russell L. Haden, M.D., chief of medicine at the Clinic, had referred Bradley to Page, a chemist and clinician, whose work had addressed the cause of high blood pressure and paved the way for treatment.

To foster the cooperation of scientists in several disciplines, Page did not permit departmentalization in the Division of Research. He favored melding patient observations, animal experimentation, and work in the chemical laboratory. His disdain of committees, excessive meetings, and other administrative distractions freed everyone to concentrate on research.

Page brought two colleagues, Arthur C. Corcoran, M.D., and Robert D. Taylor, M.D., with him from Indianapolis, where cardiovascular disease, and specifically arterial hypertension and atherosclerosis, had been their main focus. Page began his work in 1931 at New York's Rockefeller Institute after spending three years as head of the brain chemistry division of the Kaiser Wilhelm Institute (now called the Max Planck Institute) in Munich, Germany. Corcoran left Montreal's McGill University to join Page in New York, where he studied renal aspects of hypertension. His use of sophisticated methods to study kidney function in hypertensive patients opened the door to the search for effective antihypertensive drugs and animal models in which new drugs could be tested. Taylor joined Page and Corcoran after they moved to Indianapolis in 1937.

At the Clinic they developed a multidisciplinary approach aimed at solving problems in cardiovascular disease. Their unique plan called for physicians with specialized training in the basic sciences to work full time with clinical researchers. This cooperation, which continues today, is responsible for some of the most significant findings in cardiovascular medicine.

Until that time, heart disease had gone largely unstudied; with the exception of the rheumatic and syphilitic varieties, it received little attention. High blood pressure was also generally considered to be a relatively harmless consequence of aging. But by the 1940s, the incidence of heart attack, stroke and hypertension, and their interrelationship, had become evident.

During the 1920s, a number of investigators tried to produce renal hypertension in dogs with varying success. In 1934, Dr. Harry Goldblatt at Cleveland's Mt. Sinai Hospital produced the first reliable model by clamping the renal artery and partially blocking it. Page later developed a simple, practical method of causing severe hypertension by encapsulating the kidney in cellophane, making an inelastic hull that restricted normal pulsation.

As Page began to shape the Research Division, he added Dr. Arda Green, who had just crystallized phosphorylase-A in St. Louis, Georges M. C. Masson, Ph.D., from Montreal, and, in 1950, Willem J. Kolff, M.D., Ph.D., from the Netherlands. Three younger scientists, F. Merlin Bumpus, Ph.D., Harriet P. Dustan, M.D., and James W. McCubbin, Ph.D., came to the Clinic as associate staff or post-doctoral fellows and pursued illustrious careers.

Before coming to the Clinic, Page had worked on isolating a substance formed when blood is clotted, a substance known to have a strong effect on circulation. He continued this work in Cleveland and, with the collaboration of Clinic colleagues Arda A. Green, M.D., and Maurice Rapport, Ph.D., discovered a compound that proved to be 5-hydroxytryptamine. They called it "serotonin." Few biological agents have proven to have so many varied actions as serotonin; among them are profound effects on the brain as a transmitter of nerve impulses, and an active role in the formation of certain intestinal tumors.

A long series of investigations by Page and his associates led to the isolation of a substance that the group named "angiotonin" in 1939, while the group was still working in Indianapolis. Concurrently, a group directed by Braun-Menéndez in Buenos Aires isolated the same compound. Friendly dialogue between them led to an agreement on the name "angiotensin." It has formed the basis of thousands of studies worldwide, has proven to play an important role in hypertension, and is also the chief regulator of catecholamine hormone secretion from the adrenal gland. Angiotensin II became widely available for study after Bumpus, Page, and Hans Schwarz, M.D., synthesized it at the Clinic, simultaneously with Robert Schwyzer, Ph.D., in Switzerland. This major breakthrough helped spur research that led to the development of antihypertensive drugs. Bumpus theorized that blocking the renal-adrenal blood pressure control mechanisms would lower pressure. He demonstrated this by developing the first molecular antagonists to angiotensin. This encouraged pharmaceutical companies to develop angiotensin-converting enzyme inhibitors that have evolved into useful drugs for lowering blood pressure.

For many years, The Cleveland Clinic Foundation was the sole source of funds for research at the institution. Active antagonism met the prospect of accepting any government support. But in the late 1950s, increased competition, escalating costs, and the need for recognition caused the trustees to relax this policy. In 1962, the National Heart Institute of the National Institutes of Health awarded a major program grant to the Clinic instead of to individual investigators, as was customary. Since staff salaries were paid by the Clinic, the money was used to defray operating expenses. From this point on, grants became critical to growth, as did gifts from individuals and foundations, which helped to defray operating expenses, fund exploratory studies, and build an endowment fund.

Kolff had spent the war years in Holland working on an artificial kidney. With the same stubborn determination that allowed him to continue doing research while his country was under German occupation, he worked against great odds in Cleveland to obtain funds for his projects. Initially, only The Cleveland Clinic funded the artificial kidney, a project that seemed so unlikely that few wanted to invest in it. Eventually, private foundations saw its potential, and, together with the National Institutes of Health, later became prime sources of funds.

Both Page and Kolff had strong convictions, a trait that would later lead to conflict. Separation eventually became necessary, and Kolff continued his research in the Division of Surgery until Page's retirement in 1966.

While Kolff was working on applied research projects, Page and his group were establishing the Cleveland Clinic Research Division as the mecca for studies in high blood pressure. Early on, they showed how the principle of feedback participates in an intricate mechanism that controls blood pressure. After many experiments, they developed a general theory of hypertension, which they called the "mosaic theory." This theory postulated that hypertension rarely has one single cause, but rather results from shifts in the equilibria among its many component causes.

Carlos Ferrario, M.D., joined Page and McCubbin in 1966. Although Page retired soon thereafter, the investigations they had begun culminated in a brilliant series of cooperative experiments involving a former associate, Dr. D. J. Dickinson, in London. Ferrario, McCubbin, and Dickinson proved that the brain was a regulator of blood pressure. Later, Ferrario and McCubbin showed where and how angiotensin enters the brain. The blood vessels, heart, sympathetic nervous system, brain, pituitary gland, and kidneys are among the contributors to hypertension.

Under Page, one of the division's major innovations was the integration of patient care, clinical study, and laboratory investigation. This allowed an extensive study of the effects of new antihypertensive drugs on previously studied patients, and led to the development of many effective medications. A main contribution to the understanding of renal hypertension was made with the collaboration of Clinic urologist Eugene F. Poutasse, M.D., who showed that surgical removal of an obstruction in a renal artery produced a cure. Radiologist Thomas F. Meaney, M.D., provided the angiograms that were critical to the visualization and evaluation of these obstructions.

Hemodynamics, the study of flow and pressure within the cardiovascular system, has been one of the cornerstones of hypertension research. High blood pressure is a hemodynamic abnormality, and an understanding of its problems requires accurate evaluation of hemodynamic patterns associated with a rise in arterial pressure. Frederick Olmsted, a biomedical engineer assisting Page and McCubbin, was instrumental in the early design, development, and application of electromagnetic flowmeters to measure cardiac output, regional blood pressure, and other facets of circulation in healthy animals. This did much to advance understanding of the highly complex mechanisms controlling blood flow to each organ. Cardiac enlargement has always been a problem in uncontrolled hypertension. Robert C. Tarazi, M.D., and Subha Sen, Ph.D., were the first to show the effectiveness of various antihypertensive drugs in reversing cardiac hypertrophy.

The Research Division has an equally long history of research in atherosclerosis. When it became apparent that increased blood fat levels were associated with atherosclerosis under certain conditions, Clinic scientists directed their efforts towards modifying fat levels by changing the diet. Promising results in the laboratory then prompted a pioneering clinical investigation: a small group of cooperative medical students consumed experimental diets under the supervision of Helen B. Brown, Ph.D. It was found that certain diets were effective in decreasing fat levels. The U.S. Public Health

Service became interested in the program and offered substantial financial assistance, eventually assuming the complete cost of a greatly expanded, expensive program. This project, called "The National Diet-Heart Study," showed the feasibility of a much larger, long-term program that would involve the cooperation of many institutions nationwide. It ultimately provided the basis for recommending that Americans change their diet to reduce cholesterol and raise polyunsaturated fats in order to prevent heart attack and stroke. This study was the forerunner of the Framingham Study.

Page was also known for his filtration theory of the deposition of lipoproteins in the blood vessels. This was the first attempt to explain how cholesterol is deposited in the blood vessel wall during the development of atherosclerosis.

Before joining Page at the Clinic, John R. Shainoff, Ph.D., was among the first to demonstrate the deposition of lipoproteins in atherosclerotic tissue. But Shainoff's interests changed, and he began approaching atherosclerosis from another angle, believing that both the initial lesion and final closure of the diseased vessel wall involved the transformation of fibrinogen to fibrin to form blood clots. Virtually nothing was known about this. He devised methods to assess the conversion based on the freeing of "fibrinopeptides," which are soluble side products of the reaction. This enabled him to discover that fibrin could be carried in a soluble form loosely linked with fibrinogen in blood, and that these complexes are normally cleared without forming clots except when produced above a critical threshold. Today, analysis of fibrinopeptides and fibrin complexes remains the principal means for diagnosing intravascular fibrin formation.

The continuing challenge of cardiovascular disease was stimulating to investigators and clinicians alike. It provided the excitement and motivation necessary for everyone to participate in the understanding of these diseases, which are statistically among the most prevalent illnesses, and in the care of patients suffering from them. As a result of the growing national interest in cardiovascular disease, Page and local businessmen founded the American Foundation for High Blood Pressure in Cleveland in 1945. It later became the Council for High Blood Pressure Research of the American Heart Association.

Without the strength of basic programs involving cooperation among scientists, the Clinic would not have attained its position as a national leader in medicine. Although project research was highly credible, the history of the Division of Research shows that coordination and cooperation have been the keys to success.

THE BUMPUS ERA, 1966-1985

From 1945 to 1966 the philosophy of the Division of Research had been steadfastly to maintain the cardiovascular program and add approved research projects from any department. After Page retired, Bumpus was named chairman of the division, a post he retained until his own retirement in 1985. He continued to serve in the Department of Cardiovascular Research, by then renamed the Department of Cardiovascular Biology, as emeritus staff, consultant, and researcher on the newly discovered substance, "human chymase," until his death in 1993.Bumpus created the departments of Immunology, Artificial Organs (including Biomechanics), Biostatistics, and Clinical Science.

Artificial Organs was actually a legacy from Kolff's time. His associate, Yukihiko Nosé, M.D., Ph.D., continued his experimental and developmental work with artificial kidneys and hearts. When Kolff left the Clinic in 1967, the laboratory joined the Division of Research. Bumpus also broke the long tradition of seeking no outside funding. Departing from tradition has proven to be more effective than anticipated. In 1995, the Division of Research had a $52 million budget, half of which was funded by the Clinic. Ensuring the continued success of the Research Institute will require maintaining an excellent record of extramural support and inaugurating new collaborations with government, industry, and biomedical scientists in academia.

During the 1970s and '80s, research at The Cleveland Clinic was divided into two categories: program research, which was done by members of the Division of Research and, until 1966, concentrated solely on cardiovascular disease; and project research, which was conducted by physicians in the clinical departments. The plan for each project had to be submitted in writing and approved by the Research Projects Committee before funds and space were made available. Each project depended on the investigator's individual interest, and was not necessarily related to any program research.

By the mid-1970s, the Division of Research contained loosely structured sections of specific research focus: Artificial Organs, Arteriosclerosis and Thrombosis, Cardiovascular Research, Immunology, and the Clinical Research Projects Committee, which evaluated projects originating in the clinical departments.

The Department of Immunology was a natural evolution in the Clinic's growing interest in organ transplantation, autoimmune diseases, and cancer. In 1974, Bumpus recruited Jack R. Battisto, Ph.D., from the Albert Einstein College of Medicine to head this department. His research focused on the immune response and immunological tolerance. He was joined by James Finke, Ph.D., who worked with cytotoxic cells. To round out immunology, he recruited Max Proffitt, Ph.D., from Harvard and Bert Del Villano, Jr., Ph.D., from the Scripps Institute to focus on leukemia; and, as a link to clinical efforts, Claudio Fiocchi, M.D., a gastroenterologist and expert in inflammatory bowel disease.

In 1981 the department's name was changed to Molecular and Cellular Biology. After Michael J. Caulfield, Ph.D., and Martha K. Cathcart, Ph.D., joined the staff, it was renamed Immunology and Cancer. In 1986, Bumpus became acting chairman, and with the addition of research laboratories unrelated to immunology, the name was changed to the Department of General Medical Sciences. Recently, it has reverted to Immunology.

THE HEALY ERA, 1985-1991

In November 1985, Bernadine P. Healy, M.D., became the first woman to chair the Division of Research. A cardiologist, experienced research investigator, and expert in science policy and funding issues, she was eager to carry on the tradition of biomedical research that was highly interactive with clinical care. To better reflect this type of collaborative investigation, she proposed that the division be renamed the Cleveland Clinic Research Institute.

An active and involved leader, Healy's philosophy was simple: impressive talent and continually better results would mean greater success in obtaining grants and other outside funding. Her leadership continued outside the institution as well, as evidenced by her presidency of the American Heart Association in 1988-9. She felt that having a superior group of interactive scientists would create an exceptional corps of experts who could provide knowledgeable contributions to many clinical research projects and, eventually, to inventions and other patentable procedures and mechanisms. But like Page, Healy emphasized the need to translate this activity into improvements in patient care.

Healy encouraged the pursuit of creative efforts within the areas of the Clinic's priorities and greatest strengths. This, she felt strongly, would not only result in competitive work of the highest quality, but would also produce interdisciplinary programs worthy of philanthropic investment.

Among her top priorities for the Research Institute was to increase its fundamental science base, particularly in molecular and cellular biology. During her chairmanship, Healy recruited Amiya K. Banerjee, Ph.D., to chair the newly established Department of Molecular Biology. Major reorganization of the Research Institute also included splitting the Department of Cardiovascular Research into (a) the Department of Brain and Vascular Research under Carlos

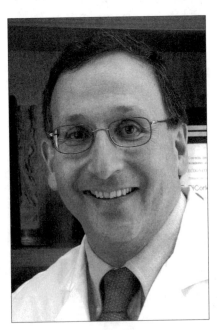

Paul E. DiCorleto, Ph.D., Chairman, Lerner Research Institute, 2002-

Ferrario, M.D., with an emphasis on neural control of blood pressure, (b) the Department of Heart and Hypertension Research under the leadership of Robert Graham, M.D., recruited from Harvard; and (c) a new Department of Vascular Cell Biology and Atherosclerosis, later called simply Cell Biology, under Paul DiCorleto, Ph.D. In addition, she created a new Department of Cancer Biology, directed by Bryan Williams, Ph.D., who came from the University of Toronto. She consolidated two departments (Artificial Organs and Musculoskeletal Research) into a Department of Biomedical Engineering and Applied Thera-

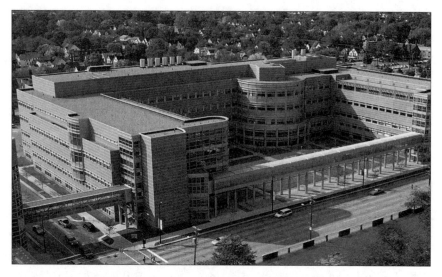

*Lerner Research Institute, 1999. Left to right: Education Wing,
Laboratories and Commons, Biomedical Engineering*

peutics, under J. Fredrick Cornhill, D.Phil., from Ohio State
University.

This was a time of major expansion for the Research Institute,
both in promising young as well as established senior research talent, reflected in substantial growth in competitively awarded
research grants. Among them were two multimillion dollar, multicenter trials: the Post-Coronary Angioplasty and Bypass Graft (Post-
CABG) study and the Bypass Angioplasty Revascularization
Investigation (BARI). NIH funds more than doubled, from seven
million dollars in 1985 to over 17 million dollars by 1991.

Recognizing that endowment funds would provide a flexible
investment for the future, Healy helped the Clinic work toward a
half-billion-dollar endowment by the year 2000. A centerpiece of
her stewardship was to be a new building complex, the Research
and Education Institute, providing 305,000 square feet of research
and education facilities encompassing laboratories, offices, classrooms, and a state-of-the-art library/telecommunications/confer-
ence facility. The first phase, named the John Sherwin Research
Building and built to house three of the eight research departments,
opened in 1991. The full Research and Education Institute complex,
renamed the Lerner Research Institute in acknowledgement of a

major donation by Alfred Lerner, President of The Cleveland Clinic Foundation Board of Trustees, opened in 1998.

To help ensure a steady stream of bright, highly motivated students, Healy seized the chance to complement the Clinic's academic partnership with Cleveland State University by affiliating formally with The Ohio State University (see Chapter 9). Healy's far-reaching ideas, dynamic personality, and outstanding professional reputation caught the attention of President George H.W. Bush, who appointed her first woman director of the National Institutes of Health in 1991.

Banerjee, vice chairman of the Research Institute, was named acting chairman upon Healy's departure. During his vice chairmanship and acting chairmanship, he reached out to other academic institutions, improving relations with Ohio State University and collaborating with Cleveland's Case Western Reserve University (CWRU) on virology projects. He continued to build his own strong program in molecular biology.

THE STARK ERA, 1992-2002

In 1992, the Board of Governors named George R. Stark, Ph.D., chairman of the Research Institute. A molecular biologist of international repute, Stark was trained at Columbia University and began his independent career at Rockefeller University, where his work centered on protein chemistry. He then went to Stanford University, where he worked on enzyme mechanisms and developed two important methods in molecular biology known as the Northern and Western blotting techniques. In 1983, he joined London's Imperial Cancer Research Fund, where he focused on gene amplification and intracellular signaling pathways modulated by interferons.

Stark's chairmanship signaled an even greater emphasis on building depth of expertise in molecular biology. However, he recognized the need to recruit excellent staff at all levels and in all fields, as well as to maintain interaction between the clinical and basic science staffs. Coincident with Stark's arrival, The Cleveland Clinic formed the Department of Neurosciences, incorporating staff from the former Department of Brain and Vascular Research. It represented the culmination of 15 years of effort to establish research programs linking the basic and clinical sciences to address the underlying mechanisms and treatment of nervous system diseases. Bruce Trapp, Ph.D., a prominent multiple sclerosis researcher from Johns Hopkins University, was recruited to chair the new department. From the outset, the program brought together clinicians from neurology, neurosurgery, neuropathology, and neuroradiology with neurobiologists, neuroimmunologists, and molecular biologists.

Stark's encouragement of new efforts that combined basic and clinical sciences included technology transfer. In 1994 this led to the Research Division's first free-standing spin-off company, BioSeiche Therapeutics, Inc. (later renamed Ridgeway Biosystems, Inc.), which was built on Robert H. Silverman, Ph.D.'s technique of using a new class of drugs, called "2-5A antisense," to target and destroy disease-causing RNA in viruses or tumor cells.

In 1994, Robert Graham returned to his native Australia, and the Board of Governors convened a committee to evaluate the Department of Heart and Hypertension Research in view of the other existing cardiovascular research programs at the Clinic. The committee recommended merging the department with the Jacobs Center for Thrombosis and Vascular Biology. The Center's director, Edward F. Plow, Ph.D., recruited from Scripps Research Institute in 1992, became chairman of the new Department of Molecular Cardiology, and Eric Topol, M.D., became vice chair. Also, Thomas A. Hamilton, Ph.D., was named chairman of the Department of Immunology, after several years as acting chair.

Stark established formal avenues for Research Institute investigators to create bridge programs with physicians in the Taussig Cancer Center, the Mellen Center for Multiple Sclerosis, the Center for Digestive Disease Research, the Urological Institute, and other clinical entities. Centers of Anesthesiology Research and Surgery Research were created, and a Department of Ophthalmic Research was started in the Cole Eye Institute. Stark also initiated a program in Structural Biology in collaboration with scientists at Case Western Reserve University and Cleveland State University.

In 1998, Stark sought a new chair of Molecular Biology, with Banerjee remaining head of the virology research program. Andrei Gudkov, Ph.D., an outstanding translational molecular biologist from the University of Illinois, assumed this role in 2000. Gudkov was instrumental in the relocation of a Chicago-based biotechnology start-up company, Quark Biotechnology, Inc., to the Clinic's campus. In September 2003, Quark announced its impending move to California to concentrate on production rather than research. But Gudkov's entrepreneurial spirit fit well with the Clinic's reinvigorated efforts to commercialize its intellectual property. Supporting these efforts was new leadership in the technology transfer office (referred to as "Cleveland Clinic Foundation Innovations") by Christopher Coburn, formerly of the Battelle Institute, in the role of administrative director and Joseph Hahn, M.D., as medical director.

In the 1990s, the Department of Biomedical Engineering had grown to be the largest in the Lerner Research Institute, with over 20 faculty members. Cornhill left the institution in 2001, and the following year Peter Cavanagh, Ph.D., a distinguished researcher in biomechanics and kinesiology, was recruited from Pennsylvania State University to chair the department. Cavanagh restructured the department, creating programmatic sections. In addition, he and Joseph Iannotti, M.D., Ph.D., created a new Orthopaedic Research Center including laboratory-based and clinical researchers from both departments.

THE DICORLETO ERA, 2002-

Stark stepped down as chair of the Lerner Research Institute in 2002 after a decade of strong leadership and dramatic growth. Paul E. DiCorleto, Ph.D., succeeded him later that year. DiCorleto received his doctorate in biochemistry from Cornell University and performed postdoctoral studies in vascular cell biology at the University of Washington. His research focused on the cellular basis of atherosclerosis and other vascular diseases. DiCorleto joined The Cleveland Clinic in 1981 and served subsequently as chairman of the Department of Cell Biology, as Associate Chief of Staff, and as a member of the Board of Governors. An important part of his plan for the Research Institute was to expand two translational research areas—human genetics/genomics and stem cell biology/regenerative medicine.

DiCorleto reaffirmed the original philosophy of the Research Division, i.e., to perform outstanding basic and applied biomedical research and to educate the next generation of biomedical researchers. The major objective remains advancement of the means of prevention, diagnosis, and treatment of disease. The research staff members receive the bulk of their support from peer-reviewed and competitively awarded external grants, the majority from the NIH. They serve as mentors to graduate students, post-doctoral fellows, medical students, and interns, and they maintain close academic ties with Case Western Reserve University, Cleveland State University, and Kent State University.

The long tradition of creative scientific interaction and innovation continues. Recent discoveries include the identification of genetic variations that are associated with premature coronary artery disease and heart attack (Eric Topol, M.D., Qing Wang, Ph.D., and Edward Plow, Ph.D.), the identification of novel diagnostics for both cardiovascular disease (Stanley Hazen, M.D., Ph.D., and Marc Penn, M.D., Ph.D.) and cancer (Andrei Gudkov, Ph.D., and Raymond Tubbs, D.O.), and the elucidation of novel genes and pathways that are involved in the pathogenesis of multiple sclerosis (Bruce Trapp, Ph.D., and Richard Rudick, M.D.) and prostate cancer (Robert Silverman, Ph.D., Graham Casey, Ph.D., and Eric Klein, M.D.). There has also been excellent progress on many fronts in applied research, such as the use of autologous stem cells to improve healing of bone fractures (George Muschler, M.D.) and the development of new imaging software for the evaluation of heart disease (Geoffrey Vince, Ph.D.). Both of these advances have opened commercialization opportunities.

Continuing in the tradition of Page, the Institute encourages scientific interactions among investigators. Program Project Grants are tangible examples of this philosophy. From these collaborations have come major program grants, including one to support atherosclerosis research headed by DiCorleto with 25 years of continuous support by the NIH, another for multiple sclerosis research headed by Richard Ransohoff, M.D., and yet another on interferons and cancer headed by Stark. Many other program grant applications are pending or in preparation. Thus, the group practice concept of research remains very much alive.

Those who have led research activity have continually renewed the principles under which the Clinic was founded: Crile understood the importance of research in providing better patient care; Page emphasized the link between basic and clinical investigation, and the importance of training the next generation; Healy's wise planning and budgeting and her personal impetus energized the initial stages of the Research and Education Institute, increased outside funding and endowment, and attracted outstanding talent. And Stark expanded these approaches and encouraged collegial and effective joint activities to strengthen the current and future base of science talent. These leaders have ensured that the Research Institute will remain on the forefront of innovation and discovery well into the next century. DiCorleto has had strong and positive interactions with all of the previous chairs, including Page (who visited the Research Institute on a regular basis until his death in 1991), and he is committed to carrying the tradition forward during his stewardship.

21. CLEVELAND CLINIC FLORIDA

By Melinda Estes, Mimi Murphy, and John Clough

Progress lies not in enhancing what is, but in advancing toward what will be.
—*Kahlil Gibran*

FLORIDA BECKONS

The Cleveland Clinic began its sixth decade in 1981 as the largest non-governmental employer in Cleveland. At that time, however, the city was in a deep recession and losing population. Regional economics and the expected effects of health care reform posed a challenge to the Clinic's continued growth in Cleveland. Nevertheless, desiring to build upon the Clinic's prior growth and success, Clinic leadership recognized the opportunity to expand the integrated, academic group practice-based delivery system beyond Cleveland. Thus, they began to explore potential locations across the United States. Because the Clinic's international reputation was strong, they also looked abroad, visiting locations in Europe, Africa, and the Far East at the invitation of local institutions or governments. The Clinic gave serious consideration to Morocco and Singapore, where stable governments offered substantial financial and hospital support. In the end, however, the logistics of staffing and running a clinic on another continent proved impractical, and the idea of overseas expansion was set aside.

The Clinic returned its attention to the United States—specifically Florida, where migration patterns from the midwest and northeast are strong. Moreover, many considered Florida to be the gateway to

Latin America. Because increasing numbers of patients from South America were traveling to Cleveland to seek medical care, Clinic leaders concluded that an affiliate in Florida would appeal to many of the international patients arriving in Cleveland by way of Miami. Therefore, southeast Florida, regionally known as "South Florida," emerged as the most favorable location for such an affiliate. Marketing studies indicated that The Cleveland Clinic enjoyed the greatest name recognition in Fort Lauderdale—an area where, despite a population of four million, no true multispecialty group practice existed. And, with the exception of the University of Miami, there was no significant institution for medical education in the region.

As the Clinic narrowed its focus to the Fort Lauderdale-Broward County area, a local broker who had had previous experience with the organization introduced Clinic leaders to administrators of the North Broward Hospital District. The introduction resulted in an offer from the District to establish a joint venture with the Clinic whereby the District would build an outpatient building adjacent to its Broward General Hospital especially for Clinic use. Specialty care staff would be recruited jointly and supplemented by Clinic staff. Although Clinic leaders and District officials approved the joint venture, the medical staff at Broward General Hospital vehemently opposed the agreement and demanded that the offer be withdrawn. Both parties gave way to staff hostility and dropped the proposal.

Contrary to the physicians' response, however, was the reaction of the Broward business community, which embraced the idea of the Clinic's entry into the area. Encouraged by Fort Lauderdale business leaders, Clinic officials grew confident that South Florida residents would welcome their new group practice and decided to open an independent, Clinic-owned group practice.

Demographic studies of South Florida (a single metropolitan area encompassing Broward, Dade, and Palm Beach Counties) showed that a location in west central Broward County where the primary road from Florida's west coast ("Alligator Alley") crossed a major north-south highway on the east coast was within a two-hour drive of more than six million people. The Clinic purchased 320 acres of land in this prime location near the community of Weston.

The Clinic next addressed the question of who would lead Cleveland Clinic Florida. The Board of Governors appointed William A. Hawk, M.D., chairman of the Department of Anatomic Pathology, to the position of chief executive officer until the new facility opened. Hawk had played a key role in the construction of the Crile Building. He was to be succeeded by Carl C. Gill, M.D., a respected cardiovascular surgeon and member of the Board of Governors, who would serve as medical director until Hawk's retirement. James Cuthbertson, secretary to the Board of Governors, was appointed chief operating officer. Hawk and Cuthbertson moved to Florida in January 1987 to begin the process of building Cleveland Clinic Florida from the ground up. Gill remained in Cleveland a few months longer to start recruiting the medical staff.

PRELIMINARY RED TAPE

As in Ohio, the corporate practice of medicine in Florida is illegal. Therefore, special legislative action was necessary to allow The Cleveland Clinic organizational structure to exist there. Moreover, the Florida licensure law required physicians who passed licensing examinations other than Florida's more than ten years earlier to take the Florida FLEX examination. This process was lengthy and arduous for mid-career physicians, especially specialists. In order to open in Jacksonville, the Mayo Clinic had gotten the state to alter both statutes. In fact, the legislature had passed a new statute, similar to that for Florida's medical schools, that permitted Florida to license 25 Mayo Clinic physicians licensed in other states without further examination. The specificity of this law to Mayo was predicated on the size of the mother institution and the amount of financial support provided for education and research, and thus excluded all other institutions. Therefore, in order to establish Cleveland Clinic Florida, both laws had to be changed again. With the help of a friendly and powerful delegation of Broward County legislators and a cadre of lobbyists, the legislature passed the needed changes on the last day of the legislative session in June 1987.

The Clinic's leaders intended to establish a campus that included an outpatient clinic, hospital, research, and education facilities. In Florida, however, hospital beds cannot be occupied without approval from the Department of Health and Rehabilitative Services through the certificate-of-need process, which is closely monitored and strenuously defended by established institutions. In March 1987, the

Clinic filed an application to build a 400-bed hospital. After a series of delays, revisions and resubmissions, the Department rejected the Clinic's bid in January 1989 on the grounds that Broward County already had too many unused hospital beds. The Clinic decided not to appeal the decision at that time.

Expecting the approval and building process to take several years, the Clinic had made arrangements for temporary outpatient and hospital facilities. Even before the statutes regarding licensure were modified, construction of a 76,000-square-foot outpatient building began 10 miles northwest of downtown Fort Lauderdale. With the expectation that it would be occupied for three years, it was designed to accommodate a staff of 40 physicians in a multispecialty setting.

Gill began recruiting staff in January 1987, but made little headway until the Florida statutes were changed in June. His first goal was to recruit the nucleus of a comprehensive clinic staff that could provide the majority of adult services. These physicians had to be the highest quality available—mature clinicians with significant patient care experience. Preference would be given to Cleveland Clinic staff and graduates as well as physicians trained and recommended by Clinic alumni. He looked for physicians with strong backgrounds in research and education. He recognized that these qualities, combined with energy, collegiality, and a dedication to excellence in patient care, would help Cleveland Clinic Florida mature the culture and maintain the model of medical practice that had always been the hallmark of the parent organization. This transfer of culture was expected to be one of the most difficult aspects of building Cleveland Clinic Florida.

Simultaneous with physician recruitment was the Clinic's search for a local hospital—a place where Clinic physicians could admit Clinic patients. The search was somewhat challenging due to local physician opposition to Clinic physicians and The Cleveland Clinic practice. Several hospitals closed their staffs in order to prevent Clinic physicians from applying for privileges. The Federal Trade Commission later investigated these hospitals for restraint of trade.

One area hospital, the North Beach Hospital, went against the tide and extended privileges to Clinic physicians. The owners of this 150-bed for-profit institution located on Fort Lauderdale's beachfront, Health Trust, Inc., had everything to gain by locking in a steady source of income. The North Beach Hospital had a small active staff and a dangerously low census. After both parties agreed on several upgrades to the hospital, the Clinic made North Beach its primary hospital.

GRAND OPENING AND PUSHBACK

Cleveland Clinic Florida opened its doors with a staff of 28 physicians on February 29, 1988—almost exactly 67 years following the opening of its parent institution in Cleveland. The Clinic's first patient was admitted to North Beach Hospital the following day. The official dedication occurred two months later, on April 8, 1988. Gill became chief executive officer, and Hawk retired, as planned. Cuthbertson remained as chief operating officer.

Although North Beach Hospital was satisfactory for most patients, it lacked the facilities and certificates of need for invasive cardiology procedures and cardiac surgery. Five hospitals in Broward County had approval to perform these services. One was Broward General, which had lost its primary team of cardiac surgeons to a competing hospital in nearby Palm Beach County. When Cleveland Clinic Florida cardiac physicians applied for privileges at this public hospital, Broward General Hospital's Medical Executive Committee postponed a review of their applications for three months. Finally, the applications were rejected as a group, and the hospital district's Board of Commissioners supported this decision. Confronted with the illegality of its action, the Board reversed its stand in January 1989 and asked the Clinic to assume control of the cardiac surgery program at Broward General. Nevertheless, the hospital's Medical Executive Committee still refused to grant privileges to the Clinic physicians. On April 27, the Commissioners were forced to import a committee of physicians from outside the state of Florida at taxpayers' expense to review the Clinic physicians' applications. They passed easily, and Gill performed Cleveland Clinic Florida's first open heart operation at Broward General on May 15, 1989, without incident, over a year after the fledgling organization's opening. Shortly thereafter, the majority of Cleveland Clinic Florida physicians obtained privileges there. Later, in 1994, a cardiac catheterization laboratory opened at North Beach Hospital, by then owned by the Clinic and renamed Cleveland Clinic Hospital, and an application for a certificate of need for open-heart surgery was filed the same year.

The struggle for privileges at Broward General made many local physicians more determined than ever to drive The Cleveland Clinic out of Broward County. Their animosity was annoying but tolerable until it began to interfere with patient care. Local physicians who interacted with Cleveland Clinic staff received threats that referrals from their non-Clinic colleagues would stop unless they severed all relationships with the Clinic. In early 1989, a terminally ill Clinic patient needed a consultation with a pulmonologist, a specialty that Cleveland Clinic Florida did not yet have on staff. Incredibly, no pulmonologist in Broward County would see the patient! The needed consultation was eventually provided by a pulmonologist from Miami, who was given temporary privileges at North Beach for this purpose.

Although the suit was eventually dropped, it caught the attention of the Federal Trade Commission. Agents began investigating selected Broward County hospitals and physicians for antitrust activity in August 1989. Sixteen months later, armed with abundant evidence, they accused local doctors of attempting to restrain trade. At the insistence of the chief of staff at Broward General Medical Center, most physicians initially resisted the commission's order to admit wrongdoing and sign a consent decree. But faced with the consequences, by May all had signed except the chief of staff. Not until faced with criminal charges did he reluctantly back down in January 1992, ending the overt hostility and the ugliest chapter in the early history of Cleveland Clinic Florida.

Practicing side by side with local physicians at North Beach Hospital was beneficial to Cleveland Clinic Florida during these troubled first years, for it helped Clinic physicians assimilate into the community while providing the hospital with a growing number of admissions from both groups. Extensive renovations had turned North Beach into an attractive, modern hospital, and the census had climbed dramatically. The Cleveland Clinic purchased North Beach Hospital in 1990 and began to merge its operations with those of the Clinic in September 1992. On January 1, 1993, its name was changed to the Cleveland Clinic Hospital.

PROGRESS

During its early years, Cleveland Clinic Florida made a remarkable impact on the face of medicine in South Florida, which was dominated by solo practitioners. Led by Gill and chief of staff, Harry K. Moon, M.D., Clinic physicians quickly demonstrated the benefits offered by a multispecialty group practice to patients and physicians alike by providing expert diagnoses and sophisticated treatments not widely available. They began performing clinical research and publishing their findings. By September 1995, 221 projects had been approved, and almost 400 articles were published the previous year alone. A basic research program began in 1994 with the recruitment of biochemist and molecular biologist Susan R. Abramson, Ph.D.

Cleveland Clinic Florida physicians initiated weekly grand rounds in 1988, and they invited community physicians to participate. Larger continuing medical education programs offered throughout the year attracted a large audience of local, regional, national, and international physicians.

Cleveland Clinic Florida's colorectal surgery residency program was the first in the state to be approved by the Accreditation Council on Graduate Medical Education (ACGME) for two residents a year. Clinic residents and fellows from the Cleveland campus rotated through through a variety of services at Cleveland Clinic Florida, and in 1996 the ACGME approved a residency program in internal medicine for Cleveland Clinic Florida as a freestanding program.

The need for educational materials to support residents and staff physicians led Cleveland Clinic Florida to open a medical library in 1990. The funds to purchase books, periodicals, and computer services were raised through donations and special events. Known as the A. Lorraine and Sigmund Goldblatt Medical Library in honor of its major benefactors, it was open to anyone who wished to use it.

By its fourth birthday, Cleveland Clinic Florida had reason to celebrate. With 300 employees and a physician staff of 63, the young medical center had doubled in size in four years. The doctors had provided for 200,000 outpatient visits, and almost 7,000 advance appointments had been booked. The Clinic's rapid growth, coupled with its unique management style, convinced the readers of the *South Florida Business Journal* to select Cleveland Clinic Florida as the Medical Business Best Outpatient Facility in 1990.

While opposition to the Clinic initially resulted in a referral boycott, local physicians soon discovered how the Clinic could assist them with patient care. A poll taken in November 1991 showed that 25% of Clinic patients were referred by their physicians.

By 1995, the Clinic staff had grown to nearly 100 physicians who practiced in a full range of adult specialties. Nevertheless, inadequate office space constricted the rapidly growing institution. Furthermore, Cleveland Clinic Hospital's small size, its distance from the outpatient clinic, and lack of sophistication presented a growing problem. The Clinic had no choice but to expand.

EXPANSION TO WESTON

As Cleveland Clinic Florida continued to operate from its temporary office space, plans to find a permanent home near Interstate Highway 75 in southwest Broward County were well under way. As previously recounted, efforts to build a medical center in Florida had begun in March 1987, when the Clinic originally filed for a certificate of need (CON) to build a 400-bed hospital. Although the application was defeated, the Clinic's determination to establish a multi-specialty medical campus was not. The Clinic filed again for a CON in 1995. Unlike the 1987 application, the intention of the Clinic's second attempt was to build a replacement hospital for the North Beach facility. The Florida Agency for Health Care Administration (AHCA) approved the 1995 application and granted the Clinic a CON to build a replacement hospital on June 6, 1997. In late 1997, Gill left Cleveland Clinic Florida and Moon succeeded him as chief executive officer. One year later, on November 12, 1998, the Clinic broke ground on a 43-acre site in Weston, Florida.

The vision for the future medical center was a fully integrated medical campus—a single location where a patient could receive all necessary medical services. It was to be a place where traditional hospital beds, an outpatient pavilion, and physician's offices were located under one roof, just as at the main campus in Cleveland. The significance of the groundbreaking in Weston was twofold. It was, on the one hand, the product of a multi-year effort to obtain a CON to build a 150-bed, $80 million hospital. On the other hand, it represented a joint venture between The Cleveland Clinic and the Santa Barbara,

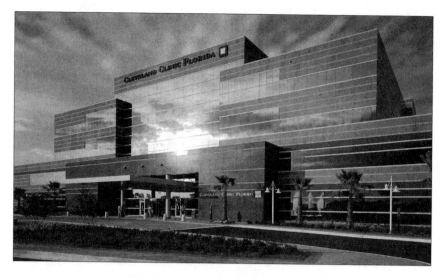

Cleveland Clinic Florida Weston, 2002

California-based Tenet Healthcare Corporation. Under the partnership, Tenet and the Clinic would co-own the hospital, and Tenet would manage its day-to-day operations. Although the hospital would bear the Clinic's name, it would become part of the Tenet South Florida Health System.

The Weston community eagerly awaited the arrival of Cleveland Clinic Florida. The proposed medical campus and hospital not only received unanimous approval from the Weston City Commission but a resounding endorsement as well. City commissioner Mark Myers characterized the Clinic's relocation as "the most exciting development in the City." At the time of the groundbreaking, it was estimated that the hospital would have more than 90 physicians on its staff, specializing in approximately 40 different areas of medicine. In addition to top-quality medical care, the hospital would focus on research and education. Already, the Clinic's residency programs were multiplying. Joining the colorectal residency program were programs in internal medicine, neurology, and geriatric medicine.

The Clinic's rapid growth was to be well supported by the future multi-specialty campus. In the new hospital, Clinic physicians and residents would have at their disposal a modern emergency room, a cardiac laboratory for diagnosis and a cardiac rehabilitation area, inpatient and out-patient surgical facilities, and a fully equipped diagnostic radiology center, all under one roof. New services at the Weston facility would include a kidney transplant program, an expanded center for minimally invasive surgery, and an expanded neurosurgery program.

As civic leaders and area residents looked forward to having a medical facility in close proximity to their work and home, Clinic physicians and administrators looked forward to working in a facility that mirrored The Cleveland Clinic in Cleveland. The facility had been specially designed to reproduce the Clinic's unique model of medicine—one that integrates inpatient and outpatient care with research and education. For Clinic physicians, the new location represented a significant milestone in the long struggle to fulfill their original mission in South Florida.

A BI-COASTAL PRESENCE

As early as 1996, Moon foresaw that the new campus would provide services to many people throughout the community, region, state, and beyond. At the time of the groundbreaking, the majority of the 220,000 patients who received care at Cleveland Clinic Florida on a yearly basis came from the southern third of the state, from Lake Okeechobee southward. Weston was an ideal location for the Clinic because of its accessibility to South Florida's three populous counties—Palm Beach, Broward, and Dade. Nevertheless, as the Clinic conducted additional demographic studies, it became evident that a growing segment of the Clinic's patient base was commuting from Florida's west coast—namely, Lee and Collier Counties.

Simultaneous with recognition of the west coast as a potential second site for the Clinic in Florida, a patient requested the Clinic to underwrite a van service to transport patients from the west coast to Cleveland Clinic Florida's Fort Lauderdale facility. This particular patient, like other patients from Naples, was so pleased with her treatment that she regularly drove from Naples to Fort Lauderdale for ongoing therapy. The Clinic funded the service and, by 1998, had transported more than 15,000 patients from Naples, Marco Island, and Fort Myers.

Clinic leaders further scrutinized Collier County's patient demographics and growth projections and determined that North Naples would be an ideal location for a multi-specialty clinic and hospital, similar to the one under construction in Weston. On August 26, 1996, Cleveland Clinic Florida filed notice with state health-care regulators of its intent to apply for a CON to build an acute-care hospital in Collier County with up to 100 hospital beds. At the same, Columbia-HCA Healthcare Corporation filed a letter of intent to make a second application to build a 150-bed hospital. The Clinic's notice followed a year after announcing plans to build a 30,000-square foot outpatient facility on a 7.6-acre parcel purchased adjacent to Interstate Highway 75.

A myriad of factors drove the Clinic's effort to build a hospital on Florida's west coast. Projected population growth, requests from current patients, and high occupancy rates in the community's two existing hospitals, especially during peak tourist season, contributed to the decision. Historically, Collier County had only one hospital provider, the Naples Community Hospital Healthcare System (NCH), which operated the 384-bed Naples Community Hospital near downtown Naples and the 50-bed North Collier Hospital, off Immokalee Road. While NCH opposed the proposal, the residents of Collier County embraced it.

A public hearing to discuss the Clinic's application was held in Naples at the request of several Cleveland Clinic supporters. An estimated 350 people attended the public forum—all in support of Cleveland Clinic Florida. Moreover, 179 letters of support were sent to the Health Planning Council of Southwest Florida, Inc. that organized the hearing. The Collier commission chairman, John Norris, speaking on behalf of the commission, stated that the board favored Cleveland Clinic provided it accepted indigent patients. Furthermore, chairman Norris pointed to the county's future growth as another factor in determining the Commission's approval and encouraged the community to view the proposed medical campus as a complement to the existing two hospitals.

The Florida Agency for Health Care Administration denied Cleveland Clinic Florida's proposal to construct a 100-bed hospital and approved Columbia-HCA's request to construct a 150-bed facility. The Cleveland Clinic and Naples Community Hospital both appealed this decision. Approximately one year later, Columbia-HCA and the Clinic negotiated a controversial settlement, later challenged by the Federal Trade Commission, and Columbia-HCA dropped its hospital plan. Naples Community Hospital remained steadfast in objecting to the construction of another local hospital. After months of litigation, NCH officials agreed to drop their opposition to the Clinic's proposal in exchange for concessions by The Cleveland Clinic regarding the amount of charity care the Clinic would provide in the new hospital. The settlement also stipulated that the Clinic could not open the new hospital before April 9, 2000.

The agreement between NCH Healthcare Systems and Cleveland Clinic Florida ended what promised to be a long-fought battle, as Clinic officials vowed to bring health-care competition to Collier County. The arrival of Cleveland Clinic Florida in Naples, particularly the hospital, marked a turning point in health care in the Collier County community that had been dominated by the NCH system with its two hospitals and array of medical services in years past. Collier County had been the last of the state's fast-growing counties to have only one health-care system, a situation that people who wanted choices for medical care found objectionable.

The Clinic decided to build the hospital on the same 37-acre parcel of land where it had already begun constructing a 190,000 square-foot medical office building. This outpatient medical center and diagnostic center, two buildings linked by a corridor, was halfway occupied in January 1999. By June of that year, the Naples Clinic opened its surgery center in the outpatient complex and by late fall, ground was broken for the 70-bed hospital.

The fall of 1999 was an especially busy time of year for Cleveland Clinic Florida. Six weeks prior to the October groundbreaking ceremony of the new Cleveland Clinic Florida Hospital in Naples, a "topping-off ceremony" was held at the Clinic's medical campus in Weston as a final steel beam was placed into the frame of the Clinic's east coast hospital. For Clinic officials, the completion of the Weston hospital signified a new milestone for Cleveland Clinic Florida. The Clinic's administration had succeeded in satisfying Florida's Agency for Health Care Administration that Broward County needed another hospital and finally obtained the much-desired CON to operate the facility. The Weston campus opened for business in July 2001.

As the finishing touches were being applied to the Weston medical facility, the dawn of a new era in hospital care was breaking on Florida's west coast. Cleveland Clinic Florida Hospital Naples celebrated its grand opening on April 2, 2001. This $57-million hospital in North Naples featured 70 private rooms and was designed with the

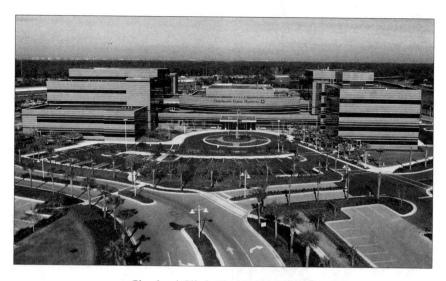

Cleveland Clinic Florida Naples, 2002

Clinic's "healing hospitality" approach to patient care. Of the 70 private rooms, six were dedicated for intensive care. The hospital, located behind the Clinic's sprawling two-year-old outpatient complex, was designed for a potential expansion to 120 beds.

The arrival of the Naples hospital ended Collier County's service by a single hospital provider, an unusual situation for a large community in Florida. There was great enthusiasm for the new hospital among community residents as well as civic and business leaders. Five hundred business leaders attended the dedication and over 6,000 residents attended the Clinic's self-guided tours the weekend before the grand opening. At the conclusion of the hospital's first week of operation, 299 patients had been treated in the emergency room, while 91 patients had been admitted to the hospital.

Much of the success in bringing the Cleveland Clinic Florida Hospital to reality in Naples was due to the accomplished administrative staff that oversaw the development and completion of the 350,000-square-foot medical campus. Fielding Epstein, formerly the radiology administrator at the Clinic's main campus in Cleveland, supervised the development of the clinic and subsequent construction of the hospital. In addition, Epstein was responsible for cultivating the political and community support for the hospital. Geoff Moebius, the former chief executive officer of Deaconess Hospital in

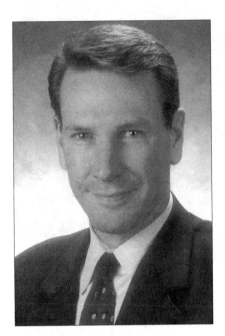

Robert Zehr, M.D., Medical Director,
Cleveland Clinic Florida, Naples, 2003-

Cleveland, was in charge of day-to-day hospital operations. The two administrators supervised the administration of the Naples medical campus, while the chief of staff, Robert J. Zehr, M.D., led the Naples professional staff.

MATURATION AND NEW LEADERSHIP

With the new Naples campus fully operational and the Weston campus nearing completion, the bi-coastal Cleveland Clinic Florida announced several changes in its administrative leadership and structural organization. Loop asked Melinda Estes, M.D., the former executive director for business development at the Cleveland Clinic and the first woman to be elected to The Cleveland Clinic's Board of Governors, to serve as the new chief executive officer of Cleveland Clinic Florida. Estes replaced Moon, who became president of the Cleveland Clinic Florida Foundation and later retired. Jerry Oliphant was named Chief Operating Officer. The new administration marked a great beginning for the future of The Cleveland Clinic in Florida. The opening of the modern, patient-centered hospital in Naples was soon to be replicated in Weston. It appeared that a new era in Cleveland Clinic Florida's history was getting under way.

Big-time healthcare arrived in western Broward County with the opening of Cleveland Clinic Florida Weston. On July 2, 2001, Cleveland Clinic Florida opened its 150-bed hospital designed to provide a full range of specialty care, including open-heart surgery, adult kidney transplantation and neurosurgery. The $150 million campus, Broward County's first new hospital since 1992, brought the Clinic's expertise in medical research to the forefront.

Shortly after its opening, Cleveland Clinic Hospital rolled out the first comprehensive heart program in Weston, which offered South Florida residents the latest and most advanced treatments in cardiac care. Services included angioplasty, cardiac catheterization, and minimally invasive robotic heart surgery. Heart catheterizations and renal transplants were performed on a regular basis and, by the end of 2001, the multi-specialty medical campus was fully operational.

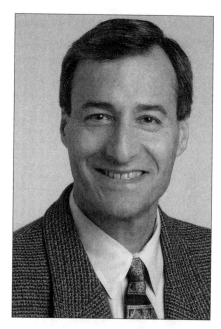

Howard Graman, M.D.,
Medical Director,
Cleveland Clinic Florida, Weston, 2003-

When Estes left the Clinic in 2003, Clinic leadership determined that the complexity of Cleveland Clinic Florida mandated separate govenance for the east- and west-coast operations and appointed Howard Graman, M.D., to lead Cleveland Clinic Weston and Robert Zehr, M.D., to lead Cleveland Clinic Naples. Another new era for Cleveland Clinic Florida had begun.

In less than 14 years, Cleveland Clinic Florida had grown from a small medical group into one of Florida's largest multi-specialty group practices. Advances in research, technology, and medical services continued at Cleveland Clinic Florida. Its leadership team, composed of physicians and administrative staff alike, directed each of the medical facilities using The Cleveland Clinic model of medicine. As such, the superior quality of the Clinic's brand of medicine supported its growth, and the population of South Florida was the beneficiary.

TRUSTEES, GOVERNORS, AND ADMINISTRATION

22. ADMINISTRATION: THE "GRAY COATS"

Our chief want in life is somebody who
shall make us do what we can.
—*Ralph Waldo Emerson*

THROUGHOUT THE HISTORY OF THE CLEVELAND CLINIC, THE ORGANIZATION'S excellence has emanated from the numerous giants of medicine, surgery, medical education, and research whose accomplishments have been chronicled in these pages. A few of these clinical pioneers have also been health industry visionaries and worthy stewards of The Cleveland Clinic's physical and monetary assets. Physician leaders Crile, LeFevre, Wasmuth, Kiser, and most recently, Loop, guided the organization through the twentieth and into the twenty-first centuries, in both good times and bad. We should, nevertheless, pause and recognize the non-clinical specialty of professional administration, without which the business accomplishments of the Clinic would not have occurred.[1]

As with its clinicians, the Clinic has enjoyed a continuing succession of skilled and capable administrators who have made countless contributions to the advancement of the institution's mission. Professional managers and administrators have worked to keep the organization viable and on course during difficult and trying financial and political times. They made the Clinic's growth potential a reality by developing the main campus, the health system, and a network of hospitals and clinics covering northeastern Ohio and both coasts of Florida. These men and women were truly "specialists," in that they brought specific and highly refined expertise in finance, operations and administration, marketing, information systems, security, foreign and governmental affairs, law, human resources, practice management, planning, construction, public relations, and entrepreneurship. The "Gray Coats" effectively complemented and supported the "White Coats" to create a healthcare organization ranking among the finest in the world.

IN THE BEGINNING

Non-physician administration at The Cleveland Clinic can be traced back to 1914, when Amy Rowland became Crile's right-hand assistant. Her duties ranged from patient care to administration. She wrote a book which turned out to be the precursor of the *To Act As a Unit* series, called simply *The Cleveland Clinic Foundation*. The William Feather Company of Cleveland published it in 1938, and the first few chapters of *To Act As a Unit* rely heavily upon it as a source.

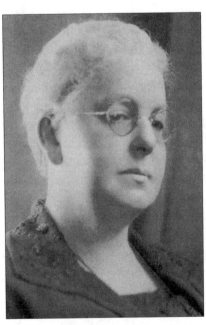

Amy Rowland, George W. Crile's assistant since 1914

Edward C. Daoust, who at times has been referred to as the fifth founder, was a professional administrator of great significance in The Cleveland Clinic's early history. Daoust, son-in-law of Bunts, was the attorney who drew up the founding documents as specified by the four founders, and who continued to serve The Cleveland Clinic Foundation, ultimately as its president, until his untimely death in 1947.

In 1921 the Clinic officially opened its doors, and Daoust, along with attorney John Marshall, figured prominently in the organization's beginnings. Perhaps the first true operations administrator was Litta Perkins, who served as business manager and handled financial matters as directed by the founders. The first hospital administrator and director of nursing was Emma Oxley, the superintendent of the Oxley Homes. These were two houses on East 93rd Street that were pressed into service as a hospital until 1924, when the first real hospital opened (see chapter 2).

Gertrude Hills was the first administrator hired for the "new" hospital that opened in 1924. In her position as manager of offices, she was responsible for hiring employees, managing banking and payroll, admitting patients, and handling other business matters as needed. She was human resources, operations, finance, and admissions all rolled into one! Charlotte Dunning was the superintendent of the new hospital for the first three years, after which Abbie Porter replaced her and served in that position until 1949. Thus, in the earliest history of The Cleveland Clinic, women played critical and prominent roles in the management of its affairs. Maynard Collier succeeded Porter. As noted in chapter 3, Litta Perkins was one of the 123 people who perished in the 1929 disaster. H. K. Whipple succeeded her as secretary later that year. He continued to serve in various administrative capacities until his death in 1940.

In 1930, John Sherwin joined the Board of Trustees. He was the first business-oriented, non-academic trustee. Sherwin took a direct and active part in Clinic affairs, serving as a precursor of today's Executive Committee of the Board of Trustees. Attorney Benjamin Fiery performed the Clinic's early patent work, a forerunner of the current office of technology transfer and innovations. In 1940, George Grill became superintendent and assistant secretary of the institution. Grill had formerly been assistant superintendent of schools in Lakewood. In 1943, he left to re-enlist in the Army with the rank of captain after his son was killed in combat.

THE POST-WAR ERA

The end of World War II brought a period of significant change and transition to the Clinic. Crile had died before the end of the war, and Lower, who had been functioning as the chief of operations, decided that it was time to retire. Daoust, still prominently

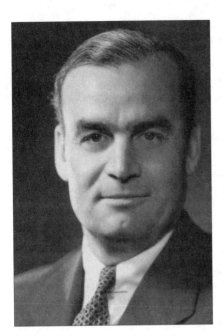
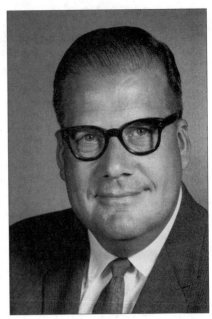

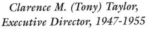

Clarence M. (Tony) Taylor,
Executive Director, 1947-1955

James G. Harding,
Hospital Administrator, 1952-1969

involved in the Clinic's business, died in a plane crash in 1947, as we have previously noted.

At that time, Sherwin stepped in and engaged the firm of Booz, Allen and Hamilton to make recommendations for the future management of The Cleveland Clinic (see chapter 5). From this engagement there emerged a design for a system of governance, headed by a non-physician executive director, modeled upon business corporations of the day. Clarence M. (Tony) Taylor left his position at Lincoln Electric and took the reins of administration, while a few physician-led committees governed medical affairs. During Taylor's tenure, from 1947 to 1955, The Cleveland Clinic ran like a corporation. In 1952, James G. Harding, a former assistant administrator at St. Luke's Hospital in Cleveland, had become The Cleveland Clinic's hospital administrator. He succeeded Ken Shoos, who in turn moved to the position of administrator at St. Luke's. In 1954, Earl J. Frederick joined the "methods department," introducing industrial engineering concepts to The Cleveland Clinic. Many believe this to have been the birth of management engineering in health care.

Toward the end of Taylor's tenure as executive director, unrest grew among the medical staff, as they desired a more active role in the management and future direction of the organization. The Clinic then engaged Hamilton and Associates to study its operations and develop a new plan, which provided for a physician-led Board of Governors to direct day-to-day activities. The Board of Trustees would retain fiduciary responsibility.

Richard Gottron assumed the position of business manager in 1958 and acted as liaison between the trustees and the Board of Governors. The first Executive Secretary to the Board of Governors was Dr. Walter Zeiter. Later, non-physician administrators, including James Lees, James Cuthbertson, Tom Bruckman, and Gene Altus, a former management engineer, would fill that position.

In 1969, LeFevre, who had become the first chairman of the Board of Governors in 1955, stepped down to be replaced by Wasmuth, an anesthesiologist with a law degree. The style of governance now changed significantly with the Board of Governors becoming much more aggressive and taking increasing responsibility for the day-to-day activities of the organization. Gottron was appointed President of the Clinic's subsidiaries (The Bolton Square Hotel Company, The Motor Center Company, and The Cleveland Clinic Pharmacy). He became despondent, however, and committed suicide at his desk in January of 1969. Later that year the Board of Governors eliminated Harding's hospital administrator position, and he left the institution.

THE TURBULENT 1960s AND 1970s

The late 1960s and early 1970s saw an increase in professional administration staffing and the differentiation of many functions into new and specialized departments. In 1968, a permanent, on-campus general counsel's office was established under the leadership of John A. ("Jack") Auble, Esq. Auble also succeeded James Nichols as secretary of The Cleveland Clinic Foundation. Nichols, with his familiar bow ties, had come to The Cleveland Clinic in 1956 from the law firm of Baker, Hostetler and Patterson, where he had done legal work for the Clinic. He served as secretary of the Foundation until 1969, when he succeeded Gottron as business

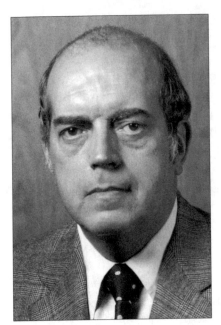

John A. "Jack" Auble,
General Counsel, 1968-1992

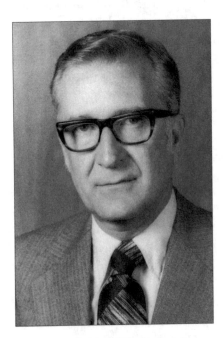

Robert J. Fischer,
Director of Finance, 1970-1985

manager after the latter's death. Nichols became director of finance early in 1970, resigning later that year. Robert Fischer succeeded him as the next head of the financial arm of the organization. In late 1970, Gerald Wolf assumed the position of controller and later was promoted to treasurer.

A creative new management concept, the administrative services coordinator, took shape in 1968 with Gilbert Cook, a former methods engineer who had become an assistant administrator, in charge. The idea was to decentralize management and business expertise to the hospital units. The purpose of this innovation was to permit nursing management to focus its energies on clinical issues. The first coordinator was Joseph Lazorchak, who later followed Harding to the Wilmington Medical Center in Delaware. At its peak, this disseminated "coordinator department" included more than 20 people, covered day and evening shifts, and provided immediate hospital unit problem-solving capabilities, as well as supply and logistics management. Many members of this entry-level administrative department later moved to positions of greater management responsibility, both inside and outside the Clinic.

After a stint as administrator of the Department of Neurology, Robert Coulton became the first administrator for the Office of Professional Staff Affairs in 1988, and Dale Goodrich was appointed administrative director of Patient Services in 1984. William Lawrence, another "coordinator department" graduate, would later move to the administrator post at St. Alexis Hospital, later known as St. Michael Hospital, then to Richmond General Hospital, known at the time as PHS Mt. Sinai East, under Primary Health Systems, Inc., before joining the University Hospitals Health System. David Posch served as executive assistant to the chief operating officer prior to leaving to accept an assistant administrator position at Ochsner Clinic in New Orleans, Louisiana.

In 1969, five individuals emerged as the key non-physician leaders, responsible for most of the day-to-day administrative operations of The Cleveland Clinic. Two of these came from the trio of James Zucker, Edmond Notebaert, and Gilbert Cook. Zucker soon left the Clinic for a position at Christ Hospital in Cincinnati, leaving Cook and Notebaert, both in their 30s. Cook had served as Harding's assistant administrator during his tenure as hospital administrator. When Harding left, and Wasmuth assumed the chairmanship of the Board of Governors, the Board determined that the hospital administrator position would remain unfilled and that Notebaert and Cook would divide responsibilities for hospital and clinic departmental operations, including nursing. Four nurse managers were appointed to oversee specific areas or zones of the hospital, and there was no single director of nursing. They aggressively and eagerly took the reins, collaboratively managing operations. They knew that in 1972, a 300-bed hospital expansion was scheduled to double the capacity of the hospital. Cook focused on nursing and many of the hospital-related patient support departments, while Notebaert managed patient access, medical records, and many of the outpatient support functions.

Two other key leaders were Paul E. Widman and James Lees. Widman, a seasoned purchasing and materials management veteran, was responsible for supplies and logistics, including the soon-to-be expanded hospital. A pharmacist by training, he came to the Clinic in 1951 from Johns Hopkins University Hospital and established what, even by today's standards, would be considered a modern materials management program. He soon added the maintenance department to his scope of responsibilities. During his career,

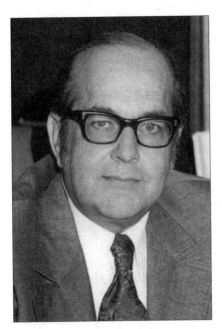

Paul E. Widman,
Head of Materials Management,
1951-1983

Widman received many honors, both for his writings as well as his innovative materials management concepts. Some refer to him as the father of hospital group purchasing, as he foresaw the benefits of combining the acquisition of supplies for groups of hospitals to create maximum bargaining power. To this day the Center for Health Affairs, formerly known as the Greater Cleveland Hospital Association, which houses a regional group-purchasing organization, periodically bestows an award in his name.

In 1970, Lees, previously charged with administration of the Research Division, took over the outpatient clinic's routine operations. Today he would be viewed as administrator of both medicine and surgery. As noted previously, Fischer held the purse strings and managed the Clinic's financial matters. These five men, Notebaert, Cook, Widman, Lees, and Fischer, formed the nucleus of non-physician, professional Cleveland Clinic operations management, as the institution was poised to begin the next period of significant growth.

Notebaert moved on to the chief executive position at Huron Road Hospital in 1978 and later to the Children's Hospital of Philadelphia. Cook took the position of hospital administrator at Lahey Clinic in Boston in 1979. Widman succumbed to thyroid cancer in 1983. Fischer retired in 1985, and Lees, then chief administrative officer, retired in 1992.

During this period, with The Cleveland Clinic on the threshold of an era of growth and development, the organization's leaders recognized the need for computerization as a management tool, at first mainly for financial applications. In the Division of Finance, Tom Keaty led early data-processing efforts in 1965, followed by Edwin

Dillahay in 1971. Howard R. (Dick) Taylor directed the fund development and public affairs functions, while Auble was accountable for legal matters.

THE CLINIC SIDE

In the early 1970s, Lees managed the outpatient clinics. When he took over the position of executive secretary to the Board of Governors in 1972 with broader responsibilities, outpatient administration bifurcated along divisional lines to medicine and surgery. Penn Behrens became administrator of the Division of Medicine in 1976 and served until Terry Bonecutter succeeded him in 1981, moving from materials management, where he was an assistant to Paul Widman. Bonecutter held that position until 1991, when Tina Kaatz took it over. Joanne Zeroske, a nurse, who later assumed department administration responsibilities in several clinical departments, succeeded Kaatz in 2000, and moved on to Radiology in 2003.

In the Division of Surgery, Kristy Kreiger was appointed administrator in 1978 and served in that capacity until 1991. Kreiger had worked in the division in various capacities since 1971. Barbara McAfee took over the administrator role, although with a somewhat different title, director of surgical division operations. Cynthia Hundorfean, a veteran surgical clinic administrator, became the division administrator in 1992.

During the 1970s, in both medicine and surgery, it became customary for departmental administrators to work in tandem with physician department chairs. For small departments, one administrator covered two departments. The growing complexity of computer systems, scheduling systems, coding and reimbursement issues, as well as increasing numbers of employees, necessitated specialized management skills, with knowledge specific to each medical and surgical specialty and department. This trend has continued, and physician/administrator collaboration in clinical departments has become the model for practice management throughout The Cleveland Clinic. These administrators have developed capabilities and expertise that earned national recognition for many of them.

ALPHABET SOUP, THE 1970s AND 1980s

In 1977, Kiser succeeded Wasmuth as chief executive officer, ushering in an era highlighted by participative management, committee governance, and more refined administrative differentiation and specialization. So began the era of the BOG, MOG, FOG, SOG, and COG. At the administrative council meeting of September 29, 1980, Kiser presented a reorganization plan. The council approved it as did the Board of Governors, and it went into effect on October 1, 1980.

BOG was an acronym for the already existing Board of Governors. The MOG, or Medical Operations Group, was formed to deal with the practice of medicine in both the clinic and hospital, and to support research and education. The areas that came under the MOG were the Divisions of Surgery, Medicine, Anesthesiology, Laboratory Medicine, Radiology, Education, Research, Nursing, and Administrative Services. Committees reporting to the MOG were hospital accreditation, professional liaison, operating room liaison, primary care liaison, manpower, equipment, quality, accreditation, and space and remodeling committees. Later, most of these functions came under the aegis of the Medical Executive Committee.

The unfortunate acronym FOG referred to the Foundation Operations Group, whose purpose was to integrate The Cleveland Clinic Foundation's resources: financial, manpower, space, and equipment. The FOG was also responsible for planning and construction, as well as certain areas of policy development. Areas reporting to the FOG were fiscal services, legal services, administrative services (also reporting to the BOG), human resources, public affairs, planning, medical staff affairs (also reporting to the BOG), fund development, and internal audit. Kiser chaired the BOG, MOG, and FOG.

The SOG, or Specialty Operations Group, was responsible for institutional advancement, communications and marketing, external affairs, legislative affairs, and international issues. Institutional advancement literally meant advancing the position and reputation of the institution and is not to be confused with the later Department of Institutional Advancement, which was responsible for fund raising. James S. Krieger, M.D., chaired the SOG.

The COG, or Combined Operations Group, which Kiser also

chaired, brought the MOG, FOG, and SOG together. The MOG became simply the Management Group in 1982, and it was chaired by chief operating officer John Eversman until it finally metamorphosed into the Medical Executive Committee (see above). The FOG and the SOG were relatively short-lived, the last meeting of the FOG having been September 27, 1984. The SOG had an even shorter duration; it very quickly became the responsibility of Frank Weaver, a portly, brash, mustachioed Texan, who arrived on the scene in 1980 (see also chapter 8). Weaver brought modern concepts of marketing, fundraising, and community affairs to the Clinic, which had not previously sought public attention, focusing rather on its clinical, educational, and research missions. He brought The Cleveland Clinic out of its shell, never again to return. Since his tenure, the Clinic has not been reluctant to put its best foot forward for the world to see. Weaver gets the credit (or the blame) for this significant change in institutional philosophy. Weaver left The Cleveland Clinic in 1989.

Widman became director of administrative services in 1977, adding human resources to his portfolio, which already included purchasing, maintenance and supplies, and logistics. In 1979, Widman became director of operations, and in 1980 he was named executive assistant to the administrative council and senior administrator of operations. At this time Lees took over as director of operations and later, chief administrative officer, a position he held until his retirement in 1993. Lees joined the Clinic in 1963 as research administrator and later became administrative assistant to the Board of Governors. His colleagues respected his wide range of knowledge and expertise in business and health care. Lees made early developmental contributions to both legislative affairs and the International Center (described later in this chapter). William Yeagley, William Lawrence, William Malensek, Dale Goodrich, and Tom Seals assisted him. Malensek, who was responsible for materials management, died in 1987, ending a 20-year battle with Hodgkin's disease. His wit, humor, fortitude, and courage inspired everyone who knew him.

This team of physician and non-physician managers shepherded the organization through a great growth spurt, adding the 300-bed G wing of the hospital and the Crile Building, designed by architect Cesar Pelli.

THE BEAN COUNTERS

The Clinic hired Remington Peck as credit and collections manager in 1934. Seven years later, Crile and Lower promoted him to assistant superintendent with a salary of $416.00 per month. He became treasurer in 1942, a position he held until his retirement in 1952. Peck gets the credit for skillfully guiding the Clinic's finances through the latter years of the Great Depression.

Milton Reinker became controller in 1952, and James Nichols became secretary of The Cleveland Clinic Foundation in 1956. Reinker turned the controller job over to Robert Fischer in 1970. Fischer, a Cleveland Clinic employee since 1953, had served as a credit interviewer, assistant credit manager, credit manager, assistant treasurer, and treasurer. Later, Gerald Wolf, who had worked at Ernst and Ernst as an auditor, joined The Cleveland Clinic as controller. Wolf subsequently moved to the position of treasurer and assistant director of finance. Daniel Harrington, another graduate of Ernst and Ernst, then became controller and later succeeded Fischer as head of finance, and eventually Chief Financial Officer. These men served The Cleveland Clinic and its financial interests with dedication, distinction, and skill for many years.

The 1970s and 1980s were times of rapid expansion. Led by the outgoing and energetic Fischer as director of the Division of Finance, the Clinic floated a $228 million bond issue in 1982 to capitalize future expansion. Savvy investors snatched the issue up in a matter of hours. The bonds received an AA rating, clearly indicating the investors' confidence in the stability of The Cleveland Clinic. During this period of high inflation, these bonds paid, on average, 12.9% per annum. It was not long until interest rates began to decline, and only one year later, the issue was replaced with a $263 million sale, refinancing the original $228 million issue. Fischer again led the effort, which saved the Clinic $99 million in interest payments over the next 30 years. These bonds paid an average interest rate of 8.9%. Again, Moody's Investor Service and Standard & Poor's Corporation rated the issue AA. From these bonds, the institution financed the Century Project (see chapter 8).

Under Fischer's leadership, with Wolf as treasurer, the financial management of The Cleveland Clinic had taken a step upward in professionalism and sophistication. Fischer was fond of calling attention, in his own inimitable way, to the fact that he was responsible for more of the institution's financial well-being than any physician! Upon his retirement in 1985, Harrington, who had succeeded Wolf as Controller, went on to follow Fischer as head of finance. Harrington eventually became the institution's first Chief Financial Officer, the position he held with distinction until his retirement in 1999. He was succeeded briefly by Dean Turner, formerly of the Meridia Hospital System, and later in 2001 by Michael O'Boyle. Wolf served as controller and later treasurer and assistant director of finance, reporting to Harrington, until his retirement in 1992. Kevin Roberts followed him as treasurer until he left the institution in 2000.

Kiser started the internal audit department, and James Cutherbertson joined the organization as its first director. Eugene Pawlowski succeeded him when Cutherbertson moved to Fort Lauderdale as Cleveland Clinic Florida's first chief administrative officer. Jon Englander, who previously had been The Cleveland Clinic's first compliance officer, succeeded Pawlowski in 1995. Donald Sinko became director of internal audit in 2000.

A NATIONAL HEALTH RESOURCE

Other administrative specialty areas emerged as the result of the need for specific administrative and management expertise. Recognition of this need accompanied The Cleveland Clinic's maturation as a large, sophisticated health system, indeed, the largest nongovernmental employer in Cleveland. With the arrival of Frank Weaver in 1980, the refinement of marketing and public affairs functions accelerated, as did the new area of fund development.

Another spin-off of the new public relations effort was the area of government affairs. In 1984, following early forays by Lees, Kiser and Weaver hired Daniel Nickelson, formerly of the Health Care Financing Administration, to serve as director of government affairs. Nickelson represented the interests of The Cleveland Clinic, and indeed, the broader field of health care in the halls of government. Thanks to Nickelson, The Cleveland Clinic had an early advantage in navigating the troubled waters of Ohio's "certificate of need" legislation. Additionally, he was able to guide the institution through the maze of interpreting and dealing with the Medicare DRG system, which today continues to be one of the modes of Medicare payment. Diagnosis-Related Groups (DRGs) were the basis of the earliest Medicare prospective payment system for hospitals. Perhaps his most visible achievement was obtaining formal recognition of the institution by Congress as a "National Health Resource." Nickelson's advocacy on the regulatory front was extremely valuable to the organization.

FURTHER EDUCATION OF THOSE WHO SERVE

Education is a prominent part of The Cleveland Clinic's mission (see chapter 19). While the initial and continued focus has been physician education, it has broadened over the years to include virtually all areas of allied health education and even management and administration. The first administrator of the Division of Education was Howard Walding. He assumed the role in 1970 under Zeiter's chairmanship. As noted previously, Walding had been director of human resources prior to his move to the Division of Education. Upon Walding's retirement in 1985, Phillip Gard was appointed as the administrator of the division. Gard began his career at the Clinic in 1974 as assistant admissions manager, transferring to the Division of Education in 1976 as manager of continuing education. He first worked with Michener and, later, with Fishleder.

The White Coats and Gray Coats came together more closely in 1990 when Dr. Philip Bailin, then chairman of the Department of Dermatology, inaugurated a practice management course. This course, taught by Clinic administrators of both the white- and gray-coat variety, and with the help of the faculty of the Weatherhead School of Management and guest speakers, was designed to improve the business acumen and performance of the Clinic's managers. Assisting Bailin with curriculum development were Terry Bonecutter and Dale Goodrich. Since the course's inception, 500 physician and non-physician managers have come together to learn and share perspectives.

The Cleveland Clinic has one of the oldest hospital-based administrative fellowship programs in the nation. Harding, hospital administrator in 1952, supervised a number of administrative fellows from his alma mater, Washington University in St. Louis. Lees continued the Clinic's commitment to the development of future healthcare managers, serving as preceptor for many graduates from the University of Pittsburgh, University of Michigan, and Ohio State University. In 1981, he passed the fellowship program to Bonecutter, who was the main preceptor until 1984. Beginning in 1984, Goodrich directed and mentored the program. It grew from one fellow to three per year, one of whom was supported by the International Center, with the intent to train a foreign-born individual who wished to return home to apply the newly learned skills. Over the years, it grew in stature and received recognition as one of the finest such programs in the country. The program trained nearly 50 individuals from 21 university programs, who completed it following receipt of their master's degrees in health administration. By 2003, The Cleveland Clinic Health System employed 14 graduates of the program.

MARKETING THE BRAND

Until Weaver's arrival, The Cleveland Clinic did not advertise or aggressively market its capabilities and services. Up to then, Howard (Dick) Taylor was responsible for nurturing what public awareness of the Foundation there was. After Weaver, the next significant head of marketing was Peter Brumleve, the first to hold the title of Chief Marketing Officer. Brumleve's tenure extended from 1994 to 1999. He advanced the Clinic's sophistication in the use of marketing techniques, increasing advertising designed to take advantage of the high regard of the medical community for The Cleveland Clinic. During this period, the Clinic's prestige and national recognition increased. In 1999, Chief Marketing Officer James Blazar took over the Clinic's marketing operation. Without these efforts to "tell the story," The Cleveland Clinic would not be as widely known as it now is.

Along with Weaver's marketing efforts came a more organized approach to public relations. After Weaver's departure, Clinic leadership sought the services of a public relations professional to guide the further development of this function, and in 1991 Holli Birrer was hired to fill the position. Birrer and her colleagues managed the relationship of the institution with both the print and electronic media and improved the public image of the organization locally, regionally, and nationally. They inaugurated a program of video news releases that helped gain national exposure for the Clinic's prominent physicians and scientists. In 2001, the organization took public awareness a step further by identifying a youthful but brilliant media executive, Angela Calman, who became the institution's first Chief Communications Officer. Calman shifted the focus of public relations from the local and regional emphasis of her predecessors to a broader national audience. Soon after her arrival she attracted a two-hour CNBC Special, which showcased The Cleveland Clinic's capabilities to the entire world. She has developed the Cleveland Clinic News Service, which provides video, audio, and print releases on a daily basis.

HUMAN RESOURCES

In the Clinic's early years, individuals who wore many hats managed the "personnel" function. Beginning shortly after the 1929 disaster, Marion Warmington and Myrtle Finnell dealt with personnel issues. In 1931, H. K. Whipple was responsible for the personnel department and some others areas as well.

The first clearly identified director of personnel was Irene Lewis, who served from 1948 until her retirement in 1958. James T. Hudson, who came to the Clinic in 1956 from General Electric, became director of personnel in May 1958 following Lewis's retirement. His tenure was short-lived, as he left the Clinic in August of that year. Robert W. Vorwerk, an Ohio State University graduate, left North American Aviation in Columbus and assumed the position of director of personnel in 1960. Vorwerk held that position until 1963, when he was promoted to director of professional ancillary services under Zeiter. Earl Prossie, who had come to the Clinic in 1961 as Vorwerk's assistant, became director of personnel in June 1963 and occupied the position until 1969, when Walding replaced him.

Relatively short tenures in this position continued with the appointment of Douglas Saarel as the director in 1975. His time at The Cleveland Clinic, though short in duration, was highly significant. He modernized human resources, yielding benefits to the organization that lasted long after his departure. The next director was Fred Buck, who held the position from 1977 to 1988.

Soon after Buck's departure, following a number of short-term and interim appointments, Robert Ivancic, who had previously been human resources director at both MetroHealth Medical Center and Hillcrest Hospital, assumed responsibility for the division and its direction. Ivancic, also an attorney, brought significant additional legal, financial, and strategic skills, which enabled him to contribute more significantly to The Cleveland Clinic than anyone previously in that position.

AUTOMATED INFORMATION

After the early days under Keaty and Dillahay, in 1983 responsibility for information technology fell to Frank R. Cope, and the Division of Foundation Information Systems was created in 1985. Cope was a seasoned information-systems professional with 15 years of experience at TRW. TRW was an aerospace company, headquartered in Cleveland at that time. His first goal was ". . . to link the many types of computer systems and devices used at the Foundation." Cope's successor was Michael Jones. Jones guided the evolution of information systems at the Clinic until his departure in 1996. At that time Dr. C. Martin Harris, recruited from the University of Pennsylvania, became the Clinic's first Chief Information Officer and chairman of the Division of Information Technology. Harris provided a unique blend of expertise in both medicine and information systems (see chapter 10).

VISITORS FROM OTHER LANDS

During the later part of the 1970s and early 1980s, The Cleveland Clinic attracted increasing numbers of international patients, particularly from the Middle East. Because of the growing importance of international patients from all parts of the world in the Clinic's patient population and their special needs, both linguistic and otherwise, Clinic leadership established an International Center in 1972 to accommodate them. Eventually, international marketing became a part of this operation as well. The International Center, located in the Clinic Plaza Hotel (later known as the Omni International) maintained a hospitality center, a staff of translators, and a concierge service for this purpose. It was part of the Division of Operations under Lees, and was ably led by the Clinic's former director of security and ex-federal marshal, Ben Hossler. All who remember "Big Ben" recall a tall, likable, fatherly man, who easily engendered trust. This persona made him a natural to win the confidence of wary foreign patients and their families. After a distinguished career as director of security at The Cleveland Clinic from 1969 to 1983, he led the International Center until 1986, when he retired. During his tenure, Hossler managed the difficult arrangements required for visits by King Khalid of Saudi Arabia and the Royal Family, Prince Charles of England, King Hussein of Jordan, the President of Brazil, and the King of Bhutan, as well as many other dignitaries. John Hutchins succeeded Hossler as director of the International Center and held the position until 1994. Cheryl Moodie, an experienced, hospitality-oriented executive, who had performed in a number of significant management roles at the Ritz-Carlton Hotels, then took the reins of the International Center. Upon Moodie's departure in 2002, Lisa Ramage returned to the Clinic from California to take over the Center, which moved physically into the Clinic's Intercontinental Hotel and administratively into the Division of Institutional Relations and Development, under Bruce Loessin.

A COMMITMENT TO CLEVELAND

The Cleveland Clinic saw the years after its founding in an affluent area known as "Millionaires' Row" slowly bring urban blight, decline, and poverty to the borders of its campus. The Hough riots of 1968 were literally at the Clinic's doorstep, and some still remember armed security guards occupying positions on rooftops, protecting the hospital and clinic. In the midst of all this, Hossler arrived at The Cleveland Clinic as security director in 1969. He introduced sophisticated, professional protection and security systems, previously not considered necessary. Some suggested that it might be best for the Clinic to move to a safer suburban location, but the Clinic's leaders made the commitment to remain within the "heart of the city." By the turn of the century, The Cleveland Clinic had become the visible and vital link between University Circle and the Midtown Corridor, as well as a key economic factor in Cleveland, employing more than 13,000 people, many from the City of Cleveland.

Hossler and his department made the Clinic's main campus safe and secure. Upon his move to the International Center, Thomas Seals arrived from the University of Alabama, Birmingham, and continued to refine and improve security systems, which are today recognized as among the best in Ohio. During Seals's tenure, which ended in 2004, there was great expansion of the use of electronic detection and surveillance systems. Seals also upgraded the qualifications of officers to the point that the Clinic's security department became a licensed "Police Force," with personnel having the requisite training and credentials of peace officers, able to carry out all responses that would be expected of any police officer.

LEGAL CONTRIBUTIONS

In 1968 the Office of General Counsel was established under the leadership of John A. Auble, Esq., as Nichols moved to the position of business manager, succeeding Gottron. Perhaps Auble's greatest and most lasting contributions were his property acquisitions adjacent to the Clinic's main campus. The purpose of this was not only to improve security, but also to provide future space for expansion. Some, during those times, questioned the value of purchasing distressed properties that seemed to be somewhat remote from the needs and the interests of The Cleveland Clinic. Were it not for Auble's efforts, the Clinic might today be facing the prospect of a landlocked campus, the plight of many urban healthcare centers. While much of the Clinic's legal work was outsourced following Aubles' retirement and the arrival of David W. Rowan (see chapter 9), Michael Meehan continues to lead the defense of Clinic physicians when needed, and to provide other needed counsel to the Clinic.

Kiser's retirement in 1989 turned the page on a period of great expansion in the history of The Cleveland Clinic while, at the same time, opening the book on a period of even greater expansion. With difficult financial times and changing reimbursement mechanisms in healthcare looming on the horizon, Dr. Floyd D. Loop assumed the position of Chief Executive Officer and chairman of the Board of Governors during a period that would truly test the mettle of the organization as well as its leadership team.

A CITY WITHIN A CITY

On approaching The Cleveland Clinic's main campus today, one is struck not only with the vastness of the property, but also with the beauty of its buildings. From a small structure on the corner of East 93rd Street and Euclid Avenue in 1921, today's campus has grown to 155 acres of land extending between Chester Avenue and Cedar Avenue from East 88th to E. 105th Street.

The Clinic's first director of planning or facilities development was Neil Carruthers. Carruthers had previously been president of the University Circle Development Foundation, vice president of the Albert M. Higley Company (General Contractor), and deputy director of production for the Atomic Energy Commission in Washington, D.C. He was involved in the beginnings of the project which led to the construction of a portion of the hospital that became known as the H Building. In 1972, during the construction of the H Building, Malcolm Cutting was recruited from Dalton, Van Dijk, and Johnson, a local architectural firm, as the first "architect-in-residence" at The Cleveland Clinic. Over the years, Cutting had been a design consultant for much of the Clinic's construction. As construction projects and planning requirements exponentially increased during the 1970s, Cutting developed a staff of architects and engineers to provide those services in-house. Initially chaired by Dr. William Hawk and later by Glen Hess, director of facilities engineering, and Dale Goodrich, administrative director in the Division of Operations, this was a multi-disciplinary team, initially known as the construction management team. Later it became the construction management committee, which was charged with fiscal oversight of all Cleveland Clinic construction projects.

Following the retirement of Malcolm Cutting, the architect's office was renamed The Office of Construction Management, and Brian J. Smith became its administrative director. Smith incorporated the function of health facility planning into the department, and documented campus facilities by using computer-assisted programs.

Kiser recruited William Frazier as the director of planning in 1974. He previously had held the director of corporate planning position at ITT Service Industries Inc. Frazier became administrator of the newly created Division of Health Affairs in 1991. One of Frazier's many contributions was the deployment and organization of the computer system serving the Department of Institutional Advancement's research efforts during the late 1990s and the early 21st Century. He served the institution for 27 years and retired in 2001. He was succeed by Rosalind Strickland, a seasoned Clinic administrator, who was also the director of community relations.

The construction of the Clinic's striking facilities, while significant and noteworthy, should not be mentioned without identifying those who, in relative anonymity and obscurity, kept the facilities operating, the facilities engineering group. Vern Blessing was the first incumbent in the position of director of facilities. Next came Bill Breyer who served from 1971 to 1976. Succeeding Breyer was Glen Hess, who had previously been in charge of campus facilities at the Ohio State University in Columbus. Hess served the organization until 1996 when he retired and was succeeded by Thomas Shepard. Shepard, starting as a painter in 1980, became the supervisor of carpentry in 1990 and in 2001 was appointed director of facilities engineering. Roland Newman, an experienced, professional construction and facilities management executive, arrived on the scene from University Hospitals of Cleveland in 1997 and brought together construction management and facilities engineering, for the first time, as a unified and coordinated entity.

EAST 93RD STREET AND BEYOND

In Cleveland, beginning in the late 1980s, approximately 30 individual freestanding, self-managed hospitals began to evolve over the next few years into four separate and distinct hospital systems. The Cleveland Clinic and University Hospitals of Cleveland were well-established, not-for-profit entities, while Columbia-HCA and Primary Health Systems, Inc. (PHS), moved in to introduce "for-profit" medicine to the greater Cleveland marketplace. Columbia-HCA was a nationally known company that had expanded rapidly throughout the country. PHS was a small, Pennsylvania-based hospital company, whose medical director was the Clinic's retired chief executive officer, William S. Kiser. Each of the four organizations aggressively pursued those community hospitals which it felt were key to insuring its future success in the greater Cleveland marketplace. Most observers assumed that the system able to attract and acquire the most highly-regarded and efficient hospitals would command market share critical to its future viability and success. Up to this time, the Clinic's practice had been largely based on referrals from independent practitioners. That was about to change dramatically.

The early 1990s might best be characterized as a period of competition, acquisition, and consolidation. In 1991, Lees retired as chief administrative officer, and Loop recruited Frank Lordeman from Meridia Hillcrest Hospital to serve as the Clinic's chief operating officer. The success of the Economic Improvement Program (see chapter 9) was instrumental in placing the Clinic on a strong financial footing, enabling what would become the greatest period of growth and expansion in its history. We have recounted much of this in chapters 9 and 10. During this period, the Intercontinental Suites Hotel was constructed on Euclid Avenue at East 89th Street, to be shortly followed by the demolition of the Omni International Hotel on Carnegie Avenue between East 96th and 100th Streets. At that location, there emerged an exquisite, 300-room, five-star Intercontinental Hotel and Conference Center, which opened in April 2003. On the drawing board and slated to be completed in the first decade of the 21st century is a one-million square-foot Heart Institute, to be located at the corner of Clinic Drive (formerly Oakdale Street, later East 93rd Street) and Euclid Avenue.

During this period, the administrative group negotiated the acquisition of Marymount, Lakewood, Fairview, Lutheran Hospitals, and the Meridia System, which included Hillcrest, Euclid, South Pointe, and Huron Road Hospitals, leading to formation of the Cleveland Clinic Health System, as we have described in chapter 10. The acquisition of these hospitals meshed nicely with the Clinic's strategy to "ring" the city with suburban outpatient clinics and surgery centers to complement the specialty medicine capabilities at the main campus. The Cleveland Clinic Health System was built without creating a new corporate entity. Within limits, member hospitals continued to manage themselves. System consolidation evolved as it made business and financial sense. Thus, the member hospitals maintained their individual community identities while achieving business integration and benefiting from Cleveland Clinic brand recognition.

After 1995, when the first family health center was established in Independence, new centers, some with ambulatory surgery, were added, as we have seen in chapter 10. Cleveland Clinic Florida, established in 1988, received renewed commitment, support, and visibility with the construction of two unified clinic and hospital campuses in Broward (Weston) and Collier (Naples) Counties. The year 2002 saw their completion and opening (see chapter 21).

The end of the twentieth century and the dawning of the twenty-first witnessed the birth of a dynamic, new Cleveland Clinic Foundation, perhaps exceeding the wildest dreams of its four founders. The Cleveland Clinic had become truly regional, national, and international in scope. The growth of the main campus, establishment of family health centers, linkages with organizations such as Kaiser Permanente, and development of the Cleveland Clinic Health System resulted in more than doubling outpatient visits and admissions, effectively blanketing northeast Ohio with The Cleveland Clinic's identity. These accomplishments came to fruition only through collaboration of The Cleveland Clinic's administrative and clinical specialists, the Gray Coats and White Coats, "acting as a unit."

---

[1] Researching and developing this chapter was difficult, primarily because of the great number of administrators who made significant contributions to The Cleveland Clinic in relative obscurity and with minimal fanfare. In this arena, there are few headlines, citations, or external recognitions of a job well done. Instead, their labors ensured that the organization gradually improved, remained solvent, expanded, and was increasingly able to serve more and more of its constituents. We fear that this characteristic of "administrative obscurity" has resulted in the omission of individuals who have made significant contributions. To those who fall in that category, we sincerely apologize. Yet we salute you and your contributions, whatever they may now be or might have been. You are, and will always be, a part of the greatness of The Cleveland Clinic.

23. TRUSTEES, GOVERNORS, AND STAFF

BY JOHN CLOUGH AND SHATTUCK HARTWELL

History never looks like history when you are
living through it. It always looks confusing
and messy, and it always feels uncomfortable.
—John W. Gardner, 1968

TRUSTEES AND GOVERNORS

THE BOARD OF GOVERNORS WAS ESTABLISHED IN 1955 AND SUBSEQUENTLY assumed increasing responsibility for the direction of the Foundation. We have recounted the stories of the four chairmen of the Board of Governors, each of whom made lasting contributions to the institution during these five decades. Dr. Fay A. LeFevre served from the beginning of the Board of Governors era through 1968, and then Dr. Carl E. Wasmuth succeeded him, serving through most of 1976. The third chairman was Dr. William S. Kiser, who served until 1989. He was followed by the present chairman, Dr. Floyd D. Loop. The challenges, issues, and opportunities of each administration characterize these periods of leadership as do the personalities of the leaders themselves.

If the establishment of the Board of Governors has generated an evolving theme, it is the role of increasing managerial responsibility assumed by the Board, which represents the professional staff. The trustees have necessarily maintained legal accountability, but they have delegated many responsibilities to the Board of

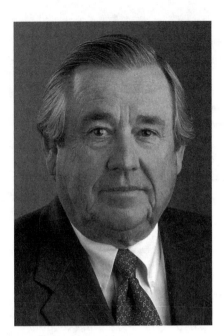

A. Malachi Mixon, III, Chairman, Board of Trustees, 1997-

Governors. Nevertheless, the ultimate responsibilities of defining institutional purpose, acquiring and selling property, staff compensation, and budgetary approval still rest with the trustees.

After nearly five decades of operation, one can look back with some amazement at the success of the plan of organization as developed by the Planning Committee in 1955. During the early years of this period only minor changes were made. The original plan stated that the chairman must be a voting member of the Board of Governors. With the recommendation of the staff, this was amended so that any member of the staff could become chairman. From its inception the Board of Governors was able to unite a group of bright, highly trained professionals so that they could work together unselfishly. This achievement can be attributed largely to a democratic system of selecting governors. The following tables list all who have served on the Board of Governors up to the time of this writing (June 2003). Table 1 lists elected members, and Table 2 includes those serving on the Board by virtue of their office.

Table 1: Elected Members of the Board of Governors

Name	Term(s)	Name	Term(s)
Fay A. LeFevre	1956-1960	Roscoe J. Kennedy	1960-1964
W. James Gardner	1956-1959	John B. Hazard	1960-1964
George Crile, Jr.	1956-1958	Guy H. Williams, Jr.	1961-1965
	1962-1966	Robert D. Mercer	1963-1967
E. Perry McCullagh	1956-1958	Charles H. Brown	1964-1968
A. Carlton Ernstene	1956-1957	Donald B. Effler	1964-1968
	1959-1963	Leonard L. Lovshin	1966-1970
Irvine H. Page	1956-1961	Ralph A. Straffon	1967-1971
Howard S. Van Ordstrand	1958-1962		1973-1976
	1965-1969	Thomas F. Meaney	1968-1972
Stanley O. Hoerr	1959-1963	James S. Krieger	1969-1973
	1965-1969	William L. Proudfit	1969-1973

Table 2: Non-elected Members of the Board of Governors

NAME	TERM(S)
Dean Turner (Chief Financial Officer)	1999-2002
Melinda Estes (Cleveland Clinic Florida)	2001-2003
Eric Topol (Chief Academic Officer[5])	2001-present
Michael O'Boyle (Chief Financial Officer)	2002-present
Karen Shobert (Recording Secretary)	2002-present

Table 3 lists chairmen of the Board of Trustees and Table 4 lists presidents of the Foundation (the president serves as chairman of the Executive Committee of the Board of Trustees) from the time the organization was founded.

Table 3: Chairmen of the Board of Trustees of The Cleveland Clinic Foundation

CHAIRMAN	TERM(S)
Henry S. Sherman	1942-1944[6]
John Sherwin, Sr.	1956-1961
George F. Karch	1966-1968
James A. Hughes	1969-1972
	1975-1984
Arthur S. Holden, Jr.	1973-1974
William E. MacDonald	1985-1990
E. Bradley Jones	1991-1992
Ralph E. Schey	1993-1997
A. Malachi Mixon, III	1997-present

Table 4: Presidents of The Cleveland Clinic Foundation

PRESIDENT	TERM(S)	PRESIDENT	TERM(S)
George Crile, Sr.	1921-1940	James A. Hughes	1974
Henry S. Sherman	1941-1942	Harry T. Marks	1975-1980
Edward C. Daoust	1943-1946	E. Bradley Jones	1981-1982
John Sherwin, Sr.	1948-1957		1990
George F. Karch	1958-1965	William E. MacDonald	1983-1984
George E. Enos	1966-1968	E. Mandell DeWindt	1985-1989
E. Tom Meyer	1969-1972	Arthur B. Modell	1991-1996
Elton Hoyt, III	1973	Alfred Lerner[7]	1996-2002

THE PROFESSIONAL STAFF

Despite the many fine physical facilities the Clinic has assembled over the years, the main asset of the Foundation is the people who work here. At the core of these is the professional staff. These physicians and scientists have been carefully chosen by their peers, and over the years have come to represent one of the finest collections of professionals in the world. The Clinic attracts them by offering the opportunity to practice their profession in an academic setting which, unlike many other academic settings, maintains a collegial, collaborative atmosphere stemming from the spirit of group practice.

Table 5: Presidents of the Staff

PRESIDENT	TERM	PRESIDENT	TERM
Robert D. Taylor	1949-1950	Caldwell B. Esselstyn, Jr.	1977-1978
Leonard L. Lovshin	1950-1951	Jess R. Young	1978-1979
Donald B. Effler	1951-1952	Froncie A. Gutman	1979-1980
John R. Haserick	1952-1953	Royston C. Lewis	1980-1981
George S. Phalen	1953-1954	William M. Michener	1981-1982
Robin Anderson	1954-1956[8]	Thomas E. Gretter	1982-1983
Richard N. Westcott	1956-1957	Russell W. Hardy	1983-1984
James S. Krieger	1957-1958	Howard Levin	1984-1985
Robert D. Mercer	1958-1959	Phillip M. Hall	1985-1986
Roscoe J. Kennedy	1959-1960	John D. Clough	1986-1987
Charles C. Higgins	1959-1960[9]	Ronald L. Price	1987-1988
Charles H. Brown	1960-1961[9]	Wilma F. Bergfeld	1988-1989
William J. Engel	1960-1962	William R. Hart	1989-1990
E. Perry McCullagh	1962-1963	George B. Rankin	1990-1991
Ray A. Van Ommen	1963-1964	Kenneth E. Marks	1991-1992
James I. Kendrick	1964-1965	Gita P. Gidwani	1992-1993
David C. Humphrey	1965-1966	Sebastian A. Cook	1993-1994
Donald E. Hale	1966-1967	George H. Belhobek	1994-1995
Arthur L. Scherbel	1967-1968	Herbert P. Wiedemann	1995-1996
Robert E. Hermann	1968-1969	Gene H. Barnett	1996-1997
Harriet P. Dustan	1969-1970	Anthony J. Thomas	1997-1998
Lawrence K. Groves	1970-1971	Martin J. Schreiber	1998-1999
Victor G. deWolfe	1971-1972	Ezra Steiger	1999-2000
Alfred M. Taylor	1972-1973	Walter G. Maurer	2000-2001
Charles B. Hewitt	1973-1974	Robert J. Cunningham	2001-2002
Thomas L. Gavan	1974-1975	Ruth K. Imrie	2002-2003
Ralph J. Alfidi	1975-1976	James F. Guttierez	2003-2004
Eugene I. Winkelman	1976-1977		

The present members of the professional staff are a culturally and ethnically diverse group representing the best physicians who could be recruited from the United States and 26 other countries. The staff is governed under a set of by-laws, which are administered by the chief of staff (an officer of the Foundation, who sits on the Board of Governors, Medical Executive Committee, and Administrative Council), and a set of elected officers (see table 5 for a historical listing of staff presidents). Since 1989 the Board of Governors has required that each new staff member be board certified in his or her specialty, either by a recognized American board or the international equivalent. Most of the physicians who joined the staff prior to 1989 are board certified as well. All staff members are periodically recredentialed by the Office of Professional Staff Affairs for the services and procedures they perform, and each staff member undergoes a detailed annual professional review of performance in the areas of patient care, research, education, administrative service, national prominence, leadership, and collegiality.

The details of the staff's activities in their various areas of expertise are outlined elsewhere in this book, but the lay media have increasingly recognized the group for its excellence. The *U.S. News and World Report* has cited several specialties for excellence, and *Good Housekeeping, The Best Doctors in America, Town and Country*, and other publications have recognized numerous individual staff members as among the best physicians in the country. Furthermore, many staff members have served as officers of their specialties' national organizations. At one time in 1993, The Cleveland Clinic staff included 13 presidents of national subspecialty societies! No other institution in the state has achieved anything approaching this, and it is a powerful endorsement of the Clinic's approach to group practice.

The Clinic's orientation to subspecialty medicine began in earnest in the 1950s with the formation of a number of subspecialty departments in internal medicine, continued in the 1960s, and accelerated in the 1970s when many of the medical subspecialty boards were organized. In one of his "State of the Clinic" addresses, then chief executive officer William S. Kiser told the staff that it was of great importance that they become "technocrats." The staff had already embraced this concept with wild abandon, and by then the only pocket of primary care remaining in the organization was the Primary Care Department, which was responsible for delivering care to Clinic employees under the Cleveland Clinic Health Plan.

In the mid-1980s, however, the health care scene began to change. Cost-based reimbursement of hospitals received a knockout blow from the Health Care Financing Administration, now known as the Center for Medicare and Medicaid Services (CMS), in the form of Diagnosis Related Groups (DRGs) reimbursement for Medicare patients. Managed care had emerged on the west coast in the 1920s, but it did not reach Cleveland until almost four decades later in the form of the Community Health Foundation, later acquired by Kaiser Permanente. Business was footing most of the bill for health care of their employees (and increasingly of their retirees as well) and was beginning to get uncomfortable with its escalating cost. Managed care, with its primary-care orientation and gatekeeping methodology, seemed to offer a reasonable possibility of controlling these costs by keeping patients away from specialists and technology, and this movement was gaining momentum. As health care costs continued to rise, it became apparent that this approach, driven by the marketplace and accelerated by potentially disastrous but ultimately abortive federal attempts at health care reform, would change the delivery system. One of the most important results of these changes would be the emergence of the primary care physician as the central player in the new order; specialists would be relegated to a supportive role. Chapters 9 and 10 describe the Clinic's responses to these forces.

The modest beginnings of the organization have been described earlier in this book, but since then the (full) staff has grown at a constant, more or less inexorable rate to the present. The Cleveland Clinic has several categories of professional staff: full, associate, and assistant, as well as clinical associate. Any combination of these gives much the same curve as in figure 1, but these numbers are for full staff. Figure 1 shows the exponential nature of the growth of the staff. Like a huge bacterial culture or a myeloma, it has followed predictable kinetics, with a doubling time of 15.6 years. Both *in vitro* and *in vivo*, constraints of space and nutrients normally cause such exponential growth curves eventually to plateau; the Clinic, however, has simply built more space each time things became tight. Though slight deflections have occurred (e.g., downward with the Great Depression and the Clinic disaster in 1929, upward with the end of World War II and the introduction of antibiotics in 1945), the

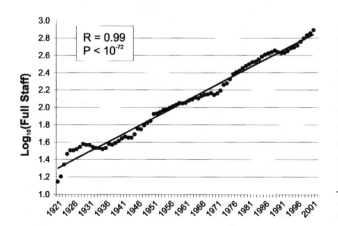

Figure 1. Exponential growth of The Cleveland Clinic's staff since the grand opening in February 1921. The ordinate shows the logarithm to the base 10 of the number of full staff on the roster at the end of each year from 1921 through 2001, as indicated on the abscissa.

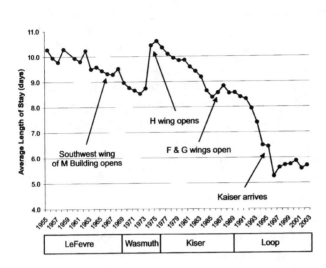

Figure 2. Average length of stay in The Cleveland Clinic Hospital shows a downward trend with upward deflections each time a new wing was opened. A final downward trend occurred in the early 1990s due to a length-of-stay reduction project to make room in the hospital for Kaiser Permanente's patients, who began arriving in 1994.

closeness of the adherence to the regression line has been remarkable over the past 82 years. For those who enjoy mathematics, the estimated staff size at any point in time can be expressed by the equation:

$$\log_{10} y = .0193x + 1.28$$

where y is the number of full staff and x is the number of years after 1921, the year the Clinic opened. This equation predicts that the number of full staff will reach 1,000 members ($\log_{10} y = 3.0$) in the year 2010, 89 years after the doors first opened. According to the Office of Professional Staff Affairs, the number was 779 at the end of 2001.

Another important trend during this tumultuous period has been the pressure to deliver increasingly complex services in the outpatient setting and to restrict hospital length of stay for those services that still require hospitalization. If we look at the Clinic's average length of stay over the years (figure 2) an interesting sawtoothed pattern appears, each "tooth" appearing at the time of hospital expansion.

Length of stay has declined still further with the addition of the Kaiser Permanente patients in 1994 and obstetrics in mid-1995. Until the marketplace applied pressure to reduce length of stay, the

Clinic's own space restrictions did it fairly effectively, and that was never more true than today.

The Clinic's staff has repeatedly shown its adaptability to adverse conditions over the years. Since the Board of Governors era began in 1955, this adaptability has continued. It will be tested mightily as reform of the health care delivery system, whether market- or government-driven, occurs over the next decade. So far the group has met the challenge and has every right to look to the future with confidence. As Loop has said, "Those who think our best years are behind us are looking the wrong direction!"

---

[1] LeFevre was elected to a 5-year term in 1955.

[2] OPSA = Office of Professional Staff Affairs. Hartwell's predecessor in this office was Leonard Lovshin (1959-1976), but he did not sit with the Board of Governors except during his elected term (1966-1970).

[3] "Present" = as of this writing, March 2004.

[4] Title of this position changed from Executive Secretary to Administrator in 1990.

[5] As a part of the preparation for the new medical school, the Board of Governors established the position of Chief Academic Officer on February 28, 2001, just 80 years after the Cleveland Clinic opened its doors.

[6] The office of Chairman of the Board was unfilled from 1945 to 1956 and from 1961 to 1966. The Trustees' Executive Committee, chaired by the president, functioned in place of the chairman during those periods.

[7] Following Lerner's death in 2002, the office of the President remained unfilled as of the present writing (March 2004). Chairman Mixon has performed the functions of president as well as chairman.

[8] Anderson served as staff president for two years during work on the Plan of Reorganization.

[9] Both Kennedy (staff president) and Hazard (staff vice president) were elected to the Board of Governors during their terms as staff officers (see Table 1). They were replaced by Higgins and Brown.

INDEX

Seek, and ye shall find...
—Matthew 7:7

A

Abdominal surgery, 63, 198, 219
Abdominoperineal resection, 197, 198
Abramson, Norman S., 116, 181
Abramson, Susan R., 339
Academic enterprise, 127, 144, 263
Academy of Medicine of Cleveland, 25, 39, 169
Access Center, 118, 121, 234
Accreditation Council on Graduate Medical Education (ACGME), 312, 339
Achkar, Edgar, 377
Acid ash diet, 212
Acquired immunodeficiency syndrome (AIDS), 166, 174
Activity Value Analysis (AVA), 108, 118
Adams, Cheryl, 296
Adelstein, David J., 254
Adenoidectomy, 204
Administrative Board, 66, 71, 72, 74-76
Administrative services coordinators, 356
Administrative Council, 114-116, 133, 150, 360, 361, 379
Adrenal gland, 62, 63, 317, 320
Adult respiratory distress syndrome (ARDS), 166
Advancement pelvic pouch anal anastomosis, 202
Aerobic exercise, special for MS patients, 242
Ahmad, Muzaffar, 116, 151, 157, 160, 161, 165, 377
Akron Children's Hospital, 122, 234
Akron City Hospital (Summa Health System), 121, 132
Albert, Debbie, 296
Alcohol and drug rehabilitation, 172
Alexander, Fred, 188
Alfidi, Ralph J., 283, 379

Allergy, 159, 166, 308
 Pediatric, 190
Alligator Alley, 334
Allogen laboratory, 253
Allograft rejection, 253
Alpha-1 antitrypsin deficiency, 166
Altus, Gene, 115, 151, 355, 377
Alumni Affairs, 150, 312
Alumni Library. *See* Library
Ambulatory care, 104, 106
Ambulatory surgery, 123, 215, 373
American Academy of Dermatology, 169
American Academy of Ophthalmology, 259
American Academy of Pediatrics, 149
American Association of Genitourinary Surgeons, 114
American Association of Tissue Banks, 252
American Board of Colon and Rectal Surgery, 203
American Board of Ophthalmology, 259
American Board of Urology, 114, 214
American Cancer Society, 218
American College of Chest Physicians, 164
American College of Mohs' Micrographic Surgery, 169
American College of Surgeons, 25, 31, 114, 213
American Contact Dermatitis Society, 169
American Foundation for High Blood Pressure. *See* American Heart Association, Council for High Blood Pressure Research
American Heart Association, 237, 323, 326
American Medical Association, 76, 310
 Council on Medical Education, 310
American Nurses Credentialing Center (ANCC), 304
American Red Cross, 271

American Society for Dermatologic Surgery, 169
American Society of Anesthesiologists, 89, 230
American Society of Clinical Pathologists (ASCP), 266
American Society of Histocompatibility and Immunogenetics, 253
American Society of Transplant Surgeons, 246
American Urological Association, 114
Amniocentesis, 184
Amputation, 211
Amyotrophic lateral sclerosis (ALS), 171
Anderson, R. John, 234
Anderson, Robin, 80, 216, 217, 379, 383
Andison, Harry M., 58
Andrish, Jack T., 190, 377
Andrology, 272
Anesthesiology, 89, 91, 107, 219
Aneurysms, 207, 219, 220, 224
Angiography, 283, 322
  Digital subtraction, 284
Angiotensin, 320, 322
Angiotonin. *See* Angiotensin
Annual Professional Review, 97, 98, 153, 312, 314, 380
Anociation, 229
Antibiotics, 197, 199, 204, 299, 381
  Penicillin, 220
  Streptomycin, 220
  Sulfonamides, 197, 204
Antilymphocyte globulin, 246
Antinuclear antibody (ANA), 168
Antisense, 2-5A, 329
Antithyroid drugs, 197, 199
Antitrust activity, 338
Antiviral susceptibility, 179
Antunez, Antonio R., 283, 287, 377
Anxiety and Mood Disorders Subspecialty Unit, 173
Appachi, Elumalai, 191
Arabian Nights, 29
Archives, 26, 99
Armed Forces Institute of Pathology, 268
Armour, Meri Beckham, 294, 295
Artery bank, 218, 219
Arthritis, 173, 209
Arthritis surgery, 211
Arthroscopic surgery, 210
Artificial organs, 139, 161, 162, 213, 324, 325
Ashtabula Clinic, 132
Ashtabula Medical Center, 132
Association of Academic Dermatologic Surgeons, 169
Association of Cardiac Anesthesiologists, 230
Association of Directors of Anatomic and Surgical Pathology (ADASP), 266

Asthma, 166, 181
Atherosclerosis, 322, 330, 331
  Blood lipids and, 322
  Diet and, 322
  Fibrinopeptides, 323
  Filtration theory, 323
Attaran, Marjan, 190
Auble, John A., 91, 105, 115, 355, 359, 369
Aultman Hospital (Canton), 122
Autism, 192
Autoantibodies, 173
Autoimmune inner ear disease, 206
Autoimmunity, 274
Automated record-keeping system (ARKS), 236
Autotransfusion, 271

B

Babies' Dispensary and Hospital, 30
Back pain, 240
Bacterial endocarditis, 71, 180
Baetz-Greenwald, Barbara, 190
Bahna, Sami, 165
Bailey, Dawn, 296
Bailin, Philip L., 168, 169, 364
Baker, Hostetler and Patterson, 355
Baldwin, J.F., 39
Ballard, Lester A., Jr., 215
Banbury, Michael K., 225, 248
Banerjee, Amiya K., 326, 328, 329
Banez, Gerard, 192
Baran, Gregory, 286
Barna, Barbara, 274
Barnes, Arthur, 233, 236, 237
Barnett, Gene H., 208, 377, 379
Battisto, Jack R., 325
Battle, John D., 175
Bauer, Thomas W., 269
Beachwood Sports Health Center, 139
Becker, Steven N., 269
Bedsores, 207
Behrens, Penn, 359
Belcher, George W., 58
Belhobek, George H., 279, 283, 379
Belinson, Jerome L., 116, 151, 215, 216
Bell, Gordon, 377
Belt, Gretchen Z., 377
Benzel, Edward C., 241
Bergfeld, John A., 136, 210
Bergfeld, Wilma F., 168, 377, 379
BeryLliosis, 164, 165
Best Doctors in America, 380
Beven, Edwin G., 219, 250
Bhat, Manju, 237
Bile duct surgery, 201
Biliary drainage, 283
Bingaman, William, 187
Biochemistry, Section of Clinical, 271
Biological Abstracts, 310

Biomaterials, 210
Biomechanics, 210, 324, 330
Biomedical engineering, 237, 314
BioSeiche Therapeutics, Inc., 329
Biostatistics, 256, 262, 324
Bipolar theory of living processes, 317
Birrer, Holli, 365
Biscotti, Charles V., 269
Blades, Brian, 111
Blakeley, Paul, 237
Blazar, James, 150, 151, 365
Blessing, Vern, 371
Blood Bank, 271, 273, 276, 277
Bloodgood, Joseph C., 39
Blue Cross of Ohio, 129, 132
Board certification of staff, 98
Board of Governors, 12, 77-80, 83-91, 93-
    99, 101, 103, 107-109, 112, 114, 116,
    119, 134, 144, 149-151, 162, 181, 202,
    225, 226, 230, 231, 239, 240, 254, 261,
    262, 268, 270, 276, 282, 283, 285, 292,
    293, 310-313, 328-330, 334, 335, 346,
    355, 357, 359, 360, 361, 370, 375, 376,
    379, 383
Board of Trustees, 12, 33, 36, 38, 46, 48,
    56, 66, 67, 70, 71, 73-75, 78-80, 83, 86,
    87, 91, 94, 96-99, 103, 107, 108, 123,
    134, 149, 316, 328, 353, 355, 378
    Executive Committee, 71-75, 96, 108,
        353, 378
Bock, Lois, 296, 297
Boland, Isabelle, 293
Bolton Estate, 143
Bolton Square Hotel Company, 45, 88,
    355
Bolwell, Brian, 247
Bond issue, 99
Bone metabolism, 167
Bonecutter, Terry, 359, 364, 365
Booz, Allen and Hamilton, 73, 74, 354
Borden, Lester S., 209, 377
Borkowski, Gregory P., 283, 377
Boumphrey, Frank, 240
Bourdakos, Demetrious, 191
Boutros, Azmy R., 231, 236
Bradley, Charles, 319
Brain Tumor Institute, 208
Brain tumors, 186, 208, 209
Brainard, Jennifer A., 270
Braun, William E., 253, 274
Bravo, Emmanuel, 161
Breast Center, 200, 201, 255
Breast surgery, 195, 200, 201, 211
Brentwood Hospital, 130-132
Breyer, William, 371
Bringelsen, Karen, 186
Brintnall, Roy A., 58
Bronchoscopy, 165, 166, 205, 298
Bronson, David L., 117, 120, 136, 151,
    177, 178, 263, 377

Broughan, Thomas, 250
Brouhard, Ben, 188, 189
Broward General Hospital, 106, 334, 337,
    338
Brown, Charles H., 169, 376, 379, 383
Brown, Helen B., 322
Brown, Mary Ann, 294
Browne, Earl Z., 217
Brownlow, William, 54
Bruckman, Thomas, 355, 377
Brumleve, Peter S., 115, 150, 365
Buck, Fred, 367
Budget process, 97, 108
Bukowski, Ronald, 176
Bumpus, F. Merlin, 161, 320, 324, 325, 377
Bunts Auditorium, 314
Bunts, Alexander T., 19, 33, 49, 55, 59, 63,
    69, 207, 309, 311
Bunts, Frank E., 11, 19, 23, 25, 28-32, 37-
    39, 41, 46, 80, 227, 280, 307, 308, 311,
    352
Bureau of Workers' Compensation, 142
Burger, Gerald A., 234
Burry, Jack, 129, 132
Bush, Betty, 295, 297
Bush, President George H.W., 328
Business manager, 85

C
Calabrese, Leonard H., 174
Call and Post, 142
Callahan, Joseph, 140
Calman, Angela, 366
Camp Ho Mita Koda, 167
Campaign, Securing the 21st Century,
    123, 140, 141
Cancer, 175, 325
    Bladder, 212
    Bone, 211
    Breast, 200, 253, 256, 281
    Cervix, 214, 256
    Colon, 170, 197, 203, 253, 256
    Head and neck, 217
    Larynx, 204
    Lung, 166, 198, 220
    Mouth, 204, 256
    Non-Hodgkin's lymphoma, 247
    Prostate, 256
    Rectum, 198, 256
    Renal, 214
    Skin, 256
    Thyroid, 281
    Tongue, 204
Cancer surgery, 200
Capital budget, 108
Caravella, Louis, 130
Cardiac assist device, 233
Cardiac surgery, 87, 103, 105, 107, 111,
    117, 123, 165, 185, 199, 215, 220, 337
    Annuloplasty ring, 223

Coronary artery bypass grafting, 221
Internal mammary artery implantation
(Vineberg), 221
Mitral valve retractor, 223
Open heart, 221
Pediatric, 187, 221
Valve surgery, 221, 223
Cardiology, 103, 117, 124, 159, 160
Invasive, 337
Pediatric, 160, 187, 190
Cardiovascular disease, 83, 87, 164, 187,
190, 218, 220, 221, 223-225, 230, 250,
319, 323, 324, 331
Cardiovascular Information Registry
(CVIR), 225
Carey, William, 250, 314
Carl Wasmuth Center for Anesthesiology
Research, 237
Carl Wasmuth Endowed Chair in
Anesthesiology and Critical Care
Medicine, 237
Carotid artery surgery, 219
Carruthers, Neil, 370
Case School of Applied Science, 39
Case Western Reserve University, 15, 119,
122, 124, 127, 144, 145, 149, 150, 152,
179, 254, 301, 302, 314, 316, 328, 329,
331
Casey, Graham, 331
Cash, Joseph M., 151, 178, 234
Cathcart, Martha K., 325
Caulfield, Michael J., 325
Cavanagh, Peter, 330
Ceccio, Cathy M., 294
Celebration of Diversity, 104
Center for Anesthesiology Education, 236
Center for Continuing Education, 315
Center for Digestive Disease Research, 329
Center for Health Affairs, 358
Center for Medicare and Medicaid Services
(CMS), 380
Center for Osteoporosis and Metabolic
Bone Disease, 174
Center for Pelvic Support, 215
Center of Oncologic Robotics and
Computer-Assisted Medicine, 257
Centers of Excellence, 113, 170, 239
Center for the Spine, 117, 142, 235, 240
Cleveland Clinic Spine Institute, 142,
240, 241
Cole Eye Institute, 117, 119, 122, 141,
234, 251, 258, 261, 329
Mellen Center for Multiple Sclerosis,
171, 242, 329
Taussig Cancer Center, 117, 141, 152,
176, 235, 253, 257, 258, 262, 287, 329
Transplant Center, 117, 201, 244, 245
Central nervous system vasculitis, 174
Century Project, 99, 101, 103, 105, 139,
293, 362

Cerebral palsy, 211
Certificate of need, 105, 121, 123, 189, 338,
340, 363
Chand, Deepa, 189
Chandler, John R., 73
Chapman, Jeffrey, 249
Charnley, Deborah Peeler, 295
Charter, The Cleveland Clinic, 36
Chemical Abstracts, 310
Chemical dependency, 172
Chemotherapy, 168, 176, 186, 257
Chicago Institute of Rehabilitation, 121
Chief Academic Officer, 144, 262, 263, 378
Chief Executive Officer, 12, 13, 88, 105,
107, 108, 115, 116, 121, 130, 152, 153,
187, 224, 226, 335, 337, 340, 345, 346,
360, 370, 372, 380
Chief Financial Officer, 12, 105, 115, 116,
148, 362, 363, 377, 378
Chief Information Officer, 116, 146, 367
Chief Marketing Officer, 115, 150, 365
Chief Nursing Officer, 151, 296, 297, 304
Chief of Medical Operations, 116
Chief of Staff, 12, 13, 75, 98, 113, 114,
116, 117, 148-150, 187, 188, 199, 295,
330, 338, 339, 346, 377, 379
Chief Operating Officer, 12, 94, 96, 97,
105, 115, 116, 131, 335, 337, 346, 357,
361, 372, 377
Children's Hospital of Philadelphia, 358
Chisolm, Guy, 377
Cholecystectomy, 195
Chou, David, 276, 277
Christ Hospital, 357
Chromosomes, 186
Chronic fatigue syndrome, 175
Chung, Sunny, 192
Church, James, 203
City Hospital, 23, 31, 170
Clayton, Elaine, 377
Clement Center. See Kenneth Clement
Family Care Center
Cleveland, 333
Cleveland Browns, 136, 210
Cleveland Clinic Ambulatory Surgery
Centers
Beachwood, 138
Lorain, 138
Strongsville, 138
Cleveland Clinic Children's Hospital,
119, 123, 131, 187, 188, 191, 297
Cleveland Clinic Children's Hospital for
Rehabilitation, 128, 131, 192
Cleveland Clinic Educational
Foundation, 80, 140, 309-312
Cleveland Clinic Florida, 101, 254, 286,
333-347, 363, 373
A. Lorraine and Sigmund Goldblatt
Medical Library, 339
Beginnings, 105, 203

Chief Executive Officer, 105, 149, 187, 224, 335
Chief of Staff, 117, 187
Chief Operating Officer, 105
Consent decree, 106
Financial performance, 107, 108, 112, 118
Health Trust, Inc., 105, 118, 336
Medical Director, 105
Medicine, 175
Neurosurgery, 207
Opening, 105, 337
Otolaryngology, 206
Outpatient building, 336
Peat Marwick Mitchell Study, 105, 106
Recruitment, 336
Weston, 106, 107, 334, 340
Cleveland Clinic Florida Hospital
Ft. Lauderdale, 105, 118, 336-338
Naples, 344, 345
Weston, 344
Cleveland Clinic Health System, 11, 192, 286, 297, 372
Central Region, 134
Eastern Region, 130, 134
Physicians' Organization, 134
Western Region, 130, 134
Cleveland Clinic Hospital, 119-121, 291, 299, 353
Expansion, 45, 73, 86, 91, 93, 103, 104
Hospital administrator, 85
Need for, 43
Original building, 45
Oxley Homes, 44, 45
Cleveland Clinic Journal of Medicine, 309, 310, 315
Cleveland Clinic Lerner College of Medicine of Case Western Reserve University, 15, 127, 144, 145, 179, 263, 316
Cleveland Clinic Quarterly. See *Cleveland Clinic Journal of Medicine*
Cleveland Clinic Reference Laboratory (CCRL), 265, 276
Cleveland Eye Bank, 251
Cleveland Foundation, 119
Cleveland General Hospital, 31
Cleveland Health Network, 129
Formation, 119, 121
Managed care organization, 122
Structure, 122
Cleveland Marshall Law School. *See* Cleveland State University
Cleveland Metropolitan General Hospital. *See* MetroHealth Medical Center
Cleveland Orchestra, 103
Cleveland State University, 89, 301, 304, 328, 329, 331
Cleveland Tomorrow, 124
Clinic Building, 282
Association Building Company, 33, 45

Connection to main Clinic Building, 59
Crowell-Little Company, 34
Description, 34
Efficiency, 41
Ellerbe and Company, 33
Move to, 39
Clinic Inn (P Building), 86
Clinical decision unit, 121, 180, 295
Clinical Pathology, 270
Clinical Trials Center, 262
Clough, John D., 11-13, 16, 95, 111, 115, 127, 151, 157, 173, 174, 274, 315, 333, 375, 377, 379
Cobalt therapy, 287
Coburn, Christopher, 330
Codman, Ernest A., 57
Cohen, Bruce, 187
Cohen, Jeffrey, 244
Cole National Corporation, 261
Cole, Jeffrey, 141
Colitis, chronic ulcerative, 185, 203
Collaborative Group of the Americas, 203
College of American Pathologists (CAP), 266
Collier, Maynard, 353
Collins, E. N., 169
Collins, Gregory B., 172
Collins, H. Royer, 210
Collinwood Eldercare Center, 93
Colorectal surgery, 103, 170, 195, 202, 215, 253, 339
Colostomy, 198, 202
Columbia University, 328
Columbia-HCA Healthcare Corporation, 128, 129, 343, 371
Combined Operations Group (COG), 360
Committee on Research Policy and Administration, 79
Communication, 108
Community relations, 93
Community-acquired infections, 180
Compensation Committee, 79, 98
Compensation philosophy, 36, 108
Compensation program, 98
Competition, 106, 118, 121
Computerized axial tomography (CAT), 284
Congenital heart anesthesia, 233, 234
Congenital heart disease, 187, 190, 220, 224
Conization, 214
Conomy, John P., 171, 242, 244
Consortium of Multiple Sclerosis Centers, 244
Construction management committee, 370
Construction management team, 370
Consultation, second-opinion, 148, 276
Contact dermatitis, 167, 168
Contingency planning, 108
Continuing medical education (CME), 312, 314, 315
Cook, Daniel J., 253

Cook, Gilbert, 356-358
Cook, Sebastian A., 288, 377, 379
Cooking, adapted for MS patients, 242
Cope, Frank R., 367
Coping strategies, for MS patirents, 242
Corcoran, Arthur C., 319
Cornea Donor Study, 251
Cornell University, 330
Cornhill, J. Fredrick, 327, 330
Coronary arteriography, 163, 221
Coronary artery disease, 166, 221, 331
Corporate practice of medicine, 36, 38, 43, 105, 335
Cosgrove, Delos M., III, 117, 153, 223, 226
Cosmetic surgery, 205
Cost containment, 92, 108, 112, 118, 222
Costin, John, 138
Coulter, Sharon J., 181, 293-395
Coulton, Robert, 357
Council of Medical Specialties, 114
Covington, Edward C., 172
Craniofacial implantation, 218
Craniofacial surgery, 217
Crile Building, 103, 104, 117, 255, 284
Crile, George (Barney), Jr., 19, 31, 33, 59, 69, 70, 80, 84, 117, 199-201, 211, 218, 253, 311, 376
Crile, George, Sr., 11, 19, 20, 23, 25, 27-31, 34, 38, 39, 43, 55, 56, 59, 62, 66, 71, 72, 161, 196, 201, 227, 229, 279, 280, 311, 317, 318, 331, 351, 353, 362, 378
Crile, Grace, 32, 62, 64, 65
Critical care. See Intensive care
Crohn's disease, 185, 202, 203
Crowe, Joseph, 201
Crown Centre, 136
Crown Centre II, 136
Cunningham, Robert J., 188, 190, 379
Curbstone consultations, 104
Current Contents, 310
Cushing, E. F., 30
Cushing, Harvey, 55
Cuthbertson, James, 105, 335, 337, 355, 377
Cutting, Malcolm, 370
Cyberknife®, 208, 257
Cyclotron, 287

D

Danielsen, Sharon, 292, 293
Daoust, Edward C., 33, 37, 38, 45, 67, 70-73, 76, 352, 353, 378
D'Arcangelo, Claudia, 157
David Jagelman Inherited Colorectal Cancer Registries, 203
Davis, Ajuah, 189
Davis, Stephen, 191
Dawson, Andrea E., 269
Day treatment, 243
Deafness, 204, 205
Deal, Chad, 174

Debt, 62, 86, 92, 99
DeCamp, Malcolm, 225, 249
Decentralization, 97, 107, 113, 298
DeGrandis, Fred, 130
Del Villano, Bert, 325
Delaney, Conor, 203
DeNelsky, Garland, 172
Dennis, Vincent W., 117, 163
Dental implantation, 218
Dentistry, 217
Deodhar, Sharad D., 164, 165, 174, 274, 275
Department of Anesthesiology.
    See Division of Anesthesiology
Department of Biomedical Engineering, 140, 210, 330
Departmental assistants, 293, 294
Dermabrasion surgery, 168
Dermatology, 103, 157, 167
    Pediatric, 190
Dermatopathology, 167, 168, 268, 269
DeWindt, E. Mandell, 378
deWolfe, Victor G., 80, 218, 379
Deyling, Cynthia, 117, 136, 137, 178
Diabetes, 157, 166, 167, 189
Diabetic renal disease, 246
Diagnosis Related Groups (DRGs), 380
Dickinson, D. J., 321, 322
Dickson, James A., 74, 209
DiCorleto, Paul E., 144, 151, 317, 326, 330-332, 377
DiFiore, John, 188
Digestive Disease Center, 170
Diggs, Lemuel W., 270, 271
Digital radiography, 286
Dillahay, Edwin, 359, 367
Dinner, Melvyn I., 217
Dinsmore, Robert S., 54, 63, 198, 199, 218, 219, 309
Disaster
    Cause, 50, 55
    Cause of death, 54
    Deaths, 49
    Liability, 57 ,59
Discharge planning, 261
Dittrick, Howard, 309, 310
Division of Anesthesiology, 89, 91, 113, 229, 230, 360
    Anesthesiology education center, 232
    Biomedical engineering center, 232
    Cleveland Clinic School of Nurse
        Anesthesia, 237
    Clinical Engineering and Information
        Technology Center, 235
    Department of Cardiothoracic
        Anesthesiology, 231, 232, 235
    Department of General Anesthesiology, 232, 236
    Department of Pain Management, 142, 232, 235, 241
    Department of Regional Practice, 232

Education Center, 236
  Research center, 232, 237
Division of Business Development, 149
Division of Education, 113, 140, 272, 307, 312, 360, 364
  Allied health education council, 312
  Center for Medical Education Research and Development (CMERAD), 315
  Continuing Medical Education Council, 312
  Educational Governing Group (EGG), 311, 313
  Management and training council, 312
  Nursing education council, 312
  Office of Alumni Affairs, 312
  Office of Faculty and Curriculum Development, 315
  Physician education council, 312
Division of Finance, 115, 358
Division of Foundation Information Systems, 367
Division of Health Affairs, 100, 115, 118, 174, 371
Division of Human Resources, 115, 297, 301
Division of Information Technology, 143
Division of Laboratory Medicine, 268, 360
Division of Marketing and Managed Care, 100
Division of Medicine, 112, 113, 116, 123, 157, 164, 165, 270, 280, 282, 359, 360
  Department of Cardiovascular Medicine, 163
  Department of Dermatology, 167
  Department of Emergency Medicine, 180
  Department of Endocrinology, 166
  Department of Gastroenterology, 169
  Department of General Internal Medicine, 176, 234
  Department of Hematology and Medical Oncology, 175
  Department of Hypertension/Nephrology, 161
  Department of Infectious Disease, 179
  Department of Neurology, 170
  Department of Psychiatry and Psychology, 172, 241
  Department of Pulmonary and Critical Care Medicine, 164
  Department of Rheumatic and Immunologic Disease, 173
Division of Nursing, 256, 291, 293
Division of Operations, 115, 295, 368, 370
Division of Ophthalmology, 122
Division of Pathology and Laboratory Medicine, 113, 174, 265, 268-270
Division of Patient Care Operations, 295
Division of Pediatrics, 119, 123, 160, 183, 192

Division of Post-Acute Care, 261
  Department of Physical Medicine and Rehabilitation, 235, 241
Division of Radiology, 113, 241, 279, 282, 360
Division of Regional Medical Practice, 117, 119, 120, 136, 263
Division of Research, 113, 161, 358, 360
Division of Surgery, 113, 114, 122, 189, 195, 199, 207, 230, 234, 259, 267, 321, 359, 360
  Department of Colorectal Surgery, 202
  Department of Dentistry, 217
  Department of General Surgery, 196
  Department of Neurological Surgery, 206
  Department of Neurosurgery, 241
  Department of Obstetrics and Gynecology, 214, 235
  Department of Orthopaedic Surgery, 209, 234, 241
  Department of Otolaryngology and Communicative Disorders, 204
  Department of Plastic and Reconstructive Surgery, 216, 234
  Department of Thoracic and Cardiovascular Surgery, 220
  Department of Urology, 212
  Department of Vascular Surgery, 218
Divisional Committees, 78, 204
Dizziness, 205
Dohn, Donald F., 189, 207, 377
Donnelly, Marlene, 294-296
Doppler echocardiography, 223
Dornette, William, 236
Dosimetry, 281
Draft impact on staff, 69, 159
Drinko, John, 242
Duke University, 163
Dumpe, Michelle, 296
Dunasky, Kathy, 13
Dunning, Charlotte E., 45, 353
Dustan, Harriet P., 161, 283, 320, 379
Dyment, Paul, 186, 187

E

E Building, 121, 180. *See* Access Center
Ebrahim, Zeyd, 236, 377
e-ClevelandClinic.com, 148
Economic Improvement Program, 101, 106, 107, 372
Education, 34, 40, 77, 80, 99, 101, 159, 161, 164, 167, 169, 173, 178-181, 184, 186-188, 190, 200, 205, 218, 241, 242, 246, 258, 285, 292, 307, 335, 339, 341, 380
  Allied health, 314
  Continuing medical (CME), 312, 314
  Graduate medical (GME), 312, 314
  Medical student, 314

Patient, 312, 314
Seminars in Clinical Teaching, 315
Education Building, 86, 311, 314
Education Governing Group, 311, 313
Educational Foundation, Cleveland
　Clinic, 80, 311
Effler, Donald B., 111, 112, 162, 220, 222,
　376, 379
Electrocoagulation, 198
Electroencephalography, 171
Electromyography, 171
Electronic image transfer, 286
Electronic medical record, 145, 147
Elson, Paul, 257
Elyria Memorial Hospital, 121
Emergency department, 295
Emergency medicine, 116, 118, 119, 121,
　180, 181
Emergency Medicine and Access Center
　Building, 234
Emerman, Charles L., 151, 181
Emory University, 250
Emphysema, 249
Empyema, 220
Endocrinology, 48, 96, 103, 117, 157, 166
Pediatric, 189
Endoscopy, 169, 170, 185, 201
Endowment, 45, 63, 79, 80, 129, 152, 201,
　239, 311, 321, 327, 332
Engel, William J., 70, 80, 84, 212, 213,
　309, 311, 377, 379
Englander, Jon, 363
Enos, George E., 90, 378
Enthoven, Alain, 137
EpiCare, 147
Epidemiology, 256
Epilepsy, 62, 171, 187, 208
Surgery, 187, 208
eRadiology, 286
Erenberg, Gerald, 186
Ernstene, A. Carlton, 70, 74, 75, 80, 84,
　157, 159, 160, 164, 376
Esfandiari, Shahpour, 234
Esophageal varices, 170
Esposito, Salvatore J., 217
Esselstyn, Caldwell B., Jr., 197, 200, 201,
　377, 379
Estafanous, Fawzy G., 107, 229, 231-233,
　236, 237, 377
Estes, Melinda L., 116, 149, 150, 269,
　333, 346, 347, 377, 378
Euclid General Hospital, 128, 130, 296, 372
Evans, Richard R., 165
Evarts, Charles M., 209, 210
Eversman, John J., 96, 361, 377
Exchange transfusion, 175
Executive Director of Managed Care, 116,
　135
Exstrophy of the bladder, 212
Eye Bank Association of America, 251

Eye Care Network, 123, 261

F
Facilities engineering group, 371
Faculty Board, 310, 311
Faiman, Charles, 117, 151, 167
Fairfax Foundation. *See* Fairfax
　Renaissance Development Corporation
Fairfax Renaissance Development
　Corporation, 93
Fairview General Hospital, 121, 128, 130
Fairview Health System, 130
Falcone, Tommaso, 151, 216
Familial polyposis, 203
Family Health Centers, 120, 211, 261, 286
Beachwood, 138
Brunswick, 139
Chagrin Falls, 139
Chardon Road/Willoughby Hills, 139
Creston, 139
Elyria, 139
Independence, 117, 120, 136, 137, 178
Lakewood, 139
Solon, 137
Strongsville, 138
Westlake, 117, 120, 137
Willoughby Hills, 117, 120, 137
Wooster, 137
Family practice, 211
Farmer, Richard G., 112, 160, 169, 172, 377
Farver, Carol F., 269
Faulkner, Willard, 270
Favaloro, René G., 112, 221, 222
Fazio, Victor W., 202, 203, 377
Federal Trade Commission, 106, 336, 338,
　343
Feldman, Mark, 234
Fellows, 308
Fellowship committee, 308
Ferchill, John, 192
Ferguson, D. Roy, 107, 377
Ferrario, Carlos M., 107, 321, 322, 326, 377
Fever of unknown origin (FUO), 180
Fibromyalgia, 175
Fiery, Benjamin F., 73, 353
Finance, 99
Financial performance, 107, 112
Finke, James, 325
Finnell, Myrtle, 366
Fiocchi, Claudio, 325
Firor, Hugh V., 188
Fischer, Jill S., 244
Fischer, Robert J., 90, 91, 99, 105, 356, 358,
　362, 363
Fischler, Diana, 269
Fishleder, Andrew J., 144, 272, 307, 313,
　314, 364, 377
Fistula, 202
Fleshler, Bertram, 169
Florida, 105

Agency for Health Care
  Administration (AHCA), 340, 343
  Broward County, 105, 334, 335, 344
  Collier County, 344
  Health Planning Council of Southwest
    Florida, 343
  Legislature, 105, 335
Flow cytometry, 273
Fluorescein angiography, 259
Foot and Ankle Center, 210
Forest City Enterprises, Inc., 107
Forest City Hospital, 93
For-profit health care, 371
Fouad, Fetnat, 161
Foundation Operations Group (FOG), 360
Founders, official designation of, 36
Fox, Joan, 262
Fractures, 211
Frances Payne Bolton School of Nursing,
  237, 301, 302
Frank E. Bunts Educational Institute, 308
Frankel, David, 192
Frazier, William, 100, 371
Frederick, Earl J., 354
Fricke, Hugo, 38, 317, 318
Friedman, Neil, 187
Fuchs, Jan, 298
Fuller, Ralph, 33
Functional electrical stimulation, 242
Fund Development. See Institutional
  Relations and Development

G

Gait analysis, 210
Galen, Robert S., 272
Gamma camera, 288
Gamma knife, 208
Garcia, Richard, 188
Gard, Phillip R., 364
Gardner, W. James, 70, 71, 74, 75, 80, 84,
  86, 206, 207, 376
Gastroenterology, 103, 107, 117, 124, 159,
  160, 169, 201
  Pediatric, 185, 190
Gastrointestinal bleeding, 185
Gastrointestinal motility, 170
Gatekeeping, 381
Gault Avon Women's Health Center, Flo
  and Stanley, 178
Gavan, Thomas L., 266, 273, 275, 276, 377,
  379
Gene amplification, 257, 328
Gene therapy, 166, 261
General Clinical Research Center (GCRC),
  262
General counsel office, 115
General Electric, 236, 366
General surgery, 103, 117, 170, 195, 196,
  217, 245
  Pediatric, 188

Genetics, 206
Geometric osteotomy, 209
George Washington University, 111, 112
Geriatrics, 117, 177
Getz, Janet W., 72, 74, 80, 85, 377
Gidwani, Gita P., 190, 379
Gifford, Ray W., Jr., 161, 162, 377
Gilkison, Conrad C., 54
Gill, Carl C., 105, 112, 187, 224, 335-337,
  339, 340, 377
Gingival hyperplasia, 218
Glasser, Otto, 48, 281, 288, 289
Glaucoma, 258
Glickman Urological Institute, 214
Go, Raymundo, 288
Goiter, 196
Goldblatt, Harry, 212, 267, 274, 319
Goldblum, John R., 151, 269, 270
Goldfarb, Johanna, 189, 190
Goldman Sachs Group, 130
Gonorrhea, 212
Gonsalves, Lilian, 377
Good Housekeeping, 380
Goodrich, Dale, 351, 357, 361, 364, 365,
  370
Goske, Marilyn, 192
Gottron, Richard A., 80, 87-90, 355, 369
Grace Hospital, 132, 261
Graft-versus-tumor effect, 247
Graham, Allen, 267
Graham, Linda M., 377
Graham, Robert, 326, 329
Graman, Howard, 138, 347
Gramlich, Terry L., 269
Grand Opening, The Cleveland Clinic, 39,
  43
Graves' disease, 196, 197
Great Depression, 59, 62, 159, 309, 362,
  381
Green, Arda A., 320
Green, Ralph G., 272
Greene, David, 206
Greenhouse, Arnold H., 171
Gretter, Thomas E., 379
Grill, George, 353
Grimberg, William, 123, 124, 140, 150
Group practice, 29, 30, 39, 41, 43, 100, 104,
  113, 331, 334
Group purchasing, 358
Groves, Lawrence K., 379
Growth, 87, 99, 101, 106, 107, 118, 159,
  165, 166, 172, 173, 176, 177, 179, 180,
  190, 215, 242, 284, 312, 381
G-suit invention, 66
Gudkov, Andrei, 329-331
Gulledge, A. Dale, 172
Gupta, Manjula K., 274
Gurd, Alan R., 190, 377
Gustafson, Barbara, 256
GUSTO trial, 164

Gutman, Froncie A., 258, 259, 377, 379
Guttierrez, James F., 379
Gynecology, 103, 116, 124, 195, 198
  Adolescent, 190

H

H. R. H. Family Foundation, 256
Haden, Russell L., 60, 63, 69, 71, 72, 75,
  76, 158, 159, 173, 175, 270, 319
Hahn, Joseph F., 66, 151, 189, 195, 199,
  207, 208, 330, 377
Hainline, Adrian, 270, 271
Hair transplantation, 168
Hale, Donald E., 230, 236, 379
Hall, Geraldine S., 274
Hall, Phillip M., 377, 379
Halle, Walter M., 63, 73
Hamby, Wallace B., 207
Hamilton and Associates, 99, 355
Hamilton, Thomas A., 174, 329
Hand surgery, 217
Hanson, Maurice R., 377
Harding, James G., 80, 87, 88, 90, 292,
  354-357, 364
Hardy, Russell W., 240, 379
Harmon, Mary, 185
Harold C. Schott Chair, 174
Harrington, Daniel J., 115, 148, 362, 363,
  377
Harris, C. Martin, 116, 146-148, 151, 367
Harris, Harold E., 204, 205
Harrison, A. Marc, 191
Hart, William R., 117, 265, 266, 268-271,
  275, 276, 379
Hartsock, Charles L., 282, 307
Hartwell, Shattuck W., Jr., 83, 89, 94-96,
  98, 103, 104, 119, 217, 375, 377, 383
Harvard Community Health Plan, 146
Harvard University, 91
Haserick, John R., 167, 168, 379
Hashkes, Philip, 175, 191
Haskell, Betty, 267
Hawk, William A., 105, 253, 268, 334,
  335, 337, 370, 377
Hayek, Salim, 237
Hazard, John Beach, 266-268, 271, 376,
  383
Hazen, Stanley, 331
Headache, 176, 186
Health care costs, 106, 380
Health Care Financing Administration.
  See Center for Medicare and Medicaid
  Services (CMS)
Health care reform, 128, 381, 383
Health Hill Hospital, 128, 131, 192
Health of the Clinic Address, 112
Health Sciences Center of the Ohio State
  University, 314
Health Systems Agency of North Central
  Ohio (HSANCO), 93

Health Ventures, Inc., 131
HealthQuest, 234
Healy, Bernadine P., 103, 119, 139, 257,
  325-328, 332
Heart Center, 143
Heart, artificial, 140, 225, 233, 324
Heart-lung machine, 221
Helipad, 180
Hematology, 117, 158, 160, 175, 254, 255
  Pediatric, 186
Hematopathology, 272, 273
Hemodialysis, 161, 162, 213, 245
Hemodynamics, 322
Hemostasis and thrombosis, 273
Henderson, J. Michael, 117, 201, 239, 245,
  246, 250
Henricks, Walter H., 277
Henry Ford Hospital (Detroit), 119
Hepatitis, 185
Hepato-biliary-pancreatic surgery, 201
Hepatology, 170
Hereditary angioneurotic edema (HANE,
  C1INH deficiency), 165
Hermann, Robert E., 200, 201, 250, 379
Hernia repair, 195
Herrick, Myron T., 25
Hertzer, Norman R., 219, 220
Herzig, Roger, 247
Hess, Glen, 370, 371
Hewitt, Charles B., 371
Hewlett, James S., 175
Hewson, Mariana, 315
Higgins, Charles C., 212, 213, 379, 383
Hillcrest Hospital, 115, 128, 130, 131, 372
Hills, Gertrude, 353
Hinnant, I. M., 165
Histocompatibility laboratory, 213, 252, 274
HLA typing, 253
Hoeltge, Gerald A., 271
Hoerr, Stanley O., 199, 200, 216, 310, 376
Hoffman, Gary S., 117, 174
Hoffman, George C., 266, 272, 377
Hofstetter, Corinne, 298
Holden, Arthur S., Jr., 86, 378
Holtzman, Ronald, 190
Home health care, 201, 261
Homi, John, 219
Hoogwerf, Byron J., 167
Horvitz Center, 176
Hospice care, 176, 256, 261
Hospital design, 104
Hospital mergers, 128, 129
Hossler, Ben, 368, 369
Howe, Charles, 39
Hoyt, Elton, III, 378
Hsi, Eric, 273
Hudson, James T., 366
Huerta, Ricky, 172
Hughes, C. Robert, 80, 282, 283
Hughes, James A., 67, 86, 90, 93, 378

Hull, Alan L., 179, 315
Hull, Tracy, 203
Human chymase, 324
Human immunodeficiency virus (HIV), 274
Humphrey, David C., 161, 379
Humphries, Alfred W., 80, 218, 219
Hundert, Edward, 144
Hundorfean, Cynthia, 359
Hunter, Edgar S., 54
Hupertz, Vera, 186
Huron Road Hospital, 128, 130, 236, 358, 372
Hutchins, John, 368
Hyatt, Roger C., 57
Hyperparathyroidism, 197
Hypertension, 103, 160-163, 166, 253, 319-322
    Mosaic theory, 321
    Pediatric, 189
    Pulmonary, 249, 350
    Renal, 213, 319, 322
Hysterectomy, 214

I

Iannotti, Joseph P., 144, 151, 211, 212, 330
Image processing, 210
Immune response, 325
Immunological tolerance, 325
Immunology, 324, 325, 329
    Pediatric, 190
Immunopathology, 164, 173, 274
Immunosuppression, 245, 247
Immunotherapy, 176, 206
Imrie, Ruth K., 137, 188, 190, 379
In vitro fertilization, 215
Inclusion body myopathy, 174
Index Medicus, 310
Infection control, 179
Infectious disease, 103, 117, 160, 177, 179
    Pediatric, 190
Infertility, 215
Inflammatory bowel disease, 169, 170, 185, 202, 203, 325
Information systems, 107, 108
Information technology, 145
Innovations, Cleveland Clinic Foundation, 199
Institute of Rehabilitation Medicine, 121, 262
Institutional Advancement, 99, 124, 140, 150
Institutional Relations and Development, 150
Instrumentation management, 236
Insulin, 44
Integrative Medicine Center, 262
Intensive care, 87, 104, 162, 165, 232, 233, 236, 300, 345
    Pediatric, 123, 189-191, 216, 297

Interferons, 244, 257, 328, 331
Intermedin, 167
Internal Audit, 99, 360, 363
Internal fixation of vertebrae, 209
Internal medicine, 94, 103, 117, 157, 159, 160, 176, 339
Internal Medicine Preoperative Assessment Consultation and Treatment (IMPACT) Center, 178, 234
International Center, 361, 368
International Hereditary Non Polyposis Colorectal Cancer Group, 203
International markets, 106
International Network for the Study of Systemic Vasculitides, 174
International patients, 334, 367
International Society of Gynecological Pathologists, 266
Internet, 13, 147, 243
Interstitial lung disease, 249
Invention of new medical equipment, 236
Ireland, 105
Isaacson, J. Harry (Bud), 179
Isotopes, 281
Ivancic, Robert, 115, 151, 367

J

Jacobs Center for Thrombosis and Vascular Biology, 329
Jagelman, David, 203
Jahnigen, Dennis, 177
Janik, Angela, 294
Jennifer Ferchill Play Deck, 191
Jennings, Martha Holden, 86, 311
Jensen, Vanessa, 192
John Weaver King School of Medical Technology, 270
John, Henry J., 38, 44, 157, 166, 167, 270
Johns Hopkins University, 151, 193, 329, 357
Johnson, E. Mary, 298
Johnson, William O., 307
Johnston, C. R. K., 165
Joint Commission on Accreditation of Hospitals, 87
Joint replacement surgery, 209, 210
Jones, E. Bradley, 108, 378
Jones, John, 220
Jones, Michael, 367
Jones, Thomas E., 38, 39, 48, 63, 69, 71, 72, 74-76, 197, 198, 202, 221
Jordan, Edwin P., 75, 310
Joyce, Michael, 252
Jules Stein Eye Institute (Los Angeles), 122

K

Kaatz, Tina, 359
Kahn, Teri A., 190, 191
Kaiser Health Plan, 120
Kaiser Hospital, 120

Kaiser Permanente, 118, 119, 146, 180, 380, 382
Kaplan, Barbara, 185
Kapural, Leonardo, 237
Karch, George F., 86, 378
Karnosh, Louis J., 170, 171
Kaufman Center for Heart Failure, 247, 248
Kay, Marsha, 185, 189
Kay, Robert, 13, 116, 120, 148, 151, 188, 295, 377
Keaty, Tom, 358, 367
Kelley, Joseph F., 165
Kendrick, James I., 209, 379
Kennedy, Marie, 70
Kennedy, Roscoe J., 70, 258, 376, 379, 383
Kenneth Clement Family Care Center, 93
Kent State University, 301, 331
Kichuk-Chrisant, Maryanne, 187
Kidney stone, 212
Kidney, artificial, 161, 213, 321, 324
Kimball, Oliver P., 38
Kimball, Sharon, 297
King, John W., 270, 271, 273
King, Martin Luther, Jr., 104
Kirklin, John W., 162
Kiser, William S., 91, 94-101, 104-109, 112, 351, 360, 363, 369, 371, 372, 375, 377, 380
Klein, Eric, 331, 377
Knee ligament reconstruction, 210
Kolczun, Michael, 138
Kolff, Willem J., 161, 162, 213, 221, 245, 320, 321, 324
Koltai, Peter, 191
Koo, Anna P., 174
Kotagal, Prakash, 187
Kottke-Marchant, Kandice, 273
Kreiger, Kristy, 359
Krieger, James S., 100, 199, 214, 215, 360, 376, 379
Krishnamurthi, Venkatesh, 246
Krupp, Neal, 173
Kuhar, Peggy, 296, 304
Kuivila, Thomas, 190
Kunkel, Robert, 176

L

L. E. cell phenomenon, 168
Laboratory Hematology and Blood Banking, 271
Laboratory medicine, 157
Laboratory Medicine Building, 266
Lahey Clinic, 358
Lakeside Hospital, 25, 30, 31, 43
Lakewood Hospital, 128, 129, 235, 372
Lakewood Hospital Association, 130
LaMotte, Thomas, 121
Lampe, John B., 183, 191
Land acquisition, 33, 87, 92, 143, 334, 370
Lang, Richard S., 151, 177, 178

Langston, Roger H. S., 251, 377
Lanza, Donald, 205
Laparoscopic surgery, 201-203
Laser surgery, 218
Latin America, 334
Latson, Larry, 187
Laurel School, 56, 58
Laurelwood Hospital, 121
Lautzenheiser, Fred, 13
Lavery, Ian, 203, 377
Lawrence, William, 357, 361
Lawson, Kathleen, 294
Lazorchak, Joseph, 356
Learning disabilities, 186
Lee, Amy, 192
Leedham, Charles L., 310
Leeds Castle Group, 203
Lees, James E., 90, 91, 355, 357-359, 361, 363, 365, 368, 372, 377
LeFevre, Fay A., 80, 83, 84, 86-88, 90, 91, 159, 310, 351, 355, 375-377, 383
Lefferts, Geoffrey, 177
Left ventricular assist device (LVAD), 225, 248
Length of stay, 226, 382
Lerner College of Medicine of Case Western Reserve University, Cleveland Clinic, 15, 127, 144, 145, 179, 263, 316
Lerner Research Institute, 119, 140, 141, 144, 151, 168, 172, 183, 220, 239, 257, 263, 316, 317, 325, 327, 330
Lerner, Alfred, 140, 144, 145, 316, 328, 378, 383
Lerner, Norma, 140, 316
Leukemia, 73, 186, 325
Level scheduling, 108
Levien, Michael, 186
Levin, Howard S., 268, 379
Levine, Michael, 151, 193
Lewicki, Linda J., 293, 294, 296
Lewis Research Laboratories (NASA), 287
Lewis, Hilel, 117, 122, 123, 141, 239, 259-261
Lewis, Irene, 366
Lewis, Richard, 241
Lewis, Royston C., 379
Library, 34, 140, 183, 236, 308, 309, 311, 316, 327, 339
Licensure, 314, 335
Linear accelerator, 257, 287
Lipid disorders, 167
Litaker, David, 178
Little, John, 207
Liver surgery, 201
Livingston, Robert B., 175
Locke, C. E., Jr., 53-55, 58, 206
Loessin, Bruce, 150, 368
London, Alan E., 116, 122, 135, 151
Long-range planning, 96, 98, 99, 101
Long-term acute care, 261

Longworth, David L., 117, 152, 179, 180
Lonsdale, Derrick, 186
Loop, Floyd D., 13, 15, 16, 109, 111-113, 115, 116, 118-121, 127, 131, 144, 149, 151-153, 222, 226, 346, 351, 369, 372, 375, 377, 383
Lorain Community Hospital, 235
Lordeman, Frank L., 115, 116, 121, 131, 132, 151, 295, 372, 377
Lovshin, Leonard L., 94, 176, 376, 379, 383
Lowenthal, Gilbert, 177
Lower, William E., 11, 19, 23, 25, 26, 28-32, 34, 36-39, 41, 43-45, 56, 57, 59-61, 67, 71-74, 195, 212, 214, 227, 280, 311, 353, 362
Loyola University, 273
Luciano, Mark S., 189
Lüders, Hans O., 117, 171
Lung abscess, 220
Lutheran General Hospital, 121, 128, 130, 235, 372
Lytle, Bruce W., 223, 224, 377

M
MacDonald, William E., 108, 378
MacIntyre, W. James, 288
Macklis, Roger, 117, 257, 287
Macknin, Michael L., 188
Macrophage function, 166
Magnet hospital designation, 304
Magnetic resonance imaging (MRI), 284
Main Clinic Building, 255
    Construction, 59
    Expansion, 73, 86
Malensek, William, 361
Managed care, 106, 118-120, 122, 124, 134, 137, 300, 380
Managed competition, 137
Management engineering, 354
Management Group, 96
Mandell, Brian, 315
Manos, Michael, 192
Marine, David, 270
Marketing, 108, 112, 113, 118
Markman, Maurie, 117, 152, 175, 239, 254
Marks, Harry T., 378
Marks, Kenneth E., 117, 136, 151, 210, 211, 379
Marshall, John, 352
Martin, Beth Anne, 192
Marymount Hospital, 122, 128, 129, 235
Masson, Georges M. C., 320
Mastectomy
    Limited, 200
    Radical, 200, 253
Master Plan, 99, 103
Mastoidectomy, 204
Mastoiditis, 204
Materials management, 357
Mather, Samuel, 57

Matzen, Richard N., 177
Maurer, Walter G., 234, 377, 379
Maxillofacial prosthetics, 217
Mayberg, Marc, 208
Mayes, James T. III, 246, 250
Maynard, Amy Caslow, 294
Mayo brothers, 196
Mayo Clinic, 25, 30, 38, 78, 162, 168, 187, 230, 335
Mayo Foundation, 38
Mayo, William J., 39, 41-43
Maytin, Edward, 168
Mazanec, Daniel J., 117, 174, 239, 240
McAfee, Barbara, 359
McBride, Sarah Tod, 63
McCann, Richard, 131, 132
McCarthy, Patrick M., 224, 248, 250
McCormack, Lawrence J., 266, 268, 274-276, 283
McCubbin, James W., 320-322
McCullagh, D. Roy, 318
McCullagh, E. Perry, 52, 71, 72, 80, 84, 157, 166, 167, 318, 376, 379
McDowell, Karen, 190
McGill University, 319
McHenry, Martin C., 179
McHugh, Michael J., 189-191
McKee, Michael, 172
McKinsey & Co., 107, 108
McMahon, James T., 269
Meaney, Thomas F., 90, 283-285, 287, 322, 376
Medical Executive Committee, 113, 114, 151, 360, 379
Medical Operations, 295
Medical Operations Group (MOG), 360
Medical students, 313
Medical Survey Committee, 77
Medicare, 380
Mee, Roger B., 188, 224
Meehan, Michael, 369
Mehta, Atul C., 249
Meisler, David M., 251
Mekhail, Nagy, 235
Mellen Center Care On-Line (MCCO), 243
Mellen Foundation, 242
Melton, Alton L., 190
Membrane oxygenator, 221
Mercer, Robert D., 183-186, 376, 379
Meridia Health System, 130
Meridia Hospital System, 130
Metabolic bone disease, 174
MetroHealth Medical Center, 120-122, 170
Metropolitan Health Planning Agency (MHPA). *See* Health Systems Agency of North Central Ohio (HSANCO)
Meyer Center for Magnetic Resonance, 285
Meyer, E. Tom, 285, 378
Michael J. Cudahy Chair for Clinical Engineering, 237

Michener, William M., 185, 311, 312, 364, 377, 379
Michota, Franklin A., Jr., 178
Microbiology, 180, 273
Microsurgery, 215
Microvascular surgery, 217, 246
Miller, Michael L., 272, 273
Miller, Samuel H., 107
Milsom, Jeffrey, 203
Minai, Omar, 249
Miner, Charles, 130, 132
Minimally invasive surgery, 201-203, 215, 220
Mion, Lorraine, 296
Mitral stenosis, 220
Mitsumoto, Hiroshi, 171
Mixon, A. Malachi, III, 153, 378, 383
Modell, Arthur B., 108, 139, 378
Modic, Michael T., 285, 286, 289, 377
Molecular and functional imaging, 288
Molecular and immunopathology, 274
Molecular biology, 326, 328, 329
Molecular microbiology, 274
Molecular pathology, 275
Montie, James E., 213
Moodie, Cheryl, 368
Moodie, Douglas S., 123, 151, 187-190, 193
Moon, Harry K., 117, 149, 339, 340, 342, 346, 377
Moore, Paul M., 204
Moore, Shirley, 293
Morledge, Thomas J., 117, 137
Morocco, 105
Morris, Harold, 171
Morrison, Stuart, 192
Mossad, Emad, 233, 234
Motor Center Company, 355
MS Learning Center, 243
MS Women's Committee, 243
Mt. Sinai Hospital, 31, 43, 53, 121, 128, 186, 319
Mullin, William V., 69, 204
Multiple sclerosis, 242
Multiple Sclerosis Society, 243
Murphy, Daniel, 187
Murphy, James, 137
Murphy, Mimi, 333
Murray, Paul, 237
Murthy, Sudish C., 225, 249
Muschler, George, 331
Musculoskeletal Tissue Bank, 252
Musculoskeletal Tissue Organization, 252
Museum of Intelligence, Power, and Personality, 63
Myers, Mark, 341
Myles, Jonathan L., 269
Myocardial infarction, 319

N

Nadzam, Deborah M., 294

Namey, Marie, 244
Naples Community Hospital, 343
Naples Community Hospital Healthcare System, 343
Nasal septum, deviated, 204
National Association of Children's Hospitals and Related Institutions (NACHRI), 123, 191
National Cancer Institute, 257
National Cancer Survivors Day, 256
National Committee for Clinical Laboratory Standards (NCCLS), 266
National Diet-Heart Study, 323
National Health Resource designation, 364
National Institutes of Health, 95, 166, 174, 218, 237, 321, 327, 328, 331
National Heart Institute, 321
National Marrow Donor Program, 247, 253
National Medical Enterprises, 116. See Tenet Healthcare Corporation.
National MS Society, 243
National Residency Match, 313
Navia, José L., 225, 248
Neonatal intensive care unit, 190, 216, 297
Neonatal nursery, 235
Neonatology, 190, 191
Nephrectomy, partial, 214
Nephrology, 103, 117, 161-163, 283
Pediatric, 188, 190
Netherton, Earl W., 74, 157, 167
Networks, alliances, mergers, 100, 101, 122
Neurofibromatosis, 186
Neurology, 103, 117, 124, 171, 208, 240, 242, 329
Pediatric, 186
Neuro-oncology, 208
Neuro-oncology Center, 208
Neuro-ophthalmology, 258
Neuropathology, 329
Neuroradiology, 329
Neurosciences, 244, 328
Neurosurgery, 48, 103, 195, 199, 206, 240, 329
Pediatric, 189
Newman, Roland, 371
Nichols, Bernard H., 38, 39, 72, 280
Nichols, Don H., 70
Nichols, James H., 88, 90, 355, 356, 362, 369
Nickelson, Daniel, 363, 364
Niezgoda, Julie, 234
Nightingale, Florence, 291
Nitrocellulose x-ray film, 49, 50, 55
Nominating Committee, 79
Norris, Donald, 186
Norris, John, 343
North Beach Hospital. See Cleveland Clinic Florida Hospital
North Broward Hospital District, 334
North Collier Hospital, 343

Northern blotting, 328
Northwestern University, 262
Nosé, Yukihiko, 324
Nosik, William A., 70
Nosocomial infections, 180
Notebaert, Edmond, 357, 358
No-touch technique, 253
Nousek, James, 258
Novick, Andrew C., 144, 213, 214, 245, 246
Nuclear medicine, 288
Nurse Executive Council (NEC), 297
Nurse-On-Call, 305
Nurses
    Ambulatory, 292
    Assistant head, 294
    Certified registered nurse anesthetists
        (CRNAs), 293
    Clinical nurse specialists, 293
    Departmental assistants, 294
    Floor hostesses, 292
    General duty, 291
    Graduate, 291
    Head, 291, 294
    Nursing assistants, 292
    Nursing unit assistant (NUA), 292
    Operating room, 291
    Patient care assistants, 292
    Practical, 292
    Private duty, 292
    Registered, 291
    Shortage, 297, 301, 303
    Unit secretaries, 292
    Ward maids, 291
Nursing, 181, 184, 243, 256
    Advanced practice, 296
    Ambulatory clinic, 298
    Capacity management, 300
    Cardiac, 294
    Cardiothoracic, 295
    Case management, 296, 300
    Center for, 295
    Clinic, 294, 298
    Clinical director, 294, 296
    Contemporary policies and procedures,
        297
    Coordinated care tracks (CCTs), 300
    Critical care, 294, 295
    Division chair, 294
    Division of Nursing, 293
    Education, 295, 296, 301
    Evolution of, 299
    Hourly differential, 304
    Information systems, 295
    Medical, 292, 294
    Medical/surgical, 295
    Neurosurgery/orthopedics/otolaryngol-
        ogy, 294
    Nurse manager, 296, 299
    Nursing administrative group, 293
    Nursing executive council, 294

Nursing management group, 294
Nursing resources, 292
    Operating room, 292-294
    Operations analyst, 296
    Operations managers, 294, 295
    Patient care technician (PCT), 300
    PIE charting system, 300
    Premium pay, 304
    Primary, 299
    Quality management, 295
    Recruitment and retention, 295, 297,
        301
    Research, 295, 296, 301, 302
    Retention bonus, 303
    Shift incentive program, 303
    Shortage, 297, 301, 303
    Sign-on bonus, 304
    Staffing and scheduling, 295
    Standards committee, 297
    Student tuition assistance program, 303
    Surgical, 292, 294
    Surgical services, 295, 297
    Systems/resources/operations, 296
Nursing Management Group, 298
Nutrition, 170, 272
Nutritional Abstracts, 310

O
O'Boyle, Michael, 148, 151, 363, 378
Obstetrics, 117, 119, 123, 184, 199, 215,
    295
    Department closing, 87, 185, 380
    Department reopening, 185
Obstetrics and Gynecology, 214
Occupational therapy, 243
Ochsner Clinic, 193, 357
Ockner, Stephen, 177
Office of Clinical Research, 144, 262
Office of Construction Management, 370
Ohio Department of Health, 118, 121
Ohio Normal School, 20
Ohio Northern University, 20
Ohio Permanente Medical Group, 119, 120
Ohio State University, 118, 119, 142, 152,
    181, 273, 314, 327, 328, 365, 366, 371
Olmsted, Frederick, 322
Omni International Hotel, 91
Oncology, 117, 175 211, 213, 215, 254, 255,
    287
    Pediatric, 186
    Radiation, 287
Operating rooms, 121, 180, 292
Operating rooms, expansion, 199
Operations, 91, 97
Ophthalmic laboratory, 259
Ophthalmology, 103, 117, 122, 195, 258
    Pediatric, 186, 258
Optometry, 259
Organs, artificial, 139, 161, 162, 213, 324,
    325

Original Clinic Building, 255
Orthopaedic Research Center, 330
Orthopedic surgery, 48, 103, 117, 123, 124, 195, 209, 215, 218, 240
Osborn Building, 23, 25, 29, 39
Osmond, John D., 25, 28
Osteomyelitis, 179, 209
Osteopathy, 174
Otolaryngology, 103, 117, 124, 195, 204
  Pediatric, 191
Otosclerosis, 204
Ouriel, Kenneth, 151, 199, 220
Oxley Homes, 353
Oxley, Emma, 353

P
P Building. *See* Clinic Inn
Page Center, 98
Page, Irvine H., 75, 80, 84, 86, 161, 318-324, 326, 331, 332, 376
Pain management, 142, 172, 241
Pain Management Center, 235
Palliative care, 176, 256, 261, 295
Palmer, Robert, 117, 177
Papanicolaou (Pap) smear, 214, 215
Papay, Frank A., 190
Parathyroid surgery, 197, 201
Parker Hannifin Building, 142
Parking, 45, 87, 91, 104
Parkinson's disease, 207
Parma Community Hospital, 121
Paschall, Velma, 190
Pathology, 117, 169, 170, 180, 283, 313
  Anatomic, 265, 268
  Clinical, 265, 270, 275
  Information Systems, 276
  Molecular, 275
Patient satisfaction, 294
Paul, Kathryn, 120
Pawlowski, Eugene, 363
Payroll, 61
Peck, Remington, 362
Pediatric intensive care, 123
Pediatrics, 103, 119, 123, 160, 169, 172, 175, 183
  Allergy, 190
  Cardiology, 190
  Gastroenterology, 190
  General, 188
  Gynecology, 190
  Immunology, 190
  Intensive care, 189, 190
  Psychology, 190, 192
  Radiology, 192
  Research, 189
  Residency program, 190
Pelli, Cesar, 103, 104, 140, 141, 258, 260, 361
Penn, Marc, 331
Pennsylvania State University, 313, 330

Peritoneal dialysis, 162
Peritonitis, 198
Perkins, Litta, 56, 352, 353
Peter Bent Brigham Hospital, 104
Petras, Robert E., 117, 269, 270
Petre, John, 235
Pettersson, Gösta, 223, 249
Phalen, George S., 209, 379
Pharmacy, 80, 295, 355
Phenylketonuria, 185
Philipson, Elliot H., 117, 123, 215
Phillips, John, 30-32, 36-38, 41, 54, 55, 58-60, 157, 158, 183, 227
Phosphorylase A, 320
Photochemotherapy, 168
Physical medicine and rehabilitation, 117, 118, 159
Physical therapy, 158, 215, 242
Physician Hospital Organization (PHO), 122, 134
Physician management, 91, 94, 96, 97, 107, 116
Pituitary ablation (Y^{90}), 207
Pituitary disorders, 167
Planning Committee, 77, 78, 80, 83, 376
Plasmapheresis, 174, 175
Plastic surgery, 94, 103, 115, 117, 195, 204, 205, 216
  Ophthalmic, 234
  Pediatric, 190, 217
Playhouse Square, 124
Plow, Edward F., 144, 329, 331
Pneumatic splint, 207
Pneumatic suit, 207
Pneumonectomy, 198, 220
Pneumonia, 220
Point-of-care testing, 272
Policy, 97, 98
Politics, 92, 118, 120
Ponsky, Jeffrey, 201
Population, 106
Portal hypertension, 201
Porter, Abbie, 292, 353
Portmann, U. V., 48, 280, 281, 287, 289
Portzer, Marietta (Del), 237
Posch, David, 357
Post-coronary artery bypass graft (post-CABG) study, 327
Potter, J. Kenneth, 230
Potts, Ronald, 119, 120
Pouch database, 202
Poutasse, Eugene F., 213, 322
Practice management course, 364
Prayson, Richard A., 269
Pre-anesthesia consultation and evaluation (PACE) clinic, 234
Pre-surgical testing, 234
Price and wage controls, 92
Price, Ronald L., 186, 379
Prieto, Lourdes, 187

Primary care, 103, 106, 124, 177, 181, 188, 380
Primary Health Systems, Inc., 357, 371
Procop, Gary W., 274
Product lines, 113
Professional Policy Committee, 75, 77
Professional staff, 378, 381
Professional Staff Affairs, Office of, 94, 98, 217, 314, 357, 379
Proffitt, Max R., 274, 325
Prossie, Earl, 366
Prostatectomy, 212
Protein chemistry, 328
Proudfit, William L., 162, 164, 308, 376
Psoriasis, 168
Psychiatry, 117, 171, 172
Psychology, 172, 184, 242
    Pediatric, 190, 192
Public Affairs, 99, 105
Public health, 42
Pulmonary disease, 103, 117, 159, 160, 164
    Pediatric, 190
Pulmonary function, 165, 166
Purdue University, 111

Q

Quality Assurance Task Force, 112
Quality management, 294
Quality Management, Office of, 234
Quiring, Daniel, 64, 65

R

Raaf, John H., 254
Radiation oncology, 287
Radiation therapy, 44, 48, 117, 167, 214, 254, 255, 257, 280, 287
Radical neck dissection, 198, 205
Radioactive iodine, 197, 199, 288
Radiology, 169, 170, 180, 257, 279
    Expansion, 284
    Pediatric, 192
Radium, 198
Radon seeds, 198
Raghavan, Derek, 152
Rainbow Babies and Children's Hospital, 186
Ramage, Lisa, 368
Rankin, George B., 379
Ransohoff, Richard, 244, 331
Rapport, Maurice, 320
Ratliff, Norman B., 269
Razavi, Mehdi, 377
Recht, Michael, 286
Recruiting process, 98
Reddy, Sethu, 151, 167
Redmond, Geoffrey, 189
Referrals, 101
Reflex Sympathetic Dystrophy Syndrome Association, 235
Regional laboratory, 275

Regional radiology, 286
Rehabilitation, 240, 261, 262
Rehm, Susan J., 377
Reid, Janet, 192
Reimbursement, cost-based, 106
Reinker, Milton, 362
Remzi, Feza, 203
Renal arteriography, 213
Renal vascular disease, 283
Renshaw, R. J. F., 169
Reproductive endocrinology, 167
Resch, Charles, 217
Research, 25, 31, 34, 39, 45, 77, 80, 95, 99, 119, 124, 161, 163-167, 170, 171, 173-176, 179, 180, 189, 203, 205, 206, 208, 210, 220, 241, 244, 257, 258, 260, 281, 307, 317, 335, 339, 380
    Bridge programs, 329
    Funding, 321
    Program-oriented, 321
Research and Education Institute, 119, 123, 327, 332
Research Building, 91, 270
    Original building, 46
Research Day, 104
Research Institute. *See* Lerner Research Institute
Research Projects Committee, 80, 324, 325
Residency Review Committee, 236
Residents, 308
Resource utilization, 108
Respiratory therapy, 165
Revenue recapture, 118
Rezai, Ali, 209
Rheumatoid arthritis, 174, 175, 211
Rheumatology, 103, 115, 117, 124, 158, 160, 173, 211, 240
    Pediatric, 190
Rhinitis, 165, 166
Rice, Frank A., 57
Rice, Thomas W., 225
Richard Fasenmyer Chair, 174
Richmond General Hospital, 357
Richter, Joel, 117, 170
Riffe, Vernal, 103
Rob, Charles, 219
Robinson Memorial Hospital, 280
Robinson, Clare, 172, 184
Robnett, Ausey H., 80, 219
Robotic modular automation laboratory system, 272
Rockefeller University, 328
Rodgers, David A., 172
Roenigk, Henry H., 168
Roentgen, Wilhelm Conrad, 281
Rogers, Douglas G., 189
Rome, Ellen, 190
Rooming in, 184
Root, Joseph C., 70
Rosenkranz, Eliot, 187

Ross, Jonathan H., 188
Rothner, A. David, 186
Rowan, David W., 115, 369
Rowland, Amy, 27, 277, 352
Rudick, Richard A., 144, 239, 242, 244, 262, 331
Ruedemann, A. D., 52, 69, 71-73, 76, 258
Rutherford, Isobel, 274
Ryan, Edward J., 70

S

S Building. *See* Main Clinic Building
Saarel, Douglas, 366
Sabella, Camille, 190
Sabik, Joseph, 223
Sahgal, Vinod, 117, 120, 262
Saphenous vein, 219
Satellites. *See* Family Health Centers
Scherbel, Arthur L., 173, 379
Schey, Ralph E., 378
Schreiber, Martin J., 377, 379
Schubert, Armin, 233
Schumacher, O. Peter, 167, 189
Schwarz, Hans, 320
Schwersenski, Jeffrey, 191
Schwyzer, Robert, 320
Scleroderma, 173
Seals, Thomas, 361, 369
Sebek, Bruce A., 268
Seitz, Valentine, 48, 281
Selden, Tom, 130
Sen, Subha, 322
Senagore, Anthony, 203
Senhauser, Donald A., 273
Sepsis, 166, 179
Serotonin, 320
Shafer, William H., 177
Shainoff, John R., 323
Shakno, Robert, 121
Shapiro, Daniel, 188
Shaughnessy, Marian K., 294
Sheldon, William C., 164, 377
Shepard, Thomas, 371
Sherman, Henry S., 66, 67, 70, 71, 73, 378
Sherrer, Edward, 53, 54
Sherwin Building, 123, 140, 327
Sherwin, John, Sr., 71-75, 86, 90, 353, 354, 378
Shobert, Karen, 378
Shofner, Nathaniel S., 307
Shoos, Ken, 354
Shumway, Sandra S., 291, 293-295
Shupe, Thomas P., 25, 38, 39
Signal transduction, 257
Silverman, Robert H., 329, 331
Singapore, 105, 333
Singsen, Bernhard, 191
Sinusitis, 166, 206
Siperstein, Allan, 201
Sister services, 103

Sivak, Michael, 170
Skillern, Penn G., 167
Skyway, 103, 104
Sleep disorders, 171
Sloan, Harry G., 25, 28, 38, 39
Smedira, Nicholas G., 225, 248, 249
Smith, Brian J., 370
Smithsonian Institution, 216, 281
Social responsibility, 92
Social work, 242, 256
Solomon, Glen, 176
Sones, F. Mason, Jr., 112, 162-164, 184, 221
Soupios, Madeline, 294
South Pointe Hospital, 128, 130, 372
Spagnuolo, Sara, 234
Specialization, 359
  Pediatrics, 185
Specialty boards, 308, 310
Specialty medicine, 42, 61, 98, 99, 101, 106, 159, 188, 195, 213, 217, 258, 380, 381
Specialty Operations Group (SOG), 360
Spinal cord stimulation, 235
Spinal surgery, 207
Sports medicine, 210
Squire, Sanders and Dempsey, 115
St. Alexis Hospital, 31, 279, 357
St. John School of Nursing, 184
St. John's Hospital, 30
St. Luke's Hospital, 83, 120, 128, 354
St. Michael Hospital, 279
St. Thomas Hospital (Summa Health System), 121, 132
St. Vincent Charity Hospital, 19, 31, 43
Staff benefits, 99
Staff, professional, 378
Stage, Miriam K., 58
Stallion, Anthony, 188
Stanford University, 328
Stanton-Hicks, Michael D., 235
Stapled ileal pouch anastomosis, 202
Stark, George R., 151, 257, 317, 328-332
Starr, Norman J., 232
Startzman, Viola, 184
Starzl, Thomas, 250
State of the Clinic Address, 100, 380
Steffen, Rita, 185
Steiger, Ezra, 379
Steinhilber, Richard M., 172, 173
Stem cell laboratory, 273
Sterba, Richard, 187
Stereotactic surgery, 207
Stewart, Bruce H., 179, 199, 377
Stewart, Robert W., 224
Stillwell, Paul C., 190
Stoler, Mark H., 269
Stoller, James K., 104
Straffon, Ralph A., 90, 95, 98, 113, 116, 148, 149, 199, 213, 245, 376, 377
Strategic planning, 113

Stress, 317
Stress management, 242
Strickland, Rosalind, 371
Strictureplasty, 202
Stroke, 319
Strome, Marshall, 117, 205, 206, 251, 252
Strong, Scott, 203
Structural Biology Program, 329
Studer, Peter, 13
Subacute care, 261
Suburban Hospital, 130
Succession planning, 66, 73, 91, 96, 109
Sullivan, Benjamin H., 169
Summa Health System, 132
Surgery, 169
    Arrhythmia surgery, 233
    Colorectal, 103, 170, 195, 202, 215,
        253, 339
    Endocrine, 201
    Hepato-biliary-pancreatic, 201
    Lung reduction surgery, 233
    Lung volume reduction, 249
    Minimally invasive, 201-203, 215, 220
    Parathyroid, 197, 201
    Thyroid, 62, 195-197, 201
    Valvuloplasty, 233
Surgical intensive care, 233
Svensson, Lars, 224
Swafford, J. H., 58
Swallowing Center, 170
Sweden, 105, 163, 283
Systemic lupus erythematosus (SLE), 167,
    173, 174

T
Tarazi, Robert C., 161, 322
Taussig Cancer Center, 141, 253
Tautkins, Barney, 288
Taylor, Alfred M., 177, 379
Taylor, Clarence M., 74, 75, 80, 354, 355
Taylor, Howard P., 184
Taylor, Howard R., 359, 365
Taylor, James S., 169, 309
Taylor, Paul C., 226
Taylor, Richard, 100
Taylor, Robert D., 161, 319, 379
Technology Leadership Council, 124
Technology transfer, 210, 329
Tefft, Melvin, 287
Telkes, Maria, 318
Tenet Healthcare Corporation, 135, 341
Tenet South Florida Health System, 341
Tesar, George E., 117, 173
Testosterone, 167
Tetzlaff, John, 229, 237
Thacker, Holly L., 178
Thiel, Karl S., 273
Thomas, Anthony J., 379
Thomas, Frank, 287
Thomas, J. Warrick, 165

Thomassen, Mary Jane, 165
Thoracic surgery, 170, 195, 198, 204, 220
Thoracoplasty, 220
Thrombosis, 325
Thrombotic thrombocytopenic purpura,
    175
Thwing, C. F., 48
Thyroid crisis, 196
Thyroid disease, 288
Thyroid function, 318
Thyroid surgery, 62, 195-197, 201
Tomashefski, Joseph F., 165
Tomer, Carol, 13
Tonsillectomy, 204
Topol, Eric J., 117, 144, 148, 164, 262,
    329, 331, 378
Tourette's syndrome, 186
Town and Country, 380
Traboulsi, Elias, 190
Transfusion, 197
    Intra-uterine, 185
Transfusion medicine, 271
Transition Team, 107
Transplantation, 179, 325
    Arterial, 218, 219
    Bone, 211, 252
    Bone marrow, 176, 247, 273
    Cornea, 251
    Heart, 187, 224, 247, 248
    Heart/Lung, 248
    Kidney, 342
    Larynx, 205, 251
    Liver, 170, 185, 201, 250
    Lung, 165, 225
    Non-myeloablative allogeneic
        hematopoietic cell, 247
    Parathyroid, 205, 252
    Renal, 163, 189, 213, 245, 252
    Renal/Pancreas, 163, 246
    Small bowel, 188
    Stem cell, 247
    Thyroid, 205, 252
Trapp, Bruce, 172, 244, 329, 331
Traquina, Diana, 191
Traumatology, 210
Tropical disease, 180
Trudell, Thomas, 129
TRW, 367
TRW Building, 143
Tubbs, Raymond R., 151, 269, 271, 272,
    274, 275, 331
Tuberculosis, 220
Tucker, Harvey M., 205
Tucker, John P., 38, 176
Tumor registry, 256
Turkey, 105
Turnbull, Rupert P., Jr., 202, 253
Turner, Dean, 363, 378
Tuthill, Ralph T., 269
Tweed, Devina, 270

U

U. S. Olympic Ski Team, 210
U.S. News & World Report survey, 124, 211, 380
Ulreich, Shawn M., 151, 296, 297, 304
Ultrafiltration, 162
Ultrasound, 170
Union Club, 90
Unitech Communications, 315
United Cerebral Palsy, 183
United Kingdom, 105
United States and Canadian Academy of Pathology (USCAP), 266
University (Wooster) Hospital, 20, 31
University Hospitals Health System, 357
University Hospitals of Cleveland, 119, 130, 142, 371
University of Alabama, 369
University of California Los Angeles, 149, 269
University of Chicago, 150
University of Cincinnati, 150, 188
University of Colorado, 177
University of Illinois, 329
University of Iowa, 231
University of Kansas, 61, 158
University of Maine, 136
University of Maryland, 95
University of Miami, 334
University of Michigan, 83, 113, 114, 150, 213, 268, 365
University of New Mexico, 311
University of Pennsylvania, 116, 146, 367
University of Pittsburgh, 89, 250, 365
University of Rochester, 220
University of Southern California, 152
University of Texas, 149
University of Toronto, 30, 326
University of Utah, 162, 275
University of Vermont, 136, 177
University of Washington, 330
University of Wisconsin, 136
Upper Extremity Center, 210
Urbain, Jean Luc, 288, 289
Urological Institute, 214, 329
Urology, 91, 95, 98, 103, 113, 116, 124, 184, 195, 199, 212, 215, 245, 255
Pediatric, 188
Uveitis, 258, 260, 261

V

Valenzuela, Rafael, 274
Van Lente, Frederick, 272
Van Ommen, Ray A., 160, 177, 179, 377, 379
Van Ordstrand, Howard S., 159, 160, 164, 165, 376
Vargo, Karen, 190
Varicose veins, 198
Vascular medicine, 84, 103, 160, 218

Vascular surgery, 103, 195, 208, 218
Vasculitis, 173, 175
Vasquez, Elizabeth, 294
Vidt, Donald G., 162, 377
Viljoen, John F., 230, 232
Vince, D. Geoffrey, 331
Virden, John C., 73
Virology, 328
Vogt, David, 250
Vorwerk, Robert W., 366

W

W.O. Walker Center, 142
Walborn, A. Mary, 117, 137
Walding, Howard, 364, 366
Walker, A. E., 20
Walker, William O., 142
Walsh, T. Declan, 256, 261, 262
Wang, Qing, 331
War
    Boxer Rebellion, 23
    Lakeside Hospital Unit, 19, 27
    Spanish-American, 23
    World War I, 25, 216, 280
    World War II, 70, 71, 159, 216, 298, 301, 318, 381
Warmington, Marion, 366
Warshawsky, Ilka, 275
Wasdovich, Andi, 296, 297
Washington University, 365
Washington, John A., 117, 271, 273-276
Wasmuth, Carl E., 89-94, 96-99, 108, 230, 236, 237, 351, 355, 357, 360, 375, 377
Waters, Jonathan, 235
Waugh, Justin M., 38, 39, 204
Weatherhead, A. Dixon, 171, 172
Weaver, Frank J., 100, 103, 105, 109, 120, 316, 361, 363, 365
WebMD, 148
Weed, Frank J., 19-21
Weekender option program, 303
Wegener granulomatosis, 174
Weick, James K., 175, 254, 255
Weise, Kathryn, 191
Westcott, Richard N., 379
Western blotting, 328
Western Reserve University, 19, 25, 30, 43, 48, 83, 183, 213, 267, 274
Weston City Commission, 341
Whipple, H. K., 353, 366
White Hospital, 280
Whitman, Gayle, 294, 295
Whitman, John F., 80
Widman, Paul E., 90, 91, 357-359, 361
Wiedemann, Herbert P., 117, 165, 377, 379
Wilbourn, Asa, 171
Wilde, Alan H., 210, 211, 377
Wilke, William S., 174
William O. Walker Center, 118, 235
Williams, Brian, 144

Williams, Bryan R. G., 257, 326
Williams, Gary, 190
Williams, Guy H. (Red), Jr., 70, 171, 376
Willis, Charles E., 271, 272
Winkelman, Eugene I., 377, 379
Wojton, Francine, 293
Wolf, Gerald E., 91, 99, 356, 362, 363
Women's Hospital, 58
Women's health, 178
Woodruff Hospital, 235, 242
Wooster Clinic, 137
Wooster University, 19, 20, 23
Work Evaluation and Rehabilitation
    Clinic (WERC), 241
Workers' compensation, 241
World Health Organization, 176, 256
Wu, James, 203
www.ccf.org, 148
Wyllie, Elaine, 187

Wyllie, Robert, 185

Y
Y2K, 146, 147
Yared, Jean Pierre, 233
Yeagley, William, 361
Yen-Lieberman, Belinda, 274
Young, Claire, 151, 305
Young, James B., 151, 161, 224, 248
Young, Jess R., 377, 379

Z
Zehr, Robert J., 346, 347
Zeiter, Walter J., 80, 311, 355, 364, 366,
    377
Zeroske, Joanne, 359
Zhou, Yihua, 174
Zins, James E., 117, 217
Zucker, James, 357